AF588333

Apolipoprotein Mimetics in the Management of Human Disease

G.M. Anantharamaiah • Dennis Goldberg
Editors

Apolipoprotein Mimetics in the Management of Human Disease

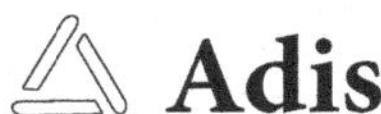

Adis

Editors
G.M. Anantharamaiah
Department of Medicine
University of Alabama School of Medicine
Birmingham, AL
USA

Dennis Goldberg
LipimetiX Development, LLC
Natick, MA
USA

ISBN 978-3-319-17349-8 ISBN 978-3-319-17350-4 (eBook)
DOI 10.1007/978-3-319-17350-4

Library of Congress Control Number: 2015942492

Springer Cham Heidelberg New York Dordrecht London

Printed on acid-free paper

Adis is a brand of Springer
Springer International Publishing AG Switzerland is part of Springer Science+Business Media (www.springer.com)

Preface

Apolipoproteins on the surface of plasma lipoproteins are responsible for not only solubilizing otherwise insoluble lipids but also are involved in the metabolism of these lipoproteins via targeting to specific cell surface receptors and activation or inhibition of lipolytic enzymes. While all of the apolipoproteins possess a common lipid-associating structural motif, the amphipathic helix, each apolipoprotein is unique in its properties and functions. Apolipoprotein A-I (apoA-1), the major protein component of high-density lipoproteins (HDL), was thought to be responsible for the much of the anti-atherogenic properties of HDL. Attention was focused on understanding the functionality of this apolipoprotein via the study of mutants that decreased atherosclerosis is some populations. Clinical studies have been performed with both recombinant human apolipoprotein A-I and certain mutants. However, this has practical limitations due to the requirement of large amounts of protein.

Although study of the model amphipathic helical peptides was initiated three decades ago, the first paper describing the ability of a small peptide consisting of only 18 amino acids to inhibit the development of atherosclerosis was published in the year 2001. Since then, the field of apolipoprotein mimetics took off as several laboratories within and outside the USA began designing and testing their peptides in animal models for not only atherosclerosis but also for other lipid-mediated diseases such as diabetes and Alzheimer's disease. Recently, the receptor binding domain of apolipoprotein E (apoE) was incorporated into the apoA-I mimetic peptides to combine the plasma cholesterol lowering properties of apoE with the anti-atherogenic properties of apoA-1. These new peptides are now considered as the apoE mimetic peptides. Both the apoA-I mimetic and apoE mimetic peptides are undergoing clinical evaluation.

This book compiles current knowledge on the studies done on apolipoprotein mimetics from leading researchers in this field. Its major aim is to present novel ideas, highly unexpected mechanisms of action in animal models and even in initial clinical studies in humans, which would lead to additional improvements in basic and clinical research in biological science. This is the first compendium of this growing field presented in the form of a book.

Birmingham, AL, USA G. M. Anantharamaiah
Natick, MA, USA Dennis Goldberg

Abbreviations

4F	Peptide Ac-D-W-F-K-A-F-Y-D-K-V-A-E-K-F-K-E-A-F-NH_2
6F	Peptide D-W-L-K-A-F-Y-D-K-F-F-E-K-F-K-E-F-F synthesized from L-amino acids
ABCA1	ATP-binding cassette, sub-family A member 1
ABCG1	ATP-binding cassette, sub-family G member 1
ACS	Acute coronary syndrome
AKT	Protein kinase B
AMPK	AMP-activated protein kinase
Apo	Apolipoprotein
ApoA-I	Apolipoprotein A-I
ApoA-II	Apolipoprotein A-II
ApoC-III	Apolipoprotein C-III
Arg1	Arginase 1
ATF3	Activating transcription factor 3
BMDM	Bone marrow-derived macrophage
CBS	Common beta subunit
CD	Cluster of differentiation
CD14	Membrane (m) or soluble (s) pattern recognition receptor (cluster of differentiation 14)
CER	Ceramide
CETP	Cholesterol ester transport protein
CHD	Coronary heart disease
CLEC4a	C-type lectin domain family 4 member A
CREB	cAMP response element-binding protein
D-4F	The 4F peptide synthesized from all D-amino acids
DCFA	Dichlorodihydrofluorescein diacetate
EM	Electron microscopy
eNOS	Endothelial constitutive nitric oxide synthase
EV	Transgenic control tomato expressing a marker protein (β-glucuronidase)
FGF	Fibroblast growth factor
HDL	High-density lipoproteins

HO-1	Heme oxygenase 1
HPETE	Hydroperoxyeicosatetraenoic acid
HPODE	Hydroperoxyoctadecadienoic acid
HSPC	Hematopoietic stem and progenitor cells
HUVEC	Human umbilical vein endothelial cell
ICAM	Intercellular adhesion molecule
IFN	Interferon
IL	Interleukin
iNOS	Inducible nitric oxide synthase
IRF-5	Interferon regulatory factor 5
IRAK1	Interleukin-1 receptor-associated kinase 1
IRF	Interferon regulatory factor
IVUS	Intravascular ultrasound
JAK2	Janus kinase 2
KLF4	Kruppel-like factor 4
L-4F	The 4F peptide synthesized from all L-amino acids
LCAT	Lecithin/cholesterol acyltransferase
LAL	Limulus amebocyte lysate
LBP	Lipopolysaccharide binding protein
LDL	Low-density lipoprotein
LDLR	Low-density lipoprotein receptor
LKB1	Liver kinase B1
LPA	Lysophosphatidic acid
LPS	Lipopolysaccharide
LXRα	Liver X receptor
Ly6C	Lymphocyte antigen 6C
MβCD	Methyl-β-cyclodextrin
MARCO	Macrophage receptor with collagenous structure
MCP-1	Monocyte chemoattractant protein-1
MDM	Monocyte-derived macrophage
MnSOD	Manganese superoxide dismutase
MPO	Myeloperoxidase
MRS	Magnetic resonance spectroscopy
NF-κB	Nuclear factor kappa-light-chain-enhancer of activated B cells
OCR	Oxygen consumption rate
OVA	Ovalbumin
PAF-AH	Platelet-activating factor acetylhydrolase
PKA	Protein kinase A
PON-1	Paraoxonase 1
PPARγ	Peroxisome proliferator-activated receptor γ
RBC	Red blood cells
RCT	Reverse cholesterol transport
ROS	Reactive oxygen species
RNS	Reactive nitrogen species
S1P	Sphingosine-1-phosphate

SAA	Serum amyloid A
SDS	Sodium dodecyl sulfate
SM	Sphingomyelin
SOCS1	Suppressor of cytokine signaling 1
STAT	Signal transducer and activation of transcription
STAT3	Signal transducer and activator of transcription 3
TF	Transferrin
Tg6F	Transgenic tomato expressing the 6F peptide
TGF	Transforming growth factor
TLR	Toll-like receptor
TLR4	Toll-like receptor 4
TNF-α	Tumor necrosis factor alpha
TRAF6	TNF receptor-associated factor 6
TTR	Transthyretin
UAB	University of Alabama at Birmingham
VCAM	Vascular cell adhesion molecule
VCAM-1	Vascular cell adhesion molecule 1
VEGF	Vascular endothelial growth factor
VLDL	Very-low-density lipoproteins
VLDL-R	VLDL receptor
WD	Western diet
XO	Xanthine oxidase

Contents

Introduction

The Structure and Function of Apolipoprotein Mimetic Peptides

Epidemiological evidence points to the cardioprotective influence of HDL and its major protein component, apoA-I. This influence has been reinforced in animal experiments involving the overexpression of apoA-I, which uniformly leads, in appropriate models, to a reduction of atherosclerosis; the chronic inflammatory process at the core of most cardiovascular diseases. So, the impact of strategies aimed at modifying HDL level and function has usually had, as its readout, effects on atherosclerosis.

Based largely on the experimental evidence, much effort has been devoted to elevating plasma HDL cholesterol, the most frequently measured indication of changes in HDL. However, attempts to raise HDL levels in patients with a variety of drug strategies have met with inconclusive results. Even when HDL was elevated by some of these strategies, the cardioprotective function was not always evident. This has led to an increasing emphasis on the importance of HDL function rather than HDL level, and this attention is ongoing. HDL and apoA-I have a multitude of functions, so it is not always clear which function is most pertinent for their cardioprotective effects. The one function that has received the most attention is reverse cholesterol transport, which involves cholesterol efflux from macrophage foam cells to the plasma and transport of the cholesterol to the liver for ultimate excretion via the bile into the feces. The role of HDL and apoA-I on the first step has received particular emphasis. But it is also clear that HDL and its components have a variety of anti-inflammatory actions that could, at least in part, account for the cardioprotective function of this lipoprotein. So attempts to marshal the potential cardioprotective influence of HDL and apoA-I must take account of these several functions.

As apoA-I is a moderate-sized protein produced by the liver and intestine and has a limited lifetime in the plasma and body fluids, its use as a feasible (cost, ease of production, and administration) therapeutic for patients is not great. It is in efforts to replicate the many biological functions of apoA-I with a smaller peptide that has led to the field of apoA-I mimetics. Indeed in some respects, the mimetics are superior to apoA-I, especially as anti-inflammatory agents. What follows is a timely and valuable collection of papers detailing the current knowledge of the utility of the mimetics.

The field of the mimetics has as its background an analysis by Segrest and colleagues of the structure of human apoA-I, which represents about 70 % of the protein components of HDL. It is a 243-amino-acid protein, containing repeating units of 22- or 11-amino-acid amphipathic alpha helices. Taking account of the physical structures of these repeating helices, he reasoned that their general function may be captured by a short 18-amino-acid prototypic peptide that represented a class A amphipathic helix, exhibiting clearly distinct segregated hydrophilic and hydrophobic faces. Although not precisely resembling the amino acid sequence of any of the apoA-I helices, this peptide duplicates the overall properties of these helices. Accordingly, Anantharamaiah in collaboration with Segrest synthesized this prototypic peptide, which has been the basis of many of the mimetic structures since studied. A variety of variants of this peptide have been constructed. The story of the "discovery" of this amphipathic peptide is told in the first chapter by Segrest (Segrest).

The original peptide, designated 18A, contained two phenylalanine residues on its hydrophobic face and hence has sometimes been called 2F. Aside from its physical properties, it was shown to promote cholesterol efflux from lipid-loaded macrophages (Tang et al. 2006). A bihelical peptide was also synthesized. It had two 2F peptides linked by a bridging proline residue—a proline residue interrupts many of the repeating units in intact apoA-I. This bihelical peptide has been designated 37pA. It too can promote cholesterol efflux from macrophages in culture.

For increased lipid binding, the peptides were end protected by acetylation and amidation. Such modified 2F was not particularly active in vivo. However, when two of the hydrophobic residues were substituted by phenylalanines, the peptide was yet more hydrophobic. In contrast to 2F, this 4F is more profoundly bioactive in vivo and is the structure most widely studied in this field. A variety of other phenylalanine variants have been synthesized, 5F, 6F, and 7F, with the first two having high bioactivity. Fogelman and colleagues (Navab et al.) have made a number of critical observations, which they have summarized in Chap. 2 of this collection. First, they showed that 4F synthesized with natural L amino acids was not stable upon oral administration. However, when synthesized from D amino acids, the peptide was stable. D-4F has been the staple peptide employed by this and other groups. It is significant that L-4F and D-4F exhibited comparable activity when administered intraperitoneally or subcutaneously, indicating that stereochemical peptide/protein interactions are probably not critical for their bioactivity. A very important finding is that these bioactive peptides have a very high affinity for oxidized fatty acids, including unsaturated lysophosphatidic acid—orders of magnitude higher than apoA-I. This argues that when this is a suggested mechanism for the anti-inflammatory action of the peptides, they would be much more effective on a molar basis than apoA-I. Of course in evaluating such a suggestion, account must be taken of the concentrations of free apoprotein and free peptide at the site of the peptide's anti-inflammatory action. An important set of studies has pointed toward the intestine as the tissue where peptide works. This is based upon the observation that the response to peptide depends on the dose administered regardless of route and not on the concentration achieved in the plasma. Indeed in some cases, the peptide may be effective even when little plasma peptide is demonstrable. Intestinal oxidized fatty acids are reduced by 4F treatment, including unsaturated lysophosphatidic acid, which is now the focus of intensive study, including its biosynthesis and degradation and relevant sites of action, including the vasculature. The relevance of lysophosphatidic acid in the clinic is strongly suggested by a recent paper reporting the elevation of the plasma concentrations of unsaturated lysophosphatidic acid species in subjects with the acute coronary syndrome but not in those with stable angina (Kurano et al. 2015).

Early in the evolution of work on the efficacy of the 18A family of peptides, it became clear that the peptides are most stable and effectively bind lipids when the end groups are modified. This requirement is an impediment for the large-scale production of peptides for therapy. So the finding that 6F is effective even without end modification opened up the possibility of transgenic organisms for the delivery of the therapeutic peptide. Indeed, an exciting potential is the use of transgenic tomato plants for the delivery of 6F peptide in the diet. Frozen tomatoes expressing the transgene included in the diet can be quite effective in vivo.

A number of subsequent chapters summarize research using 4F as a treatment in a number of experimental models. In each of these models, valuable accessory findings have been reported. In the diabetes model discussed in Chap. 4 by Abraham and colleagues (Benson et al.), using rats or ob/ob mice, 4F has a number of effects—an increase in heme oxygenase 1 expression and of adiponectin levels along with an improvement of blood glucose and a reduction in proinflammatory HDL. Also in the heme oxygenase 2—mice, 4F induces heme oxygenase 1 expression and rescues several features of the metabolic syndrome in these HO $2^{-/-}$ mice, including again an increment in adiponectin. Even the growth of model tumors, e.g., ovarian tumor cells, can be attenuated by apoA-I and 4F, perhaps by binding lysophosphatidic acid, a known tumor promoter, as described by Reddy and colleagues in their chapter (Chap. 5) (Farias-Eisner et al.). However, this may not be a universal influence of apoA-I and 4F, as in a melanoma tumor model described by Zamanian-Dayoush et al. (2013), attenuation of tumor growth was achieved without any change in the plasma concentration of many isomers of lysophosphatidic acid.

In the chapter (Sharifov et al.) by Gupta and colleagues, various mechanisms have been proposed for the attenuation of LPS-induced inflammation. Like apoA-I, it directly binds LPS though with somewhat higher affinity. It also is thought to reduce the cell surface expression of Toll-like receptors (TLRs) including TLR4, the cell surface receptor for LPS, with a consequent reduced expression of proinflammatory cytokines. It functions as an antioxidant and binds oxidized lipids that may be generated by LPS. 4F also has the capacity to modify pulmonary inflammation as described by Pritchard (Pritchard). ApoA-I deficiency adversely affects pulmonary inflammation in several models, while 4F improves pulmonary function in these by several potential mechanisms—binding of proinflammatory lipids and improvement of the function of HDL as well as the binding of interferon-regulating factor with a reduction of inflammation, perhaps by influencing the polarity of macrophages. In Chap. 8, White and colleagues (Usmar et al.) discuss the role of apoA-I and A-I mimetics in biasing the phenotype of macrophages to the M2 anti-inflammatory state with the production of cytokines such as IL-10, an action that could make an important contribution to the utility of the mimetic peptides in the treatment of inflammatory disorders.

The work summarized so far suggests that two major mechanisms of action are at play in the treatment of the variety of inflammatory diseases to which the mimetic peptide has been applied. The high affinity of these peptides resulting in the binding and attenuation of the activity of proinflammatory oxidized lipid intermediates including unsaturated lysophosphatidic acid represents one such mechanism. Second, the capacity of some of the peptides to promote cholesterol efflux may be an important mechanism in some cases. These two mechanisms are not always separate from one another. Cholesterol efflux may induce an anti-inflammatory state. This could be the result of two distinct anti-inflammatory pathways. Tang and Oram (Navab et al.) noted that 2F, D-2F, 4F, and 37pA all interacted with ABCA-1, promoting efflux and stimulating Janus kinase 2 phosphorylation and Stat 3 phosphorylation with the activated Stat 3 entering the nucleus and suppressing the transcription of proinflammatory cytokines. Given the activity of 2F and 37pA in this response in cultured cells, it is unlikely that this is a major mechanism for in vivo attenuation of inflammation as these peptides are not highly active in vivo (Getz et al. 2010). An alternative anti-inflammatory mechanism attendant on cholesterol efflux relates to the enrichment of lipid rafts in cholesterol-loaded cells. TLR receptors are concentrated in lipid rafts in such conditions, resulting in proinflammatory signaling. The removal of cholesterol from lipid rafts will deplete them of TLRs and reduce this signaling. This could in part account for the attenuation of LPS activity by peptide influence on the cholesterol content of rafts. It could also contribute to the polarization of macrophages to the M2 phenotype.

In Chap. 3, Remaley and colleagues (Li et al.) describe the variants of the bihelical peptide 37pA, in which the first helix is identical to 18A linked by a proline residue to a second amphipathic helix in which five of the hydrophobic residues are substituted with alanine residues. This reduces the hydrophobicity of the second helix in accord with the observation that in intact apoA-I, the neighboring helices do not exhibit the same hydrophobicity. This bihelical peptide, designated 5A, promotes cholesterol efflux in vivo and reduces atherosclerosis extent in apoE$^{-/-}$ mice.

Like apoA-I, apoE is a multifunctional protein that has amphipathic helices as a core structural element. Much of the focus on the function of apoE has depended on its capacity to promote the plasma clearance of "atherogenic" lipoproteins. In Chap. 9, Robert Raffai (Raffai) reviews the pleiotropic functions of apoE that extend beyond lipoproteins, particularly its antioxidative and anti-inflammatory activities. ApoE also has a cell endogenous influence on stem cell proliferation mediated by the regulation of cholesterol homeostasis and limits monocytosis that represents a risk factor for atherosclerosis. Unlike apoA-I, apoE is synthesized in many cell types.

ApoE contains two domains, an N-terminal domain which includes the LDL receptor-binding domain and a lipid-binding domain. In Chap. 10, Garber and colleagues (Garber et al.) review the utility of the minimal human apoE sequence that binds to the receptor linked by its carboxyl group to 18A and thus is a hybrid peptide that contains apoE- and apoA-I-related sequences. It is designated hE18A, and like 4F, its efficacy can be enhanced by end modification. The short apoE sequence also binds heparin sulfate proteoglycan (HSPG). Because of the interaction with these two cell surface molecules, this peptide can facilitate the clearance of apoB-containing lipoproteins with reduction in both plasma cholesterol and triglyceride, a reduction which may also occur in animal models lacking the LDL receptor, suggesting the implication of HSPG. Clinical studies are ongoing using the product designated AEM-28.

Among the human apoE isoforms, apoE4 is a well-recognized risk factor for Alzheimer's disease. While apoE is produced in the astrocytes and microglia of the central nervous system, the delivery of apoE proteins from the blood does not occur readily because of the relative impermeability of the blood–brain barrier. Any attempt to deliver apoE sequences that may be protective for the development of Alzheimer's disease, particularly in those carrying at least one apoE4 allele. Vitek and colleagues (Vitek et al.) have used a peptide approach to the delivery of such sequences to the brain, developing peptides that cross the blood–brain barrier. Two peptides encompassing residues 133–149 of apoE (COG 133) have been modified to attain better penetration. The first couples this sequence with the protein transduction domain, antennapedia, to generate COG 112. The second derives from residues 138–149 of apoE, in which position 3(H) and position 8(R) are substituted with amino isobutyric acid, and is designated COG 1410. Both are end modified. In mouse models of Alzheimer's disease, these two peptides reduced the pathology, including amyloid burden, tau fibrils, and cognitive memory and behavior. The peptides also reduced inflammatory cytokine production by peritoneal macrophages and enhanced neurite outgrowth in culture.

Though it is just over 20 years that the first synthetic apoA-I-related mimetic peptide (18A) was reported by Anantharamaiah and Segrest and colleagues, the field has grown greatly in insights and potential mechanisms of action. With the improving ease of peptide delivery and the ready capacity of synthetic chemists to fabricate variants of these peptides, it is now possible to develop improved potential therapeutics which takes advantage of our understanding of the multifunctionality of the apoproteins A-I and E. Furthermore, the probing of the mechanisms of action of these peptides has revealed new biology that enhances the analysis of inflammation attenuation and cardioprotection. Much more can be expected in the years to come. This collection provides a platform to think about these possibilities.

Godfrey S. Getz
Donald N. Pritzker
Distinguished Service Professor Emeritus
University of Chicago, Department of Pathology
Chicago, IL, USA

Bibliography

Benson M, Peterson SJ, Mehta P, Abraham NG, ApoA-I mimetic peptides and diabetes

Farias-Eisner R, Su F, Anantharamaiah GM, Navab M, Fogelman AM, Reddy ST, Apolipoprotein A-I mimetic peptides in mouse models of cancer

Garber DW, Goldberg D, Anantharamaiah GM, Apolipoprotein E mimetic peptides cholesterol dependent and independent properties

Getz GS, Wool GD, Reardon CA (2010) HDL apolipoprotein related peptide in treatment of atherosclerosis and other inflammatory disorders. Curr Pharm Design 16(25):3173–3184

Kurano M, Suzuki A, Inoue A, Tokuhara Y, Kano K, Matsumoto H, Igarashi K, Ohkawa R, Nakamura K, Dohi T, Miyauchi K, Daida H, Tsukamoto K, Ikeda H, Aoki J, Yatomi Y (2015) Possible involvement of minor lysophospholipids in the increase in plasma lysophosphatidic acid in acute coronary syndrome. Arterioscler Thromb Vasc Biol 35:463–470

Li D, Gordon S, Schwendeman A, Remaley AT, Apolipoprotein mimetic peptides for stimulating cholesterol efflux

Navab M, Reddy ST, Meriwether D, Fogelman SI, Fogelman AM, ApoA-I mimetic peptides: a review of the present status

Pritchard KA, Apolipoprotein mimetics in the amelioration of respiratory inflammation

Raffai RL, Apolipoprotein E & atherosclerosis: beyond lipid effects

Segrest JP, HDL and the amphipathic helix

Sharifov OF, Anantharamaiah GM, Gupta H, Effects of ApoA-I mimetic peptide L-4F in LPS-mediated inflammation

Tang C, Vaughan AM, Anantharamaiah GM, Oram JF (2006) Janus kinase 2 modulates the lipid removing but not protein stabilizing interaction of amphipathic helices with ABCA1. J Lipid Res 47(1):107–113

Usmar VD, Gjordano S, White CR, Regulation of macrophage polarity by HDL, apolipoproteins and apolipoprotein mimetic peptides

Vitek MP, Li F, Colton CA, Apolipoprotein-E and mimetics as targets and therapeutics for Alzheimer's disease

Zamanian-Daryoush M, Linder D, Tallant TC, Wang Z, Buffa J, Klipfell E, Parker Y, Hatala D, Parsons-Wingerter P, Rayman P, Yusufishaq MSS, Fisher EA, Smith JD, Finke J, DiDonato JA, Hazen SL (2013) The cardioprotective protein apolipoprotein A1 promotes potent anti-tumorigenic effects. J Biol Chem 288:21237–21252

The Editors

G.M. Anantharamaiah, PhD Dr. Anantharamaiah is a Professor of Medicine, Biochemistry, and Molecular Genetics at the University of Alabama at Birmingham, where he has served as a faculty for the last 33 years. He was recruited by Dr. Jere P. Segrest in 1982 as an Assistant Professor at a time when the amphipathic helix theory required additional experimental support. It was a chance matter that Dr. Ananth had studied the shorter bioactive analogues of ACTH for his Ph.D. thesis, which were 18 residues in length. When he joined UAB, he decided to reduce the size of an apoA-I mimetic peptide design to 18 residues in length, which led to the design of several active peptide analogues, all of which were studied for the first 15 years for their apoA-I mimetic properties in vitro. When he suggested in one of the external scientific advisory meetings that these peptides may mimic apoA-I in vivo and may even inhibit atherosclerosis, most of the scientists in the gathering suggested that 18A sequence had nothing to do with the apoA-I sequence and thus is not relevant to the studies of apoA-I and HDL. However, he and his colleague Dr. David Garber (who is an animal physiologist and still collaborates closely with Dr. Ananth) were fortunate that Dr. Don Small, a famous scientist in the field of lipoproteins, sided with Dr. Ananth by stating "…after all atherosclerosis is a lipid imbalance. Ananth should be given chance to determine if analogs of 18A, which are membrane active and mimicked several properties of full length human apoA-I, can tilt this imbalance to exhibit beneficial effects in inhibiting atherosclerosis." Due to lack of funds, instead of transgenic dyslipidemic mouse models which are highly expensive, C57BL6/J mice on the Paigen diet were administered 20 μg/mouse/day for 12 weeks. The results showed inhibition of atherosclerosis with 5F analogue. Since there was no change in the plasma cholesterol levels, Dr. Ananth discussed these results with Visiting Professor Dr. Alan Fogelman, who showed high enthusiasm in collaborating with Dr. Ananth. As discussed in Chap. 2 by Dr. Fogelman and coworkers, an 18A analogue called 6F has been genetically expressed in tomatoes, and concentrates of tomato when fed to atherosclerosis-sensitive animals inhibit not only atherosclerosis but also several forms of tumor proliferation.

Since our initial observations with 18A analogues and other analogues developed in other laboratories did not reduce plasma cholesterol levels despite inhibiting atherosclerosis, it was thought that development of analogues with both anti-inflammatory and plasma cholesterol–reducing properties was needed to enable risk reduction in patients with hypercholesterolemia and who are resistant to statin treatment. Since apoE (which was originally referred to as Arg-rich apolipoprotein), the protein component of VLDL and HDL, has been shown to bypass the LDL receptor and clears atherogenic lipoproteins via the HSPG pathway, Dr. Ananth started designing peptide analogues to mimic the apoE structural motif that has now been shown to also exhibit cholesterol-independent antiatherogenic effects. Only ten amino acid residues from apoE which are highly enriched in Arg and Lys residues (residues 141–150) were directly linked to the 18A described earlier. As described in Chap. 10 by Drs. Garber, Goldberg, and Ananth, the resulting peptide exhibited not only potent cholesterol-reducing properties but also anti-inflammatory properties analogous to full-length apoE. Thanks to Dr. Goldberg's enthusiasm and interest, despite initial setbacks, Dr. Goldberg advanced rapidly the clinical trials of this peptide. Drs. Goldberg and Ananth have collaborated closely and published several exciting papers on the antiatherogenic effects of apoE mimetics. Over the years, Dr. Ananth has been an author in more than 200 original publications, and several patents, most of which are related to the studies of apolipoprotein mimetics.

Dennis Goldberg, PhD, FAHA Dr. Goldberg has 30 years of experience in the pharmaceutical and biotechnology industries, ranging from drug discovery at a Fortune 25 company to Chief Executive Officer of "virtual" biotechnology companies. Dr. Goldberg is Founder and President of LipimetiX Development, LLC., and has served as President, CEO, and Founder of Transport Pharmaceuticals, Inc.; President, CEO, and Founder of neXus therapeutics, Inc., a biotechnology management and consulting company; and President, CEO, and Director of BZL Biologics, a company developing monoclonal antibodies for the treatment of prostate cancer. The BZL antibody technology was licensed by Millennium Pharmaceuticals (NASDAQ:MLNM). Dr. Goldberg was President, CEO, and Cofounder of Talaria Therapeutics, which developed the large unilamellar vesicle (LUV) technology. Talaria Therapeutics was acquired by Esperion Therapeutics (NASDAQ:ESPR) less than 2 years after its formation.

Dr. Goldberg was also Vice President of Product Development and Regulatory Affairs at GelTex Pharmaceuticals (NASDAQ:GELX), where he was responsible for all biological and clinical development activities at the company leading to the discovery and approval of Renagel® and Welchol®. He was also Cofounder of Transcend Therapeutics, a spinout of Clintec Nutrition Co. (a joint venture between Baxter and Nestle), where he was Vice President of Research and Development and Science Coordinator for the Atherosclerosis Research Program at Pfizer Central Research. Dr. Goldberg holds a Ph.D. in physiology and biochemistry from Temple University and received postdoctoral training at the University of Pennsylvania and at the Specialized Center of Research on Atherosclerosis, University of California, San Diego. He is a Fellow of the American Heart Association. He has published extensively in basic and clinical sciences and is the inventor of 12 US patents.

As described in various chapters in this book, several scientists all over the country have immensely contributed to the studies of apolipoprotein mimetics, which has become a separate field of study. Since there was no compendium for describing the fast-growing number of research publications in this branch of study, Dr. Goldberg suggested to Dr. Ananth to initiate the editing of a textbook. We thank all of the authors who enthusiastically contributed to this.

HDL and the Amphipathic Helix

Jere P. Segrest

Abstract High-density lipoproteins (HDL) are a population of apolipoprotein A-I-containing particles inversely correlated with the risk of coronary heart disease (CHD) (Linsel-Nitschke and Tall 2005), but lower HDL cholesterol levels are not uniformly associated with excess cardiovascular risk, nor do they always confer a protective benefit (Mahdy Ali et al. 2012). Further, HDL has biological functions that transcend its antiatherogenic role; to paraphrase Einstein, "God" did not create HDL to prevent atherosclerosis. In this chapter, I will present a brief history of HDL, focusing on the discovery of the amphipathic helix, a concept that led to the development of HDL peptide mimetics.

Discovery, Isolation, and Characterization of HDL

The first clear evidence for the existence of HDL in blood was a publication in 1929 in which M. A. Macheboeuf described the precipitation with acidified ammonium sulfate of what we now know to be HDL (Gotto et al. 1986). He later showed that this blood component possessed electrophoretic α-mobility. In the late 1940s, John Gofman and colleagues use analytical ultracentrifugation to quantify individual lipoproteins and reported that LDL was a positive risk factor for atherosclerosis (Gofman and Lindgren 1950). In 1951, Howard Eder and colleagues first described HDL as a negative risk factor for atherosclerosis (Barr et al. 1951), an observation that was largely ignored at the time.

J.P. Segrest
Atherosclerosis Research Unit, Department of Medicine, Center for Computational and Structural Dynamics, University of Alabama at Birmingham, Birmingham, AL 35294-0012, USA
e-mail: shahp@cshs.org

G.M. Anantharamaiah, D. Goldberg (eds.), *Apolipoprotein Mimetics in the Management of Human Disease*, DOI 10.1007/978-3-319-17350-4_1

In 1955, Richard Havel and colleagues used sequential flotation to isolate HDL (Havel et al. 1955).

In the mid-1960s, John Glomset and colleagues described Lecithin/cholesterol acyltransferase (LCAT) and its activation by HDL and hypothesized reverse cholesterol transport by HDL (Glomset 1968), a process whereby HDL is thought to be atheroprotective via removal of cholesterol deposits from atherosclerotic lesions.

In the 1960s, attention was focused on the protein components of the lipoproteins, the apolipoproteins. These proteins were shown to be heterogeneous, and the currently accepted A, B, C, etc. nomenclature was proposed by Alaupovic and colleagues (Gustafson et al. 1965) in 1965. A few years later, Shore and Shore isolated two major proteins from HDL that they named apoHDL that were later called apolipoprotein A-I (apoA-I) and apoA-II (Shore and Shore 1968). Finally, HDL-C was rediscovered in the mid-1970s by several groups as a negative risk factor for atherosclerosis (Rhoads et al. 1976; Castelli et al. 1977; Gordon et al. 1977; Miller et al. 1977; Goldbourt and Medalie 1979).

Early History of HDL Structure

The ability to isolate large amounts of HDL opened the door to an understanding of HDL structure. In a seminal paper published in 1960, Scanu and Hughes (1960) showed that apoHDL is taken up by HDL and forms complexes with phospholipid. The obvious question then was: what is unique about the proteins of HDL that allow them to associate with lipid? A series of publication in the next decade provided part of the answer.

The next major advance toward understanding the molecular nature of apoHDL was by Camejo and colleagues (1968) who in 1968 showed that apoHDL inserts into phospholipid monolayers with a high surface activity, meaning that the protein of HDL inserted itself between the phospholipid headgroups of membrane surfaces. A second piece of the puzzle was the publication the next year by Gotto showing that intact HDL has a high α-helical content (1969). A couple of years later, Forte and colleagues (1971) used negative stain EM to demonstrate that the incubation of apoHDL with phospholipid vesicles breaks the large vesicles into smaller disk-shaped particles the thickness of a phospholipid bilayer. Finally, in 1972 Lux and colleagues showed that binding of apoHDL to lipid resulted in an increase in α-helical content of the protein.

Thus, in 1972 it was clear that the proteins of HDL associate strongly with phospholipid, disrupt the phospholipid upon binding, and when lipid-bound, are α-helical. In the same year, Angelo Scanu gave a talk to the New York Academy, entitled "Structure of human serum lipoproteins." At the end of the talk, he was asked the following question:

> "I had hoped you would come to grips with the question why one kind of protein interacts with phospholipid to form a membrane and another kind of protein interacts with phospholipid to form a highly dispersed lipoprotein…"

He answered: "I am not sure that I am in the position of providing a meaningful answer to your question. At present, we do not have sufficient information on the nature of the proteins in membranes and circulating lipoproteins to allow for a careful comparison of their properties."

Discovery of the Amphipathic Helix: An Untold Story

At this point in time, unbeknownst to Scanu, the first part of the question about membrane proteins had already been answered. As a postdoctoral fellow at NIH with Vincent Marchesi, I had shown that the RBC transmembrane glycoprotein, glycophorin, interacted with the plasma membrane bilayer through a transmembrane α-helix (Segrest et al. 1972). With this concept and the development of Sodium dodecyl sulfate (SDS) gel electrophoresis that allowed analysis of the otherwise water-insoluble transmembrane proteins, the field of membrane research took off.

Lipoprotein research initially lagged somewhat behind membrane research. As a postdoc at NIH, I became a newly minted expert on protein-lipid interactions with several of the researchers in the laboratory of Don Fredrickson at NIH; I remember having lengthy discussions with both Sam Lux and Peter Herbert. At this point, three apolipoproteins had been sequenced, apoA-II, apoC-I, and apoC-III, called then by the cumbersome names, Apo LP-Gln II (HDL), Apo LP-Ser (VLDL), and Apo LP-Ala (VLDL), respectively. The latter two are minor components of the HDL proteome. During these discussions, it was clear that the same lipid-binding motif found in membrane proteins, the hydrophobic α-helix generally recognized by a continuous run of predominantly hydrophobic but otherwise non-charged amino acids (Segrest and Feldmann 1974), was not present in these three apolipoproteins. I filed the problem away for later consideration.

A few months later, I was privileged to join T. Gulik-Krzywicki for 2–3 months at the CNRS Institution in Gif-sur-Yvette, France–near Paris–to study the transmembrane protein glycophorin (Segrest et al. 1974a; Lea et al. 1975). As luck would have it, Richard Jackson, who had worked a year with me in Marchesi's lab and had now jointed Tony Gotto at the Baylor School of Medicine, flew with me to Europe for the 21st Colloquium of the "Protides of the Biological Fluids" organized by H. Peters in Bruges, Belgium, where we both were speakers. On the long flight, Richard and I had a detailed conversation about ways that apolipoproteins might associate with lipid. We decided that α-helical structures with stretches of charged residues might be involved; I still have a drawing made on the plane of a helix with charged residues arranged along one side.

After the Bruges meeting, I took a train to Paris. When I arrived at the CNRS, my host, Gulik-Krzywicki, was away at another meeting and I had a couple of days free. The lab chief, V. Luzzati, showed me to my office where I opened up a bag full of space-filling corey pauling koltun (CPK) models (this was before personal computers). I had lugged these models with me to use to see if I could identify the apolipoprotein lipid-binding motif in three apolipoprotein sequences that Richard had given me.

After contemplating the sequences for a while, I noticed an interesting pattern in the linear sequence of apoA-II; there was one stretch, residues 18–30, in which extremely hydrophobic residues alternated in a predictable way with positive and negative residues. Since Richard and I had decided the lipid-binding regions might be α-helical, I used the CPK models to construct a helix with this sequence, and I saw for the first time the amphipathic helical motif: fully half of one side of the helix was hydrophobic, and the other side was highly charged. The clinching feature was the distribution of the charged residues on the polar face. To quote from the subsequent publication (Segrest et al. 1974b), "The negatively charged residues, Glu and Asp, invariably occur[ed] in a narrow strip along the center of the polar face, while the positively charged residues, Lys and Arg [were] located on the lateral edge of the polar faces, alternating from side to side." This was later called a class A amphipathic helical pattern (Segrest et al. 1990).

Okay, I told myself, calm down. This is just one sequence; maybe the others are different. However, I could see the charge-hydrophobic residue pattern in several places in the other apolipoproteins. The next morning, after little sleep, I built the other two sequences with the CPK models and was incredibly excited to see that the next apolipoprotein that I modeled, apoC-I, had three class A amphipathic helical pattern sequences, varying from 8 to 21 residues in length. The clincher, however, was that apoC-III had a perfect amphipathic helix toward its C-terminus that was 28 residues long. In this helix alone, there were four positive and five negative residues on the polar face in class A pattern (Fig. 1a). Of the other residues on the polar face, six were polar (Ser and Thr) and two were Gly. The hydrophobic face, equally impressive, contained 11 entirely hydrophobic residues, seven that were aromatic (Fig. 1b). I was convinced.

Since neither the Internet nor the fax machine existed, I placed a long distant phone call to Richard Jackson in Houston to describe what I had found. Richard and Tony Gotto thought the idea promising, so I worked with a photographer at CNRS to take photos of the models. I then used transparent paper to trace the structure of the six amphipathic CPK models and mailed the images to Richard and Tony.

We made the decision to meet at the 1973 International Biochemistry Conference on my way back to the USA. There Richard, Tony, Joel Morrisett, and I wrote a manuscript and submitted it to Nature, where it was summarily rejected. We ended up publishing our initial description of the theory of the amphipathic helix in FEBS Letters in 1974 (Segrest et al. 1974b). This, then, was the answer to the second part of the question to Angelo Scanu: how do apolipoproteins interact "with phospholipid to form a highly dispersed lipoprotein[s]" (Fig. 2).

After moving to UAB in late 1974, I decided to test the theory of the amphipathic helix by designing, synthesizing, and determining the lipid affinity of an 18 amino acid "generic" amphipathic helical peptide (subsequently named 18A). I wrote the grant and submitted it to NIH. To paraphrase Montaigne, it was not funded because "it was not true."

I then spent time showing it was true and submitted a revised application to NIH. Again, to paraphrase Montaigne, it was not funded because "while surely true, it was not important." Upon resubmission where I showed it was true and important, paraphrasing Montaigne once more, it was surely true, it was surely important, but "it has already been done," NIH disallowed the grant.

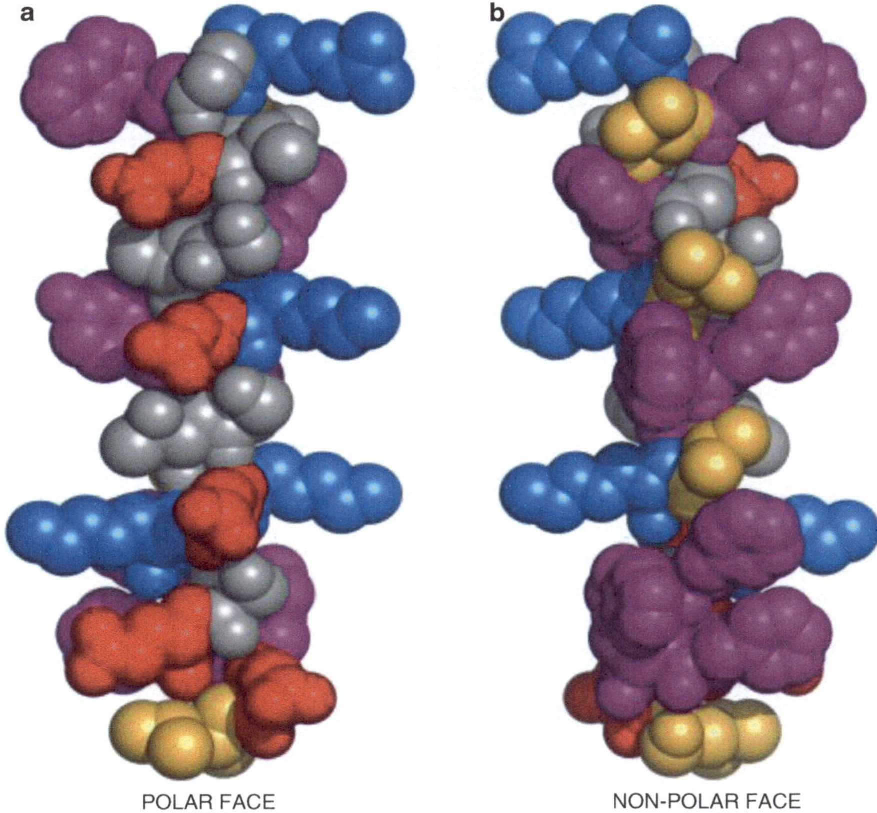

Fig. 1 Space-filling CPK model of single 28-residue-long amphipathic helix, residues 40–67, in apoC-III. (**a**) Polar face. (**b**) Nonpolar face. Positively charged residues, *blue*; negatively charged residues, *red*; aromatic residues, *magenta*; aliphatic residues, *gold*; serine/threonine/glycine, *gray*

Okay, so the third time I actually got funded by NIH, but it took a lot of "blood, sweat and tears," to quote Winston Churchill. In a series of subsequent publications (Kanellis et al. 1980; Segrest et al. 1983; Anantharamaiah et al. 1985), my lab created and used the first HDL peptide mimetic, named 18A by my colleague G. M. Anantharamaiah (1985), to confirm the validity of the amphipathic helix concept.

The Amphipathic Helix and HDL

Using 18A, we were able to show that the amphipathic α-helix is a common secondary structural motif in biologically active peptides and proteins. In a review article from this laboratory (Segrest et al. 1990), naturally occurring amphipathic α-helixes

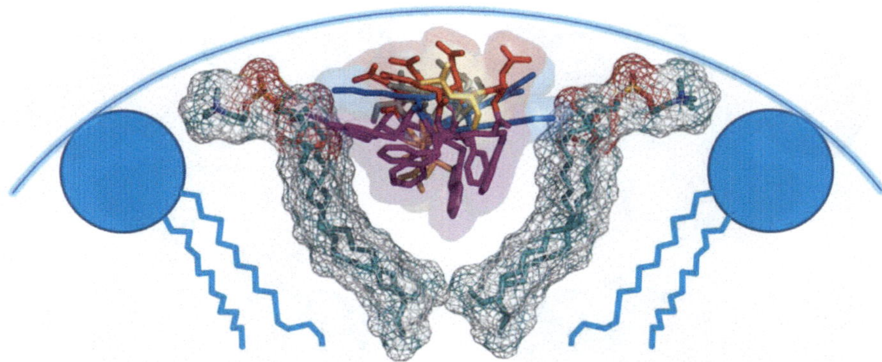

Fig. 2 Model of the detergent effect of the amphipathic helix in apoC-III on phospholipid. The amphipathic helix, upon insertion into a phospholipid monolayer surface, creates surface curvature. The amphipathic helix is in combination stick and transparent surface mode. Positively charged residues, *blue*; negatively charged residues, *red*; aromatic residues, *magenta*; aliphatic residues, *gold*; uncharged, polar residues, *gray*. The two phospholipids adjacent to the amphipathic helix are in combination stick and mesh representation

were grouped into seven distinct classes: A, apolipoproteins; H, polypeptide hormones; L, lytic polypeptides; G, globular proteins; K, calmodulin-regulated protein kinases; C, coiled-coil proteins; and M, transmembrane proteins. These groupings were based upon a detailed analysis of physical, chemical, and structural properties using helical wheel projections. The primary determinant of class was found to be a characteristic of the polar face: charge, charge density, charge distribution, and angle subtended.

Class A amphipathic α-helixes represent the lipid-associating amphipathic α-helical domains of the exchangeable apolipoproteins (Segrest et al. 1990). As already noted, the most distinctive feature of the class A amphipathic α-helix is a unique clustering of positively charged residues at the polar-nonpolar interface and negatively charged amino acid residues at the center of the polar face. We have suggested that the amphipathic basic residues, when associated with PL, extend ("snorkel") toward the polar face of the helix to insert their charged moieties into the aqueous milieu (Segrest et al. 1992, 1994). The snorkel hypothesis is supported by the results of a number of experimental studies from our laboratory (Kanellis et al. 1980; Segrest et al. 1983; Anantharamaiah et al. 1985; Mishra et al. 1994), as well as from others (Rozek et al. 1995).

Current History of HDL Structure

ApoA-I dominates the surface of most particles that fall in the HDL density range. Mature human apoA-I has 243 amino acid residues and is encoded by exons 3 and 4 of the gene in chromosome 11. Exon 3 encodes residues 1–43, commonly called the "globular" domain (Segrest et al. 1992). It contains an N-terminal segment of ten residues, designated G0, followed by three 11-mer amino acid tandem repeats, G1, G2, and G3. The common lipid-associating motif in apoA-I is the amphipathic α-helix (Segrest et al. 1974b, 1994), which is encoded by exon 4 and is often punctuated by proline residues. While there is wide agreement that apoA-I's structure is dominated by 11- and 22-mer helical domains, the three-dimensional organization of these segments has been vigorously debated for years (Li et al. 2002; Bhat et al. 2007; Silva et al. 2008; Gu et al. 2010; Jones et al. 2010; Huang et al. 2011; Segrest et al. 2013a). The situation is made more complex because apoA-I commonly exists in different states: lipid-free, lipid-poor, and discoidal or spheroidal lipoproteins of different sizes (Linsel-Nitschke and Tall 2005). Our current understanding of the structure of apoA-I in each state remains incomplete.

The first tangible evidence for the conformation of apoA-I on dHDL was reported by Borhani et al. (1997); their X-ray structure for residues 44–243 of lipid-free apoA-I suggested a double belt model. The first experimental test of the belt model was by Axelsen et al. (Koppaka et al. 1999) using PATIR-FTIR. Theoretical considerations of the geometric and physical chemical nature of the apoA-I double belt resulted in publication by my lab (Segrest et al. 1999) of an atomic resolution antiparallel double belt amphipathic helical model for dHDL with an LL5/5 registry. Five laboratories that studied apoA-I/HDL using a variety of physical chemical methods obtained results consistent with this model (Li et al. 2000, 2002; Bhat et al. 2005, 2007; Maiorano and Davidson 2000; Tricerri et al. 2000, 2001; Panagotopulos et al. 2001; Davidson and Hilliard 2003; Oda et al. 2003; Maiorano et al. 2004; Silva et al. 2005; Martin et al. 2006; Wu et al. 2007).

Current Thoughts on the Biomedical Implications of HDL

Recent studies have called into question the hypotheses that elevating HDL-C is necessarily therapeutic (Alwaili et al. 2010; Rader and Tall 2012). One reason for this conundrum is that HDL particles are heterogeneous in shape, density, size, composition, and function (Linsel-Nitschke and Tall 2005). Shotgun proteomics has shown that HDL particles contain, at last count, 84 proteins (Shah et al. 2013), including many correlating with antioxidant, anti-inflammatory, and antiatherogenic properties (Vaisar et al. 2007; Davidson et al. 2009). Complicating our understanding of its function, the HDL platform is a complex of lipid and protein easily deformable by thermal fluctuations (Zlotnick 2004) whose study requires diverse and innovative approaches.

The Segrest laboratory pioneered the use of computer methods for the study of HDL: (1) We combined this approach with experimentation to understand the dynamic interactions of apoA-I with itself and with the "soft" lipid components of dHDL (Gu et al. 2010; Jones et al. 2009a, b, 2010) and sHDL (Jones et al. 2009a). (2) Using sophisticated sequence alignment algorithms, we established the importance of individual amino acid residues for the structure and function of apoA-I (Bashtovyy et al. 2011).

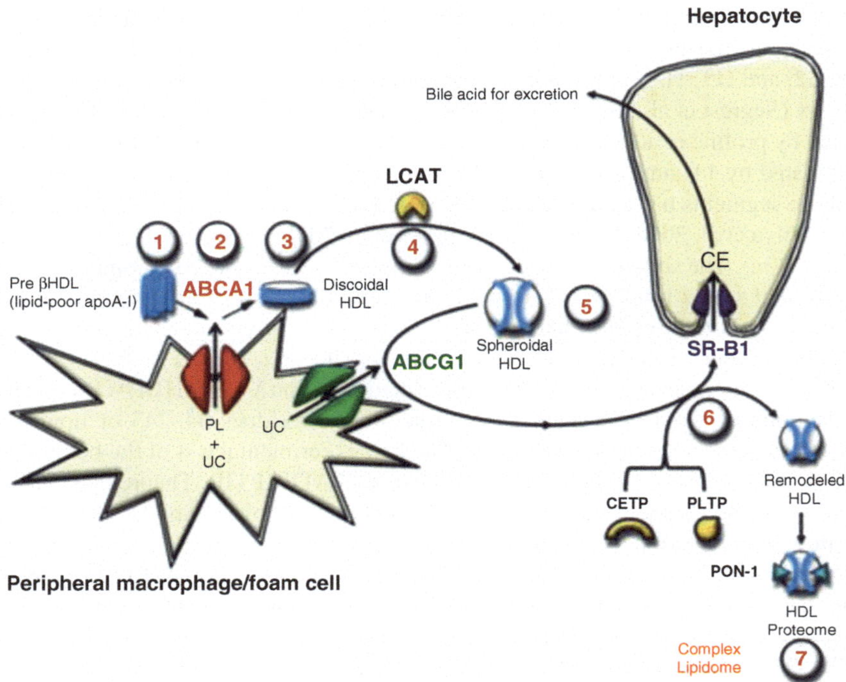

Fig. 3 Relationship of HDL assembly and remodeling to reverse cholesterol transport and the anti-inflammatory HDL proteome

The antiatherogenic nature of HDL is most firmly related to reverse cholesterol transport, a process coupled to HDL assembly and remodeling (Fig. 3). Assembly of nascent dHDL from lipid-poor apoA-I is driven by ABCA1, which acts as a PL pump transporting PL from the inner to the outer membrane monolayer. The structure and function of **lipid-poor apoA-I ❶** and **ABCA1❷** and the physical mechanism involved in the formation of nascent **dHDL❸** are not known (Fig. 1). Cells overexpressing ABCA1 in the absence of apoA-I extrude small vesicles from their membrane surfaces into the cell media (Wang et al. 2000; Duong et al. 2006). Assembly of HDL continues with the action of **LCAT❹** to create **circulating sHDL** containing a core of CE ❺; in animal models, LCAT deficiency reduces HDL and increases CVD (Fazio and Linton 2011). A certain subset of plasma sHDL particles, called Lp(A-I and A-II), contains the apoA-II. Another subset, called Lp(A-I), contains apoA-I without apoA-II (Segrest et al. 2013a, b; Cheung et al. 1987; Silva et al. 2010). Circulating HDL contains two to five (Segrest et al. 2013b) apoA-I arranged in an unknown fashion on the particle. Circulating HDL is remodeled though interactions with the transfer proteins ❻ **CETP** and **PLTP** (Segrest et al. 2013a). Remodeling of sHDL continues with interaction of the particles with other members of the proteome, e.g., **PON1❼**. ABCG1 interacts with sHDL to transfer UC to sHDL. Finally, sHDL interacts with SR-B1, stimulating CE uptake for excretion as bile acids and UC.

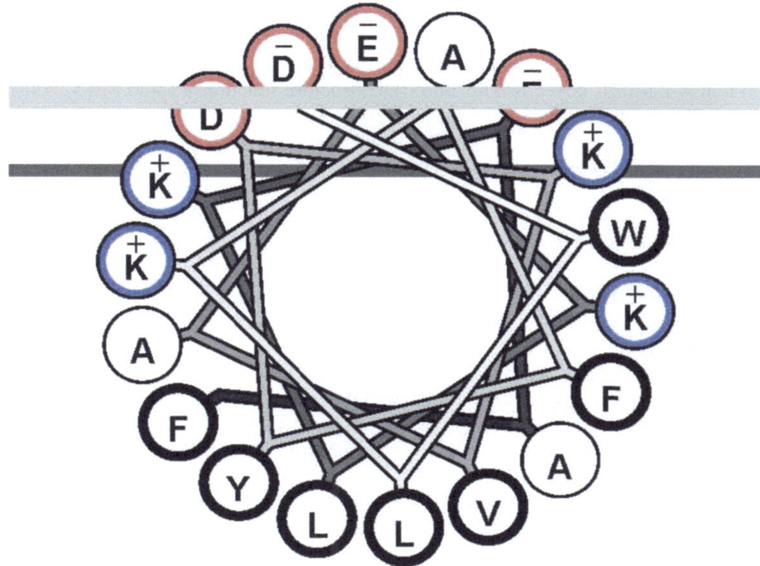

Fig. 4 Helical wheel diagram of the 18A amphipathic helical peptide mimetic. Made using the Λα WHEEL program (Segrest et al. 2002). The lines in front (*thicker gray*) and back (*thinner gray*) mark the calculated tilt of the plane of a membrane monolayer relative to the helix

What Are Peptide Mimetics and Should I Care?

An emerging area in the field of HDL therapy is the development of apolipoprotein mimetic peptides. The initial mimetics were based upon the nonhomologous sequence of the initial synthetic peptide model of the amphipathic helix, 18A (Fig. 4) (Anantharamaiah et al. 1985). Synthetic apoA-I mimetics that emerged from the principles elucidated in our research have been reported to stimulate an increase in plasma HDL concentration and/or PON-1, an antioxidant enzyme that hydrolyzes oxidized phospholipids associated with a decrease in atheroma formation in apoE null and LDL-receptor null mice. As addressed in the chapters that follow, studies of peptide analogs have yielded unique and often unexpected information about and treatment of human diseases.

References

Alwaili K, Awan Z, Alshahrani A, Genest J (2010) High-density lipoproteins and cardiovascular disease: 2010 update. Expert Rev Cardiovasc Ther 8:413–423

Anantharamaiah GM, Jones JL, Brouillette CG, Schmidt CF, Chung BH, Hughes TA, Bhown AS, Segrest JP (1985) Studies of synthetic peptide analogs of the amphipathic helix. Structure of complexes with dimyristoyl phosphatidylcholine. J Biol Chem 260:10248–10255

Barr DP, Russ EM, Eder HA (1951) Protein-lipid relationships in human plasma. II. In atherosclerosis and related conditions. Am J Med 11:480–493

Bashtovyy D, Jones MK, Anantharamaiah GM, Segrest JP (2011) Sequence conservation of apolipoprotein A-I affords novel insights into HDL structure-function. J Lipid Res 52:435–450

Bhat S, Sorci-Thomas MG, Alexander ET, Samuel MP, Thomas MJ (2005) Intermolecular contact between globular N-terminal fold and C-terminal domain of ApoA-I stabilizes its lipid-bound conformation: studies employing chemical cross-linking and mass spectrometry. J Biol Chem 280:33015–33025

Bhat S, Sorci-Thomas MG, Tuladhar R, Samuel MP, Thomas MJ (2007) Conformational adaptation of apolipoprotein A-I to discretely sized phospholipid complexes. Biochemistry 46:7811–7821

Borhani DW, Rogers DP, Engler JA, Brouillette CG (1997) Crystal structure of truncated human apolipoprotein A-I suggests a lipid-bound conformation. Proc Natl Acad Sci U S A 94: 12291–12296

Camejo G, Colacicco G, Rapport MM (1968) Lipid monolayers: interactions with the apoprotein of high density plasma lipoprotein. J Lipid Res 9:562–569

Castelli WP, Doyle JT, Gordon T, Hames CG, Hjortland MC, Hulley SB, Kagan A, Zukel WJ (1977) HDL cholesterol and other lipids in coronary heart disease. The cooperative lipoprotein phenotyping study. Circulation 55:767–772

Cheung MC, Segrest JP, Albers JJ, Cone JT, Brouillette CG, Chung BH, Kashyap M, Glasscock MA, Anantharamaiah GM (1987) Characterization of high density lipoprotein subspecies: structural studies by single vertical spin ultracentrifugation and immunoaffinity chromatography. J Lipid Res 28:913–929

Davidson WS, Hilliard GM (2003) The spatial organization of apolipoprotein A-I on the edge of discoidal high density lipoprotein particles: a mass specrometry study. J Biol Chem 278:27199–27207

Davidson WS, Silva RA, Chantepie S, Lagor WR, Chapman MJ, Kontush A (2009) Proteomic analysis of defined HDL subpopulations reveals particle-specific protein clusters. Relevance to antioxidative function. Arterioscler Thromb Vasc Biol 29:870

Duong PT, Collins HL, Nickel M, Lund-Katz S, Rothblat GH, Phillips MC (2006) Characterization of nascent HDL particles and microparticles formed by ABCA1-mediated efflux of cellular lipids to apoA-I. J Lipid Res 47:832–843

Fazio S, Linton MF (2011) Low levels of high-density lipoprotein cholesterol due to lecithin: cholesterol acyltransferase mutations increase carotid atherosclerosis. J Am Coll Cardiol 58:2488–2490

Forte TM, Nichols AV, Gong EL, Levy RI, Lux S (1971) Electron microscopic study on reassembly of plasma high density apoprotein with various lipids. Biochim Biophys Acta 248:381–386

Glomset JA (1968) The plasma lecithins: cholesterol acyltransferase reaction. J Lipid Res 9:155–167

Gofman JW, Lindgren F (1950) The role of lipids and lipoproteins in atherosclerosis. Science 111:166–171

Goldbourt U, Medalie JH (1979) High density lipoprotein cholesterol and incidence of coronary heart disease–the Israeli Ischemic Heart Disease Study. Am J Epidemiol 109:296–308

Gordon T, Castelli WP, Hjortland MC, Kannel WB, Dawber TR (1977) High density lipoprotein as a protective factor against coronary heart disease. The Framingham study. Am J Med 62:707–714

Gotto AM Jr (1969) Recent studies on the structure of human serum low-and high-density lipoproteins. Proc Natl Acad Sci U S A 64:1119–1127

Gotto AM Jr, Pownall HJ, Havel RJ (1986) Introduction to the plasma lipoproteins. Methods Enzymol 128:3–41

Gu F, Jones MK, Chen J, Patterson JC, Catte A, Jerome WG, Li L, Segrest JP (2010) Structures of discoidal high density lipoproteins: a combined computational-experimental approach. J Biol Chem 285:4652–4665

Gustafson A, Alaupovic P, Furman RH (1965) Studies of the composition and structure of serum lipoproteins: isolation, purification, and characterization of very low density lipoproteins of human serum. Biochemistry 4:596–605

Havel RJ, Eder HA, Bragdon JH (1955) The distribution and chemical composition of ultracentrifugally separated lipoproteins in human serum. J Clin Invest 34:1345–1353

Huang R, Silva RA, Jerome WG, Kontush A, Chapman MJ, Curtiss LK, Hodges TJ, Davidson WS (2011) Apolipoprotein A-I structural organization in high-density lipoproteins isolated from human plasma. Nat Struct Mol Biol 18:416–422

Jones MK, Catte A, Li L, Segrest JP (2009a) Dynamics of activation of lecithin:cholesterol acyltransferase by apolipoprotein A-I. Biochemistry 48:11196–11210

Jones MK, Catte A, Patterson JC, Gu F, Chen J, Li L, Segrest JP (2009b) Thermal stability of apolipoprotein A-I in high-density lipoproteins by molecular dynamics. Biophys J 96: 354–371

Jones MK, Zhang L, Catte A, Li L, Oda MN, Ren G, Segrest JP (2010) Assessment of the validity of the double superhelix model for reconstituted high density lipoproteins: a combined computational-experimental approach. J Biol Chem 285:41161–41171

Kanellis P, Romans AY, Johnson BJ, Kercret H, Chiovetti R Jr, Allen TM, Segrest JP (1980) Studies of synthetic peptide analogs of the amphipathic helix. Effect of charged amino acid residue topography on lipid affinity. J Biol Chem 255:11464–11472

Koppaka V, Silvestro L, Engler JA, Brouillette CG, Axelsen PH (1999) The structure of human lipoprotein A-I. Evidence for the "belt" model. J Biol Chem 274:14541–14544

Lea EJ, Rich GT, Segrest JP (1975) The effects of the membrane-penetrating polypeptide segment of the human erythrocyte MN-glycoprotein on the permeability of model lipid membranes. Biochim Biophys Acta 382:41–50

Li H, Lyles DS, Thomas MJ, Pan W, Sorci-Thomas MG (2000) Structural determination of lipid-bound apo A-I using fluorescence resonance energy transfer. J Biol Chem 275:37048–37054

Li HH, Lyles DS, Pan W, Alexander E, Thomas MJ, Sorci-Thomas MG (2002) ApoA-I structure on discs and spheres. Variable helix registry and conformational states. J Biol Chem 277:39093–39101

Linsel-Nitschke P, Tall AR (2005) HDL as a target in the treatment of atherosclerotic cardiovascular disease. Nat Rev Drug Discov 4:193–205

Mahdy Ali K, Wonnerth A, Huber K, Wojta J (2012) Cardiovascular disease risk reduction by raising HDL cholesterol–current therapies and future opportunities. Br J Pharmacol 167:1177–1194

Maiorano JN, Davidson WS (2000) The orientation of helix 4 in apolipoprotein A-I-containing reconstituted high density lipoproteins. J Biol Chem 275:17374–17380

Maiorano JN, Jandacek RJ, Horace EM, Davidson WS (2004) Identification and structural ramifications of a hinge domain in apolipoprotein A-I discoidal high-density lipoproteins of different size. Biochemistry 43:11717–11726

Martin DD, Budamagunta MS, Ryan RO, Voss JC, Oda MN (2006) Apolipoprotein A-I assumes a "looped belt" conformation on reconstituted high density lipoprotein. J Biol Chem 281: 20418–20426

Miller NE, Thelle DS, Forde OH, Mjos OD (1977) The Tromso heart-study. High-density lipoprotein and coronary heart-disease: a prospective case-control study. Lancet 1:965–968

Mishra VK, Palgunachari MN, Segrest JP, Anantharamaiah GM (1994) Interactions of synthetic peptide analogs of the class A amphipathic helix with lipids. Evidence for the snorkel hypothesis. J Biol Chem 269:7185–7191

Oda MN, Forte TM, Ryan RO, Voss JC (2003) The C-terminal domain of apolipoprotein A-I contains a lipid-sensitive conformational trigger. Nat Struct Biol 10:455–460

Panagotopulos SE, Horace EM, Maiorano JN, Davidson WS (2001) Apolipoprotein A-I adopts a belt-like orientation in reconstituted high density lipoproteins. J Biol Chem 276:42965–42970

Rader DJ, Tall AR (2012) The not-so-simple HDL story: is it time to revise the HDL cholesterol hypothesis? Nat Med 18:1344–1346

Rhoads GG, Gulbrandsen CL, Kagan A (1976) Serum lipoproteins and coronary heart disease in a population study of Hawaii Japanese men. N Engl J Med 294:293–298

Rozek A, Buchko GW, Cushley RJ (1995) Conformation of two peptides corresponding to human apolipoprotein C-I residues 7–24 and 35–53 in the presence of sodium dodecyl sulfate by CD and NMR spectroscopy. Biochemistry 34:7401–7408

Scanu A, Hughes WL (1960) Recombining capacity toward lipids of the protein moiety of human serum alpha 1-lipoprotein. J Biol Chem 235:2876–2883

Segrest JP, Feldmann RJ (1974) Membrane proteins: amino acid sequence and membrane penetration. J Mol Biol 87:853–858

Segrest JP, Jackson RL, Marchesi VT, Guyer RB, Terry W (1972) Red cell membrane glycoprotein: amino acid sequence of an intramembranous region. Biochem Biophys Res Commun 49:964–969

Segrest JP, Gulik-Krzywicki T, Sardet C (1974a) Association of the membrane-penetrating polypeptide segment of the human erythrocyte MN-glycoprotein with phospholipid bilayers. I. Formation of freeze-etch intramembranous particles. Proc Natl Acad Sci U S A 71:3294–3298

Segrest JP, Jackson RL, Morrisett JD, Gotto AM Jr (1974b) A molecular theory of lipid-protein interactions in the plasma lipoproteins. FEBS Lett 38:247–258

Segrest JP, Chung BH, Brouillette CG, Kanellis P, McGahan R (1983) Studies of synthetic peptide analogs of the amphipathic helix. Competitive displacement of exchangeable apolipoproteins from native lipoproteins. J Biol Chem 258:2290–2295

Segrest JP, De Loof H, Dohlman JG, Brouillette CG, Anantharamaiah GM (1990) Amphipathic helix motif: classes and properties. Proteins 8:103–117

Segrest JP, Jones MK, De Loof H, Brouillette CG, Venkatachalapathi YV, Anantharamaiah GM (1992) The amphipathic helix in the exchangeable apolipoproteins: a review of secondary structure and function. J Lipid Res 33:141–166

Segrest JP, Garber DW, Brouillette CG, Harvey SC, Anantharamaiah GM (1994) The amphipathic alpha helix: a multifunctional structural motif in plasma apolipoproteins. Adv Protein Chem 45:303–369

Segrest JP, Jones MK, Klon AE, Sheldahl CJ, Hellinger M, De Loof H, Harvey SC (1999) A detailed molecular belt model for apolipoprotein A-I in discoidal high density lipoprotein. J Biol Chem 274:31755–31758

Segrest JP, Jones MK, Mishra VK, Anantharamaiah GM (2002) Experimental and computational studies of the interactions of amphipathic peptides with lipid surfaces. Curr Top Membr 52:391–429

Segrest JP, Jones MK, Catte A (2013a) MD simulations suggest important surface differences between reconstituted and circulating spherical HDL. J Lipid Res 54:2718–2732

Segrest JP, Cheung MC, Jones MK (2013b) Volumetric determination of apolipoprotein stoichiometry of circulating HDL subspecies. J Lipid Res 54:2733–2744

Shah AS, Tan L, Long JL, Davidson WS (2013) The proteomic diversity of high density lipoproteins: our emerging understanding of its importance in lipid transport and beyond. J Lipid Res 54:2575–2585

Shore V, Shore B (1968) Some physical and chemical studies on two polypeptide components of high-density lipoproteins of human serum. Biochemistry 7:3396–3403

Silva RA, Hilliard GM, Li L, Segrest JP, Davidson WS (2005) A mass spectrometric determination of the conformation of dimeric apolipoprotein A-I in discoidal high density lipoproteins. Biochemistry 44:8600–8607

Silva RA, Huang R, Morris J, Fang J, Gracheva EO, Ren G, Kontush A, Jerome WG, Rye KA, Davidson WS (2008) Structure of apolipoprotein A-I in spherical high density lipoproteins of different sizes. Proc Natl Acad Sci U S A 105:12176–12181

Silva RAGD, Gauthamadasa K, Venkatesan S, Rye KA, Jerome WG, Davidson WS (2010) Site-specific interactions of apolipoprotein A-I and apolipoprotein A-II in discoidal versus spherical high-density lipoprotein particles. Arterioscler Thromb Vasc Biol 30:E280–E280

Tricerri MA, Behling Agree AK, Sanchez SA, Jonas A (2000) Characterization of apolipoprotein A-I structure using a cysteine-specific fluorescence probe. Biochemistry 39:14682–14691

Tricerri MA, Behling Agree AK, Sanchez SA, Bronski J, Jonas A (2001) Arrangement of apolipoprotein a-i in reconstituted high-density lipoprotein disks: an alternative model based on fluorescence resonance energy transfer experiments. Biochemistry 40:5065–5074

Vaisar T, Pennathur S, Green PS, Gharib SA, Hoofnagle AN, Cheung MC, Byun J, Vuletic S, Kassim S, Singh P, Chea H, Knopp RH, Brunzell J, Geary R, Chait A, Zhao XQ, Elkon K, Marcovina S, Ridker P, Oram JF, Heinecke JW (2007) Shotgun proteomics implicates protease inhibition and complement activation in the anti-inflammatory properties of HDL. J Clin Invest 117:746–756

Wang N, Silver DL, Costet P, Tall AR (2000) Specific binding of ApoA-I, enhanced cholesterol efflux, and altered plasma membrane morphology in cells expressing ABC1. J Biol Chem 275:33053–33058

Wu Z, Wagner MA, Zheng L, Parks JS, Shy JM 3rd, Smith JD, Gogonea V, Hazen SL (2007) The refined structure of nascent HDL reveals a key functional domain for particle maturation and dysfunction. Nat Struct Mol Biol 14:861–868

Zlotnick A (2004) Viruses and the physics of soft condensed matter. Proc Natl Acad Sci U S A 101:15549–15550

ApoA-I Mimetic Peptides: A Review of the Present Status

Mohamad Navab, Srinivasa T. Reddy, David Meriwether, Spencer I. Fogelman, and Alan M. Fogelman

Abstract ApoA-I mimetic peptides were designed to function similar to apoA-I, the main protein in HDL. These peptides were found to be efficacious in a large number of animal models of disease. Because it was thought that HDL and apoA-I act primarily in the circulation, it was thought that these peptides also acted primarily in the circulation. Consequently, it was thought that the plasma concentration of peptide must be the major determinant of efficacy. Disparate results in human clinical trials of one apoA-I mimetic peptide, 4F, led to additional studies in mice where it was found that plasma peptide levels do not predict efficacy. Regardless of the route of administration, the small intestine was found to be the critical compartment for determining efficacy. Levels of unsaturated lysophosphatidic acid (LPA) in the small intestine were found to significantly correlate with systemic inflammation and the extent of aortic atherosclerosis in mouse models. The levels of unsaturated LPA in

M. Navab • S.I. Fogelman • A.M. Fogelman, MD (✉)
Division of Cardiology, Department of Medicine, David Geffen School of Medicine at UCLA, 10833 Le Conte Avenue, Box 951736, Los Angeles, CA 90095-1736, USA
e-mail: afogelman@mednet.ucla.edu

S.T. Reddy
Division of Cardiology, Department of Medicine, David Geffen School of Medicine at UCLA, 10833 Le Conte Avenue, Box 951736, Los Angeles, CA 90095-1736, USA

Department of Obstetrics and Gynecology, David Geffen School of Medicine at UCLA, 10833 Le Conte Avenue, Box 951736, Los Angeles, CA 90095-1736, USA

Department of Molecular and Medical Pharmacology, David Geffen School of Medicine at UCLA, 10833 Le Conte Avenue, Box 951736, Los Angeles, CA 90095-1736, USA

D. Meriwether
Division of Cardiology, Department of Medicine, David Geffen School of Medicine at UCLA, 10833 Le Conte Avenue, Box 951736, Los Angeles, CA 90095-1736, USA

Department of Molecular and Medical Pharmacology, David Geffen School of Medicine at UCLA, 10833 Le Conte Avenue, Box 951736, Los Angeles, CA 90095-1736, USA

G.M. Anantharamaiah, D. Goldberg (eds.), *Apolipoprotein Mimetics in the Management of Human Disease*, DOI 10.1007/978-3-319-17350-4_2

the tissue of the small intestine were reduced by the administration of the 4F peptide leading to reduced systemic inflammation and aortic atherosclerosis in mice. The dose required for efficacy was found to be on the order of 40–100 mg/kg/day, making the cost of such peptides prohibitively high because they can only be produced by chemical synthesis. However, a related peptide, 6F, did not require end-blocking groups for efficacy as is the case for the 4F peptides. Consequently, the 6F peptide could be produced in transgenic tomatoes. Feeding these tomatoes at only 2.2 % by weight in a Western diet to LDLR-null mice reduced aortic atherosclerosis similar to the 4F and 5F peptides opening the possibility of treating a variety of diseases with oral apoA-I mimetic peptides expressed in transgenic edible plants.

ApoA-I Mimetic Peptides Were Designed to Mimic a Plasma Apolipoprotein

To understand the interactions of lipoproteins in the artery wall, LDL and HDL were studied in a human artery wall model. The oxidation of human LDL by human artery wall cells in culture was associated with increased production of monocyte chemoattractant protein-1 (MCP-1). Human apoA-I removed seeding molecules from human LDL and thus rendered the LDL resistant to oxidation by human artery wall cells and decreased MCP-1 production by the artery wall cells. The apoA-I-associated seeding molecules included hydroperoxyoctadecadienoic acid (HPODE) and hydroperoxyeicosatetraenoic acid (HPETE). LDL from mice genetically susceptible to diet-induced aortic atherosclerosis was (1) highly susceptible to oxidation by human artery wall cells, (2) induced the production of high levels of MCP-1 by the cells, (3) was rendered resistant to oxidation after incubation in vitro with human apoA-I, and (4) induced much lower levels of MCP-1 production after incubation with human apoA-I. Injection of human apoA-I (but not human apoA-II or murine serum albumin) into mice within 3 h of injection rendered their LDL resistant to oxidation and decreased its ability to induce MCP-1 production by human artery wall cells. Infusion of human apoA-I into humans rendered their LDL resistant to oxidation and decreased its ability to induce MCP-1 production by human artery wall cells within 6 h of infusion (Navab et al. 2000).

ApoA-I is a plasma apolipoprotein which contains 243 amino acids and is the most abundant apolipoprotein in HDL. Almost three decades ago, peptides with 18 amino acid residues were designed to mimic apoA-I (Anantharamaiah et al. 1985). While these peptides have no sequence homology to apoA-I, they were designed to form a class A amphipathic helix and mimic the ability of apoA-I to bind non-oxidized lipids. By blocking the end groups of these peptides with an acetyl group and an amide group, their lipid binding was improved. The prototypic peptide contained 2 phenylalanine residues on the hydrophobic face and was named "2F" (Anantharamaiah 1986). Despite the ability of 2F to bind non-oxidized lipids similar to apoA-I, the peptide was ineffective in a mouse model of atherosclerosis (Datta et al. 2001).

In contrast, a peptide with 18 amino acid residues containing 5 phenylalanine residues on the hydrophobic face significantly reduced aortic lesions in a mouse model of diet-induced atherosclerosis (Garber et al. 2001).

A series of apoA-I mimetic peptides each containing 18 amino acid residues was tested for the ability to prevent LDL from inducing MCP-1 production in cultures of human artery wall cells. Peptides containing 4, 5, or 6 phenylalanine residues (4F, 5F, or 6F, respectively) on the hydrophobic face were significantly more effective than peptides containing 2 or 7 phenylalanine residues (2F or 7F, respectively) (Datta et al. 2001). The peptides 4F, 5F, and 6F were equally effective in this assay (Datta et al. 2001).

Based on the results of this in vitro assay and solubility characteristics that were thought to favor absorption and would result in higher plasma levels after oral administration, the peptide 4F was selected, and it was synthesized from all D-amino acids (D-4F) to prevent degradation of the peptide by digestive enzymes (Navab et al. 2005a). While the dose of D-4F required to achieve efficacy was significantly less than that of the same peptide synthesized from all L-amino acids (L-4F) when the peptides were administered orally (Navab et al. 2002), when the peptides were administered by injection, they were equally efficacious (Van Lenten et al. 2007).

The Peptides Were Effective in a Large Number of Animal Models of Disease

The 4F and 5F peptides were found to be efficacious in a wide variety of animal models of disease including: *air pollution-induced inflammation of the small intestine* (Li et al. 2014), *air pollution-induced changes in lipid metabolism and HDL antioxidant function* (Li et al. 2013), *Alzheimer's disease* (Handattu et al. 2009), *arthritis* (Charles-Schoeman et al. 2008), *asthma* (Nandedkar et al. 2011), *atherosclerosis* (Navab et al. 2002, 2005b, 2009; Li et al. 2004; Morgantini et al. 2010; Wool et al. 2011; Ou et al. 2012; Qin et al. 2012), *chronic rejection of transplanted hearts* (Hsieh et al. 2007), *cancer* (Gao et al. 2011, 2012; Ganapathy et al. 2012; Su et al. 2010, 2012; Neyen et al. 2013), *hepatic fibrosis* (DeLeve et al. 2008), *hyperlipidemia-induced platelet aggregation* (Buga et al. 2010), *hyperlipidemia and sickle cell-induced vascular dysfunction* (Ou et al. 2003, 2005), *hyperlipidemia inhibition of parathyroid hormone activity* (Sage et al. 2011), *hypertension-induced inflammatory changes in the cerebral circulation* (Rodrigues et al. 2013), *influenza A pneumonia* (Van Lenten et al. 2002), *pulmonary hypertension* (Sharma et al. 2014), *renal inflammation* (Buga et al. 2008; Vaziri et al. 2010), *scleroderma* (Weihrauch et al. 2007; Xu et al. 2011, 2012), *tissue injury in sepsis* (Zhang et al 2009; Dai et al. 2010; Datta et al. 2011; Kwon et al. 2012; Sharifov et al. 2013; Moreira et al. 2014), *systemic lupus erythematosus* (Woo et al. 2010), *tissue injury in hyperglycemia and myocardial infarction* (Baotic et al. 2013), *type I diabetes* (Kruger et al. 2005; Peterson et al. 2007), *type II diabetes and obesity* (Peterson et al. 2008, 2009; Ruan et al. 2011; Vecoli et al. 2011; Vanella et al. 2012; Cao et al. 2012; Marino et al. 2012), and *vascular dementia* (Buga et al. 2006).

The 4F peptide has also been incorporated into nanoparticles for the detection of atherosclerosis (Marrache and Dhar 2013) and into a peptibody that generated HDL-like particles in mice (Lu et al. 2012).

The 4F Peptide Was Tested in Human Clinical Trials

The first clinical trial (Bloedon et al. 2008) administered a single oral dose of D-4F of 0.43–7.14 mg/kg or placebo to high-risk cardiovascular patients. Doses of 4.3 mg/kg or 7.14 mg/kg significantly improved HDL function in the cell-based assay used to screen the peptides (i.e., the ability of HDL to inhibit LDL-induced MCP-1 activity in cultures of human aortic endothelial cells was significantly improved at these doses compared to placebo). Doses of 0.43 and 1.43 mg/kg were ineffective. The maximum plasma concentration (Cmax) achieved with the lower doses was 1.62 ± 1.92 ng/mL and 7.75 ± 6.43 ng/mL, respectively. The maximum plasma concentration achieved with the higher doses was 8.13 ± 5.66 ng/mL and 15.9 ± 6.53 ng/mL, respectively.

The second study (Dunbar et al. 2007) administered 13 daily doses of D-4F at 1.43 mg/kg, or 4.3 mg/kg, or 7.14 mg/kg or placebo to high-risk cardiovascular patients. Doses of 4.3 and 7.14 mg/kg significantly improved the HDL function in the cell-based assay compared to placebo. Again, the dose of 1.43 mg/kg was ineffective. The maximum plasma concentrations achieved were 3.6, 9.2, and 37.1 ng/mL, respectively, for the 1.43, 4.3, and 7.14 mg/kg doses.

The third study (Watson et al. 2011) was designed to maximize the plasma peptide levels while minimizing the dose required. The reasons for this strategy were as follows: (1) the cost of manufacturing the peptide is high because of the need for solid phase synthesis and chemical addition of end groups and (2) it was thought that the critical success factor was the plasma peptide level. Consequently, L-4F peptide was administered by subcutaneous injection or by intravenous infusion at doses ranging between 0.042 and 1.43 mg/kg. None of the tested doses improved HDL function compared to placebo despite achieving maximum plasma levels of peptide of 3,255 ± 640 ng/mL.

Reconciling the Divergent Results from the Clinical Trials

The first two studies used oral D-4F and the third used injected L-4F. There is a difference in the dose required for efficacy between D-4F and L-4F when administered orally (Navab et al. 2002). Much higher doses of L-4F are required when administered orally (Navab et al. 2002, 2009; Su et al. 2010). However, when administered by injection, there does not appear to be a significant difference in the dose required for efficacy (Van Lenten et al. 2007). Additionally, the plasma levels in these studies were determined by mass spectral analysis, and the plasma levels reported were for the intact peptide. It was noted that the maximal dose used in the third study was lower than that of the reported to be efficacious in the first two studies and was also lower than that used successfully in mice (Navab et al. 2002), rabbits (Van Lenten et al. 2007), and normolipidemic monkeys (Navab et al. 2004, 2005b). Therefore, mouse studies were conducted to determine whether the dose or plasma levels of peptide better determined efficacy.

ApoE-null mice were administered the peptide D-4F either orally or subcutaneously (SQ) at doses of 0.15, 0.45, 4.5, or 45 mg/kg per day (Navab et al. 2011). The plasma peptide levels were ~1,000-fold higher when administered SQ compared with oral administration. However, regardless of the route of administration, doses of 4.5 mg/kg and 45 mg/kg significantly reduced serum amyloid A (SAA) plasma levels and improved HDL function as measured by the cell-based assay for MCP-1 activity, while doses of 0.15 mg/kg and 0.45 mg/kg were ineffective regardless of the route of administration. A dose of 45 mg/kg/day administered to LDLR-null mice on a Western diet (WD) reduced aortic atherosclerosis by 50 % ($p<0.0009$) whether administered orally or SQ and also significantly reduced plasma SAA levels ($p<0.002$) and plasma lysophosphatidic acid (LPA) levels ($p<0.0009$). Despite the enormous difference in plasma levels when the peptide was administered orally compared to SQ, at each dose administered, the concentration and amount of peptide in the feces were similar regardless of whether the peptide was administered orally or SQ. It was concluded that (1) the dose of 4F administered and not the plasma level achieved determines efficacy and (2) the intestine may be a major site of action for the peptide regardless of the route of administration.

Another study in LDLR-null mice provided further support for these conclusions. In this study, (Navab et al. 2012) LDLR-null mice were fed WD and administered D-4F orally or SQ. Plasma and liver peptide levels were 298-fold and 96-fold higher, respectively, after SQ administration, while peptide levels in the small intestine varied by only 1.66 ± 0.33-fold. Levels of metabolites of arachidonic and linoleic acids that are known to bind with high affinity to D-4F were significantly reduced in the small intestine, liver, and hepatic bile to a similar degree whether the peptide was administered orally or SQ. In contrast, levels of 20-HETE, which is known to bind the peptide with low affinity, did not change with peptide administration. Peptide administration significantly reduced plasma SAA and triglyceride levels and increased HDL-cholesterol levels similarly whether the peptide was administered orally or SQ. The plasma levels of metabolites of arachidonic and linoleic acids significantly correlated with plasma SAA levels ($p<0.0001$). The results of these two studies (Navab et al. 2011, 2012) clearly demonstrated that plasma peptide levels did not predict efficacy, but levels of peptide in the intestine did predict efficacy. Since the highest dose of peptide used in the human clinical trial that did not demonstrate efficacy (Watson et al. 2011) was below any dose shown to be effective, it was concluded that despite the high plasma levels achieved in these clinical trials, even if all of the administered peptide would have reached the small intestine (which is not likely), the dose reaching the small intestine would have been inadequate and, thus, likely explained the negative results.

Overcoming the Barrier of the High Cost of Production of Chemically Synthesized ApoA-I Mimetic Peptides

The studies discussed above indicate that there is no advantage to administering these apoA-I mimetic peptides by any route other than by the oral route since the critical level to be achieved appears to be in the small intestine. These studies also indicate that high doses of peptide, preferably in the 40–100 mg/kg/day range, will be required for maximum efficacy. Unfortunately, the 4F and 5F peptides require end-blocking groups that can only be added by chemical synthesis. As a consequence, the chronic administration of these peptides would be prohibitively expensive. To overcome this problem, Chattopadhyay et al. (2013) looked for an apoA-I mimetic peptide that would be efficacious without having to add end-blocking groups. They found that the peptide 6F, which was previously found to be equally as effective as 4F and 5F in the cell-based assay (Datta et al. 2001), did not require end-blocking groups for efficacy (Chattopadhyay et al. 2013). This allowed these investigators to construct transgenic tomato plants that expressed the 6F peptide (Tg6F) or a control marker protein, β-glucuronidase (EV). These transgenic tomatoes were harvested, lyophilized, ground into powder, added to WD at 2.2 % by weight, and fed to LDLR-null mice providing the mice with 45 mg/kg/day of 6F peptide. After 13 weeks, the mice receiving Tg6F had a greater than 50 % decrease in aortic atherosclerosis ($p=0.0134$) compared to WD alone; the mice receiving the control tomatoes did not have a significant reduction in aortic atherosclerosis. Body weights did not differ among the treatment groups, but plasma SAA, total cholesterol, and triglyceride levels were significantly lower in the mice receiving Tg6F. Plasma HDL-cholesterol levels and paraoxonase-1 activity were significantly higher in the mice receiving Tg6F. After feeding Tg6F intact 6F peptide was found in the small intestine but not in the plasma. Moreover, after feeding Tg6F LPA levels were decreased in the tissue of the small intestine, and the levels of unsaturated LPA in the tissue of the small intestine significantly correlated with the extent of aortic atherosclerosis. It was concluded that 6F acts in the small intestine and transgenic expression of 6F in edible plants may be a novel approach to oral apoA-I mimetic therapy (Chattopadhyay et al. 2013; Getz and Reardon 2013).

Subsequent to the report by Chattopadhyay et al. (2013), Zhao et al. (2014) reported that an apoA-I mimetic peptide with a completely different structure from the 4F, 5F to 6F peptides was equally effective when administered by injection or given orally despite the inability to detect peptide in the plasma after oral administration and the findings of very high peptide plasma levels after injection. These findings suggested that the site of action of multiple apoA-I mimetic peptides with completely different structures might be in the intestine regardless of the route of administration (Wool et al. 2014).

Determining the Mechanism of Action of Oral ApoA-I Mimetic Peptides

Following up on the observation that LPA levels in the tissue of the small intestine significantly correlated with the extent of aortic atherosclerosis (Chattopadhyay et al. 2013), Navab et al. (2013) reported that feeding LDLR-null mice WD resulted in increased levels of unsaturated LPA in the tissue of the small intestine, but did not alter the levels of saturated LPA in the small intestine. Adding Tg6F to WD significantly decreased the WD-mediated increase in small intestine unsaturated LPA levels and did not alter the levels of saturated LPA in the small intestine. Moreover, adding Tg6F to WD prevented many WD-mediated changes in the expression of genes in the small intestine. Remarkably, if instead of feeding WD, unsaturated LPA was added to low-fat mouse chow (1 μg unsaturated LPA per gram mouse chow) and fed to the mice, the levels of LPA in the tissue of the small intestine were similar to those seen after feeding WD. Moreover, the WD-mediated changes in gene expression in the small intestine were mimicked by feeding low-fat mouse chow supplemented with unsaturated LPA. Most interestingly, feeding low-fat mouse chow supplemented with unsaturated (but not saturated) LPA produced changes in plasma levels of SAA, total cholesterol, triglycerides, and HDL-cholesterol and also resulted in a fast-performance liquid chromatography lipoprotein profile that was strikingly similar to that seen after feeding the mice WD. Adding Tg6F (but not control tomatoes) to LPA-supplemented chow prevented the LPA-induced changes. It was concluded that WD-mediated systemic inflammation and dyslipidemia may be in part due to WD-mediated increases in the levels of unsaturated LPA in the tissue of the small intestine. It was further concluded that Tg6F reduces WD-mediated systemic inflammation and dyslipidemia by preventing the WD-mediated increase in unsaturated LPA levels in the tissue of the small intestine (Navab et al. 2013; Remaley 2013).

Other Peptides

In addition to the peptides described by Zhao et al. (2014), Bielicki et al. (2010) described a single-helix peptide (ATI-5261) that stimulates cellular cholesterol efflux with an efficiency approximating native apolipoproteins. Daily intraperitoneal injection of fat-fed LDLR-null mice at a dose of 30 mg/kg for 6 weeks reduced atherosclerosis by 30 %. In apoE-null mice, administering the peptide every other day by intraperitoneal injection at a dose of 30 mg/kg for 6 weeks reduced atherosclerosis by ~45 %. Amar et al. (2010) designed a bihelical amphipathic peptide (5A) that mediated a 3.5-fold increase in ABCA1-mediated efflux from cells and an additional 2.5-fold increase after the peptide was incorporated into phospholipid complexes. Twenty-four hours after intravenous injection of the peptide-phospholipid complex at a dose of 30 mg/kg in apoE-null mice, there was a 181 % increase in HDL-cholesterol and a 219 % increase in the content of HDL phospholipid. There was an associated 29–53 % decrease in aortic plaque surface area. Wool et al. (2011) demonstrated that injection of 4F or a tandem 4F peptide containing a proline linker caused increased production of antibodies against oxidation-specific epitopes, including a disproportionate induction of the IgM natural antibody E06/T15 to oxidized phospholipids. Interestingly, only the 4F peptide reduced atherosclerosis of early lesions in chow-fed apoE-null mice. At the doses administered (1.19 mg/kg 4F peptide or 2.38 mg/kg of the tandem peptide), neither peptide reduced more advanced lesions.

Conclusions

ApoA-I mimetic peptides were designed to mirror the functions of apoA-I, the main protein in HDL. ApoA-I mimetic peptides were found to be efficacious in a large number of animal models of disease. It was thought that these peptides acted primarily in the circulation as we imagine is the case for HDL and apoA-I. As a result, it was thought that the plasma concentration of peptide must be the major determinant of efficacy. Through an accident of disparate results from clinical trials of one apoA-I mimetic peptide, 4F, it was found that plasma peptide levels do not predict efficacy. Remarkably, regardless of the route of administration, the critical compartment for determining efficacy appears to be in the small intestine. The levels of unsaturated LPA in the small intestine were found to significantly correlate with systemic inflammation and the extent of aortic atherosclerosis in mouse models. The 4F peptide was found to reduce the level of unsaturated LPA in the small intestine and reduce systemic inflammation and aortic atherosclerosis in mice. However, the dose required for efficacy was found to be on the order of 40–100 mg/kg/day, which makes the cost of producing such peptides by chemical synthesis prohibitively high. Fortunately, a related peptide 6F was found to not require end-blocking groups, which can be only added by chemical synthesis. As a result, the 6F peptide was produced in transgenic tomatoes and was found to be efficacious in a mouse model of atherosclerosis similar to the 4F and 5F peptides. These studies open the possibility to treatment of a variety of diseases with oral apoA-I mimetic peptides expressed in transgenic edible plants.

Funding This work was supported in part by US Public Health Service Grants HL-30568 and the Laubisch, Castera, M.K. Grey Funds at UCLA and the Leducq Foundation.

Disclosures AMF, STR, and MN are principals in Bruin Pharma, and AMF is an officer in Bruin Pharma.

References

Amar MJ, D'Souza W, Turner S, Demosky S, Sviridov D, Stonik J, Luchoomun J, Voogt J, Hellerstein M, Sviridov D, Remaley AT (2010) 5A apolipoprotein mimetic peptide promotes cholesterol efflux and reduces atherosclerosis in mice. JPET 334:634–641

Anantharamaiah GM (1986) Synthetic peptide analogs of apolipoproteins. Methods Enzymol 128:627–647

Anantharamaiah GM, Jones JL, Brouillette CG, Schmidt CF, Chung BH, Hughes TA, Brown AS, Segrest JP (1985) Studies of synthetic peptide analogs of amphipathic helix I: structure of peptide/DMPC complexes. J Biol Chem 260:10248–10255

Baotic I, Ge ZD, Sedlic F, Coon A, Weihrauch D, Warltier DC, Kersten JR (2013) Apolipoprotein A-1 mimetic peptide D-4F enhances isoflurane-induced eNOS signaling and cardioprotection during acute hyperglycemia. Am J Physiol Heart Circ Physiol 305:H219–H227

Bielicki JK, Zhang H, Cortez Y, Zheng Y, Narayanaswami AP, Johansson J, Azhar S (2010) A new HDL mimetic peptide that stimulates cellular cholesterol efflux with high efficiency greatly reduces atherosclerosis in mice. J Lipid Res 51:1496–1503

Bloedon LT, Dunbar R, Duffy D, Pinell-Salles P, Norris R, DeGroot BJ, Movva R, Navab M, Fogelman AM, Rader DJ (2008) Safety, pharmacokinetics, and pharmacodynamics of oral apoA-I mimetic peptide D-4F in high-risk cardiovascular patients. J Lipid Res 49:1344–1352

Buga GM, Frank JS, Mottino GA, Hendizadeh M, Hakhamian A, Tillisch JH, Reddy ST, Navab M, Anantharamaiah GM, Ignarro LJ, Fogelman AM (2006) D-4F decreases brain arteriole inflammation and improves cognitive performance in LDL receptor-null mice on a Western diet. J Lipid Res 47:2148–2160

Buga GM, Frank JS, Mottino GA, Hakhamian A, Narasimha A, Watson AD, Yekta B, Navab M, Reddy ST, Anantharamaiah GM, Fogelman AM (2008) D-4F reduces EO6 immunoreactivity, SREBP-1c mRNA levels, and renal inflammation in LDL receptor-null mice fed a Western diet. J Lipid Res 49:192–205

Buga GM, Navab M, Imaizumi S, Reddy ST, Yekta B, Hough G, Chanslor S, Anantharamaiah GM, Fogelman AM (2010) L-4F alters hyperlipidemic (but not healthy) mouse plasma to reduce platelet aggregation. Arterioscler Thromb Vasc Biol 30:283–289

Cao J, Puri N, Sodhi K, Bellner L, Abraham NG, Kappas A (2012) ApoA-I mimetic rescues the diabetic phenotype of HO-2 knockout mice via an increase in HO-1 adiponectin and LKBI signaling pathway. Int J Hypertens 2012:628147

Charles-Schoeman C, Banquerigo ML, Hama S, Navab M, Park GS, Van Lenten BJ, Wagner AC, Fogelman AM, Brahn E (2008) Treatment with an apolipoprotein A-1 mimetic peptide in combination with pravastatin inhibits collagen-induced arthritis. Clin Immunol 127:234–244

Chattopadhyay A, Navab M, Hough G, Gao F, Meriwether D, Grijalva V, Springstead JR, Palgnachari MN, Namiri-Kalantari R, Su F, Van Lenten BJ, Wagner AC, Anantharamaiah GM, Farias-Eisner R, Reddy ST, Fogelman AM (2013) A novel approach to oral apoA-I mimetic therapy. J Lipid Res 54:995–1010

Dai L, Datta G, Zhang Z, Gupta H, Patel R, Honavar J, Modi S, Wyss JM, Palgunachari M, Anantharamaiah GM, White CR (2010) The apolipoprotein A-I mimetic peptide 4F prevents defects in vascular function in endotoxemic rats. J Lipid Res 51:2695–2705

Datta G, Chaddha M, Hama S, Navab M, Fogelman AM, Garber DW, Mishra VK, Epand RM, Epand RF, Lund-Katz S, Phillips MC, Segrest JP, Anantharamaiah GM (2001) Effects of increasing hydrophobicity on the physical–chemical and biological properties of a class A amphipathic helical peptide. J Lipid Res 42:1096–1104

Datta G, Gupta H, Zhang Z, Mayakonda P, Anantharamaiah GM, White CR (2011) HDL mimetic peptide administration improves left ventricular filling and cardiac output in lipopolysaccharide-treated rats. J Clin Exp Cardiolog 2(172). doi: 10.4172/2155-9880.1000172

DeLeve LD, Wang X, Kanel GC, Atkinson RD, McCuskey RS (2008) Prevention of hepatic fibrosis in a murine model of metabolic syndrome with nonalcoholic steatohepatitis. Am J Pathol 173:993–1001

Dunbar RL, Bloedon LT, Duffy D, Norris RB, Movva R, Navab M, Fogelman AM, Rader DJ (2007) Daily oral administration of the apolipoprotein A-I mimetic peptide D-4F in patients with coronary heart disease or equivalent risk improves high-density lipoprotein anti-inflammatory function. J Am Coll Cardiol 49(Suppl A):366A, Abstract 1014–123

Ganapathy E, Su F, Meriwether D, Devarajan A, Grijalva V, Gao F, Chattopadhyay A, Anantharamaiah GM, Navab M, Fogelman AM, Reddy ST, Farias-Eisner R (2012) D-4F an apoA-I mimetic peptide inhibits proliferation and tumorigenicity of epithelial ovarian cancer cells by upregulating the antioxidant enzyme MnSO. Int J Cancer 130:1071–1081

Gao F, Vasquez SX, Su F, Roberts S, Shah N, Grijalva V, Imaizumi S, Chattopadhyay A, Ganapathy E, Merriwether D, Johnston B, Anantharamaiah GM, Navab M, Fogelman AM, Reddy ST, Farias-Eisner R (2011) L-5F, an apolipoprotein A-I mimetic, inhibits tumor angiogenesis by suppressing VEGF/basic FGF signaling pathways. Integr Biol (Camb) 3:479–489

Gao F, Chattopadhyay A, Navab M, Grijalva V, Su F, Fogelman AM, Reddy ST, Farias-Eisner R (2012) Apolipoprotein A-I mimetic peptides inhibit expression and activity of hypoxia-inducible factor 1a in human ovarian cancer cell lines and a mouse ovarian cancer model. J Pharmacol Exp Ther 342:255–262

Garber DW, Datta G, Chaddha M, Palgunachari MN, Hama SY, Navab M, Fogelman AM, Segrest JP, Anantharamaiah GM (2001) A new synthetic class A amphipathic peptide analogue protects mice from diet-induced atherosclerosis. J Lipid Res 42:545–552

Getz GS, Reardon CA (2013) ApoA-I mimetics: tomatoes to the rescue. J Lipid Res 54:878–880

Handattu SP, Garber DW, Monroe CE, van Groen T, Kadish I, Navvar G, Cao D, Palgunachari MN, Li L, Anantharamaiah GM (2009) Oral apolipoprotein A-I mimetic peptide improves cognitive function and reduces amyloid burden in a mouse model of Alzheimer's disease. Neurobiol Dis 34:525–534

Hsieh GR, Schnickel GT, Garcia C, Shefizadeh A, Fishbein MC, Ardehali A (2007) Inflammation/oxidation in chronic rejection: apolipoprotein A-I mimetic peptide reduces chronic rejection of transplanted hearts. Transplantation 84:238–243

Kruger AL, Peterson S, Turkseven S, Kaminski PM, Zhang FF, Quan S, Wolin MS, Abraham NG (2005) D-4F induces heme oxygenase-1 and extracellular superoxide dismutase, decreases endothelial cell sloughing, and improves vascular reactivity in rat model of diabetes. Circulation 111:3126–3134

Kwon WY, Suh GJ, Kim KS, Kwak YH, Kim K (2012) 4F apolipoprotein AI mimetic peptide attenuates acute lung injury and improves survival in endotoxemic rats. J Trauma Acute Care Surg 72:1576–1583

Li X, Chyu K-Y, Faria JR, Yano J, Nathwani N, Ferreira C, Dimayuga PC, Cercek B, Kaul S, Shah PK (2004) Differential effects of apolipoprotein A-I-mimetic peptide on evolving and established atherosclerosis in apolipoprotein E-null mice. Circulation 110:1701–1705

Li R, Navab M, Pakbin P, Ning Z, Navab K, Hough G, Morgan TE, Finch CE, Arajuo JA, Fogelman AM, Sioutas C, Hsiai T (2013) Ambient ultrafine particles alter lipid metabolism and HDL anti-oxidant capacity in LDLR-null mice. J Lipid Res 54:1608–1615

Li R, Navab K, Hough G, Daher N, Zhang M, Mittelstein D, Lee K, Pakbin P, Saffari A, Bhetraratana M, Sulaiman D, Beebe T, Wu L, Jen N, Wine E, Tseng CH, Araujo JA, Fogelman AM, Sioutas C, Navab M, Hsiai TK (2015) Effect of exposure to atmospheric ultrafine particles on production of free fatty acids and lipid metabolites in the mouse small intestine. Environ Health Perspect 123:34–41

Lu SC, Atangan L, Won Kim K, Chen MM, Komorowski R, Chu C, Han J, Hu S, Gu W, Veniant M, Wang M (2012) An apoA-I mimetic peptibody generates HDL-like particles and increases alpha-1 HDL subfraction in mice. J Lipid Res 53:643–652

Marino JS, Peterson SJ, Li M, Vanella L, Sodhi K, Hill JW, Abraham NG (2012) ApoA-1 mimetic restores adiponectin expression and insulin sensitivity independent of changes in body weight in female obese mice. Nutr Diabet 12:e33

Marrache S, Dhar S (2013) Biodegradable synthetic high-density lipoprotein nanoparticles for atherosclerosis. Proc Natl Acad Sci U S A 110:9445–9450

Moreira RS, Irigoyen M, Sanches TR, Volpini RA, Camara NO, Malheiros DM, Shimizu MH, Seguro AS, Andrade L (2014) Apolipoprotein A-I mimetic peptide 4F attenuates kidney injury, heart injury, and endothelial dysfunction in sepsis. Am J Physiol Regul Integr Comp Physiol 307:R514–R524

Morgantini C, Imaizumi S, Grijalva V, Navab M, Fogelman AM, Reddy ST (2010) Apolipoprotein A-I mimetic peptides prevent atherosclerosis development and reduce plaque inflammation in a murine model of diabetes. Diabetes 59:3223–3228

Nandedkar SD, Weihrauch D, Xu H, Shi Y, Feroah T, Hutchins W, Rickaby DA, Duzgunes N, Hillery CA, Konduri KS, Pritchard KA Jr (2011) D-4F, an apoA-I mimetic, decreases airway hyperresponsiveness, inflammation, and oxidative stress in a murine model of asthma. J Lipid Res 52:499–508

Navab M, Hama SY, Cooke CJ, Anantharamaiah GM, Chaddha M, Jin L, Subbanagounder G, Faull KF, Reddy ST, Miller NE, Fogelman AM (2000) Normal high density lipoprotein inhibits three steps in the formation of mildly oxidized low density lipoprotein: step 1. J Lipid Res 41:1481–1494

Navab M, Anantharamaiah GM, Hama S, Garber DW, Chaddha M, Hough G, Lallone R, Fogelman AM (2002) Oral administration of an apoA-I mimetic peptide synthesized from D-amino acids dramatically reduces atherosclerosis in mice independent of plasma cholesterol. Circulation 105:290–292

Navab M, Anantharamaiah GM, Reddy ST, Van Lenten BJ, Ansell BJ, Fonarow GC, Vahabzadeh K, Hama S, Hough G, Kamranpour N, Berliner JA, Lusis AJ, Fogelman AM (2004) The oxidation hypothesis of atherogenesis: the role of oxidized phospholipids and HDL. J Lipid Res 45:993–1007

Navab M, Anantharamaiah GM, Reddy ST, Hama S, Hough G, Grijalva VR, Yu N, Ansell BJ, Datta G, Garber DW, Fogelman AM (2005a) Apolipoprotein A-I mimetic peptides. Arterioscler Thromb Vasc Biol 25:1325–1331

Navab M, Anantharamaiah GM, Hama S, Hough G, Reddy ST, Frank JS, Garber DW, Handattu S, Fogelman AM (2005b) D-4F and statins synergize to render HDL anti-inflammatory in mice and monkeys and cause lesion regression in old apolipoprotein E-null mice. Arteroscler Thromb Vasc Biol 25:1426–1432

Navab M, Ruchala P, Waring AJ, Lehrer RI, Hama S, Hough G, Palgunachari MN, Anantharamaiah GM, Fogelman AM (2009) A novel method for oral delivery of apolipoprotein mimetic peptides synthesized from all L-amino acids. J Lipid Res 50:1538–1547

Navab M, Reddy ST, Anantharamaiah GM, Imaizumi S, Hough G, Hama S, Fogelman AM (2011) Intestine may be a major site of action for the apoA-I mimetic peptide 4F whether administered subcutaneously or orally. J Lipid Res 52:1200–1210

Navab M, Reddy ST, Anantharamaiah GM, Hough G, Buga GM, Danciger J, Fogelman AM (2012) D-4F mediated reduction in metabolites of arachidonic and linoleic acids in the small intestine is associated with decreased inflammation in low-density lipoprotein receptor-null mice. J Lipid Res 53:437–445

Navab M, Hough G, Buga GM, Su F, Wagner AC, Meriwether D, Chattopadhyay A, Gao F, Grijalva V, Danciger JS, Van Lenten BJ, Org E, Lusis AJ, Pan C, Anantharamaiah GM, Farias-Eisner R, Smyth SS, Reddy ST, Fogelman AM (2013) Transgenic 6F tomatoes act on the small intestine to prevent systemic inflammation and dyslipidemia caused by Western diet and intestinally derived lysophosphatidic acid. J Lipid Res 54:3403–3418

Neyen C, Mukhopadhyay S, Gordon S, Hagemann T (2013) An apolipoprotein A-I mimetic targets scavenger receptor A on tumor-associated macrophages: a prospective anticancer treatment? Oncoimmunology 2:e24461

Ou J, Ou Z, Jones DW, Holzhauer S, Hatoum OA, Ackerman AW, Weihrauch DW, Gutterman DD, Guice K, Oldham KT, Hiller CA, Pritchard KA Jr (2003) L-4F, an apolipoprotein A-I mimetic, dramatically improves vasodilation in hypercholesterolemia and sickle cell disease. Circulation 107:2337–2341

Ou J, Wang J, Xu H, Ou Z, Sorci-Thomas MG, Jones DW, Signorino P, Densmore JC, Kaul S, Oldham KT, Pritchard KA Jr (2005) Effects of D-4F on vasodilation and vessel wall thickness in hypercholesterolemic LDL receptor-null and LDL receptor/apolipoprotein A-I double knockout mice on Western diet. Circ Res 97:1190–1197

Ou ZJ, Li L, Liao XL, Wang YM, Hu XX, Zhang QL, Wang ZP, Yu H, Zhang X, Hu P, Xu YQ, Liang QL, Ou JS, Luo G (2012) Apolipoprotein A-I mimetic peptide inhibits atherosclerosis by altering plasma metabolites in hypercholesterolemia. Am J Physiol Endocrinol Metab 303:E683–E694

Peterson SJ, Husney D, Kruger AL, Olszanecki R, Ricci F, Rodella LF, Stacchiotti A, Rezzani R, McClung JA, Aronow WS, Ikehara S, Abraham NG (2007) Long-term treatment with the apolipoprotein A1 mimetic peptide increases antioxidants and vascular repair in type I diabetic rats. J Pharmacol Exp Ther 322:514–520

Peterson SJ, Drummond G, Kim DH, Li M, Kruger AL, Ikehara S, Abraham NG (2008) L-4F treatment reduces adiposity, increases adiponectin levels, and improves insulin sensitivity in obese mice. J Lipid Res 49:1658–1669

Peterson SJ, Kim DH, Li M, Positano V, Vanella L, Rodella LF, Piccolomini F, Puri N, Gastaldelli A, Kusmic C, L'Abbate A, Abraham NG (2009) The L-4F mimetic peptide prevents insulin resistance through increased levels of HO-1, pAMPK, and pAKT in obese mice. J Lipid Res 50:1293–1304

Qin S, Kamanna VS, Lai JH, Liu T, Ganj SH, Zhang L, Bachovchin WW, Kashyap ML (2012) Reverse D4F, an apolipoprotein-AI mimetic peptide inhibits atherosclerosis in apoE-null mice. J Cardiovasc Pharmacol Ther 17:334–343

Remaley AT (2013) Tomatoes, lysophosphatidic acid, and the small intestine: new pieces in the puzzle of apolipoprotein mimetic peptides? J Lipid Res 54:3223–3226

Rodrigues SF, Vital SA, Granger DN (2013) Mild hypercholesterolemia blunts the proinflammatory and prothrombotic effects of hypertension on the cerebral circulation. J Cereb Blood Flow Metab 33:483–489

Ruan X, Li Z, Zhang Y, Yang L, Pan Y, Wang Z, Feng GS, Chen Y (2011) Apolipoprotein A-I possesses and antiobesity effect associated with increase of energy expenditure and upregulation of UCP1 in brown fat. J Cell Mol Med 15:763–772

Sage AP, Lu J, Tetradis S, Ascenzi MG, Adama DJ, Demer LL, Tintut Y (2011) Hyperlipidemia induces resistance to PTH bone anabolism in mice via oxidized lipids. J Bone Miner Res 26:1197–1206

Sharifov OF, Xu X, Gaggar A, Grizzle WE, Mishra VK, Honaar J, Litovsky SH, Palgunachari MN, White CR, Anantharamaiah GM, Gupta H (2013) Anti-inflammatory mechanisms of apolipoprotein A-I mimetic peptide in acute respiratory distress syndrome secondary to sepsis. PLoS ONE 8:e64486

Sharma S, Umar S, Potus F, Iorga A, Wong G, Meriwether D, Breuils-Bonnet S, Mai D, Navab K, Ross D, Navab M, Provencher S, Fogelman AM, Bonnet S, Reddy ST, Eghbali M (2014) Apolipoprotein A-I mimetic peptide 4F rescues pulmonary hypertension by inducing microRNA-193-3p. Circulation 130:776–785

Su F, Kozak KR, Imaizumi S, Gao F, Amneus MW, Grijalva V, Ng C, Wagner A, Hough G, Farias-Eisner G, Anantharamaiah GM, Van Lenten BJ, Navab M, Fogelman AM, Reddy ST, Farias-Eisner R (2010) Apolipoprotein A-I (apoA-I) and apoA-I mimetic peptides inhibit tumor development in a mouse model of ovarian cancer. Proc Natl Acad Sci U S A 107:19997–20002

Su F, Grijalva V, Navab K, Ganapathy E, Meriwether D, Imaizumi S, Navab M, Fogelman AM, Reddy ST, Farias-Eisner R (2012) HDL mimetics inhibit tumor development in both induced and spontaneous mouse models of colon cancer. Mol Cancer Ther 11:1311–1319

Van Lenten BJ, Wagner AC, Anantharamaiah GM, Garber DW, Fishbein MC, Adhikary L, Nayak DP, Hama S, Navab M, Fogelman AM (2002) Influenza infection promotes macrophage traffic into arteries of mice that is prevented by D-4F, an apolipoprotein A-I mimetic peptide. Circulation 106:1127–1132

Van Lenten BJ, Wagner AC, Navab M, Anantharamaiah GM, Hama S, Reddy ST, Fogelman AM (2007) Lipoprotein inflammatory properties and serum amyloid A levels but not cholesterol levels predict lesion area in cholesterol-fed rabbits. J Lipid Res 48:2344–2353

Vanella L, Li M, Kim D, Malfa G, Bellner L, Kawakami T, Abraham NG (2012) ApoA1: mimetic peptide reverses adipocyte dysfunction in vivo and in vitro via an increase in heme oxygenase (HO-1) and Wnt10b. Cell Cycle 11:706–714

Vaziri ND, Kim HJ, Moradi H, Farmand F, Navab K, Navab M, Hama S, Fogelman AM, Quiroz Y, Rodriguez-Iturbe B (2010) Amelioration of nephropathy with apoA-1 mimetic peptide in apoE-deficient mice. Nephrol Dial Transplant 25:3525–3534

Vecoli C, Cao J, Neglia D, Inoue K, Sodhi K, Vanella L, Gabrielson KK, Bedia D, Paolocci N, L'abbate A, Abraham NG (2011) Apolipoprotein A-I mimetic peptide L-4F prevents myocardial and coronary dysfunction in diabetic mice. J Cell Biochem 112:2616–2626

Watson CE, Weissbach N, Kjems L, Ayalasomayajula S, Zhang Y, Chang I, Navab M, Hama S, Hough G, Reddy ST, Soffer D, Rader DJ, Fogelman AM, Schecter A (2011) Treatment of patients with cardiovascular disease with L-4F, an apoA1 mimetic, did not improve select biomarkers of HDL function. J Lipid Res 52:361–373

Weihrauch D, Xu H, Shi Y, Wang J, Brien J, Jones DW, Kaul S, Komorowski RA, Csuka ME, Oldham KT, Pritchard KA Jr (2007) Effects of D-4F on vasodilation, oxidative stress, angiostatin, myocardial inflammation, and angiogenic potential in tight skin mice. Am J Physiol Heart Circ Physiol 293:H1432–H1441

Woo JM, Lin Z, Navab M, Van Dyck C, Trejo-Lopez Y, Woo KM, Li H, Castellani LW, Wang X, Iikuni N, Rullo OJ, Wu H, La Cava A, Fogelman AM, Lusis AJ, Tsao BP (2010) Treatment with apolipoprotein A-1 mimetic peptide reduces lupus-like manifestations in a murine lupus model of accelerated atherosclerosis. Arthritis Res Ther 12:R93

Wool GD, Cabana VG, Lukens J, Shaw PX, Binder CJ, Witztum JL, Reardon CA, Getz GS (2011) 4F peptide reduces nascent atherosclerosis and induces natural antibody production in apolipoprotein E-null mice. FASEB J 25:290–300
Wool GD, Reardon CA, Getz GS (2014) Mimetic peptides of human apoA-I helix 10 get together and ameliorate atherosclerosis: is the action in the gut? J Lipid Res 55(10):1983–1985
Xu H, Zaidi M, Struve J, Jones DW, Krolikowski JG, Nandedkar S, Lohr NL, Gadicherla A, Pagel PS, Csuka ME, Pritchard KA, Weihrauch D (2011) Abnormal fibrillin-1 expression and chronic oxidative stress mediate endothelial mesenchymal transition in a murine model of systemic sclerosis. Am J Physiol Cell Physiol 300:C550–C556
Xu H, Krolikowski JG, Jones DW, Ge ZD, Pagel PS, Pritchard KA Jr, Weihrauch D (2012) 4F decreases IRF5 expression and activation in hearts of tight skin mice. PLoS ONE 7:e52046
Zhang Z, Datta G, Zhang Y, Miller AP, Mochon P, Chen YF, Chatham J, Anantharamaiah GM, White CR (2009) Apolipoprotein A-I mimetic peptide treatment inhibits inflammatory responses and improves survival in septic rats. Am J Physiol Heart Circ Physiol 297:H866–H673
Zhao Y, Black AS, Bonnet DJ, Maryanoff BE, Curtiss LK, Leman LJ, Ghadiri MR (2014) In vivo efficacy of HDL-like nanolipid particles containing multivalent peptide mimetics of apolipoprotein A-I. J Lipid Res 55:2053–2063

Apolipoprotein Mimetic Peptides for Stimulating Cholesterol Efflux

Dan Li, Scott Gordon, Anna Schwendeman, and Alan T. Remaley

Abstract Apolipoprotein mimetic peptides are short synthetic peptides that have many of the same biological properties of ApoA-I, the main protein component of high-density lipoproteins (HDL). They have been shown to have beneficial effects in a wide variety of animal disease models, including atherosclerosis. One of the better understood properties of apolipoprotein mimetic peptides is their ability to promote the efflux of excess cellular cholesterol by the ABCA1 transporter and by other mechanisms. In this chapter, we will compare and contrast six different apolipoprotein mimetic peptides that are being investigated as possible therapeutic agents, particularly in regard to those features that are important in the cholesterol efflux process and in the overall reverse cholesterol transport pathway.

Introduction

Apolipoprotein mimetic peptides were first developed to investigate the structural features that enable apolipoproteins to bind to lipids and lipoproteins (Anantharamaiah et al. 1985). Most are based on sequences related to ApoA-I, the main protein component of high-density lipoproteins (HDL), but peptides based on the other exchangeable-type apolipoproteins found on HDL have also been described, as well as peptides that have no significant homology to any known apolipoprotein but form

D. Li • A. Schwendeman
Department of Pharmaceutical Sciences and Medicinal Chemistry, Biointerfaces Institute, College of Pharmacy, University of Michigan, Ann Arbor, MI 48109, USA

S. Gordon • A.T. Remaley, MD PhD (✉)
Lipoprotein Metabolism Section, Cardio-Pulmonary Branch, National Heart, Lung, and Blood Institute, National Institutes of Health, Bethesda, MD 20892, USA
e-mail: aremaley1@nhlbi.nih.gov; aremaley1@mail.nih.gov

G.M. Anantharamaiah, D. Goldberg (eds.), *Apolipoprotein Mimetics in the Management of Human Disease*, DOI 10.1007/978-3-319-17350-4_3

an amphipathic helix. Interest in these peptides as possible therapeutic agents developed as a consequence of promising results from early-stage clinical trials of reconstituted HDL in patients with acute coronary syndrome (ACS) (Krause et al. 2013). In these trials, purified or recombinant ApoA-I is combined with phospholipid to form lipoprotein particles similar to pre-β HDL, the discoidal form of HDL that is particularly good at promoting cholesterol efflux from cells. Reconstituted HDL (rHDL) was intravenously infused once a week for up to 5 weeks, and by intravascular ultrasound (IVUS), a significant decrease was found in coronary plaque volume compared to baseline (Krause et al. 2013). The rationale for such a therapy is that the HDL infusion treatment, following ischemic heart attack, would quickly stabilize patients and prevent them from developing another cardiovascular event in the near term. Patients with ACS are routinely started on statins, but statins take several months before they show benefit in reducing cardiovascular events.

Apolipoprotein mimetic peptides are being considered as possible alternatives to full-length ApoA-I protein for making rHDL for several reasons. First, they appear to mediate many of the beneficial antiatherogenic functions of HDL, such as cholesterol efflux and antioxidant activities (Shah et al. 2005; Sethi et al. 2007; Navab et al. 2005a, b). Thus, it may be less expensive and perhaps safer in regard to the use of recombinant or plasma purified ApoA-I to use synthetic peptide mimetics in the preparation of rHDL. In addition, alternative routes of delivery besides intravenous infusion may be possible with the use of peptides, particularly small peptides synthesized with D-amino acids, thus potentially allowing for the chronic treatment of cardiovascular disease.

Two main strategies have been employed in the design of therapeutic apolipoprotein mimetic peptides. The first is based on maximizing the ability of these peptides to promote cholesterol efflux by the reverse cholesterol transport (RCT) pathway (Fig. 1). The second strategy is based on optimizing one of the other beneficial features of ApoA-I and HDL, such as its ability to bind and sequester proinflammatory oxidized lipids. In this chapter, we will first review how ApoA-I and HDL mediate cholesterol efflux and participate in the RCT pathway. Next, we will review all of the apolipoprotein mimetic peptides undergoing drug development listed in Table 1, with an emphasis on those features related to the cholesterol efflux properties of these peptides.

Reverse Cholesterol Transport Pathway

One of the major cardioprotective mechanisms for HDL is its ability to help maintain cellular cholesterol homeostasis by the RCT pathway (Rosenson et al. 2012) (Fig. 1). This process involves the removal of excess cholesterol from peripheral tissues and its delivery to the liver where it can be excreted into the bile or recycled. RCT begins with the transfer or "efflux" of excess cellular cholesterol to an extracellular lipoprotein acceptor. In regard to atherosclerosis protection, cholesterol efflux is most relevant to the removal of excess cholesterol from macrophage foam cells in vascular lesions. The movement of unesterified "free" cholesterol from the outer leaflet of the plasma

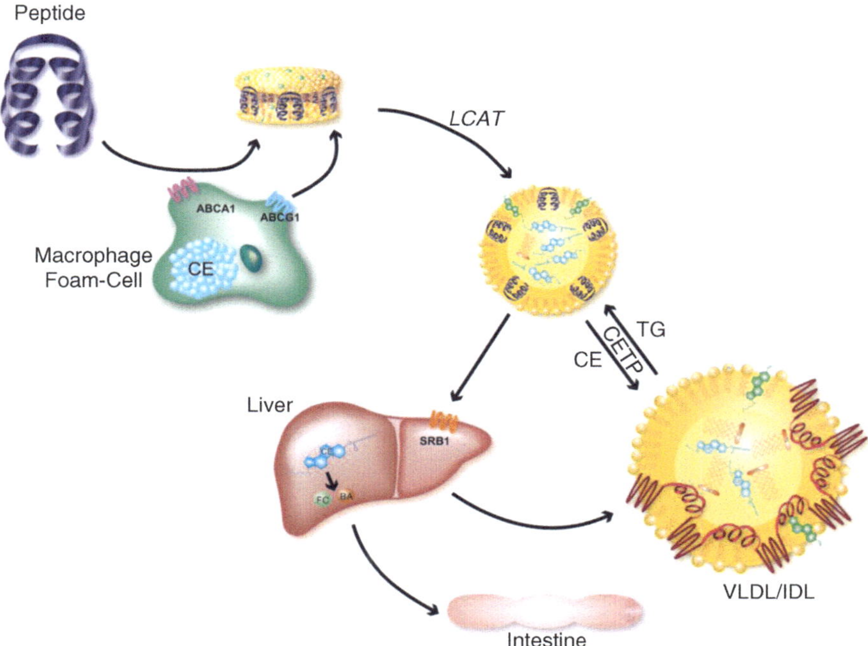

Fig. 1 Reverse cholesterol transport by apolipoprotein mimetic peptides. In the RCT pathway, circulating mimetic peptides accumulate phospholipid (*yellow*) and free cholesterol (*FC*, *green spheres*) from macrophage foam cells via the transmembrane transporters *ABCA1* and *ABCG1*. *LCAT* mediates the transesterification of an acyl chain from phospholipid to FC, forming cholesterol ester (*CE*, *blue*). The hydrophobic CE moves to the core of the particle forming mature spherical particles. CE can then be exchanged for triglyceride (*TG*) from *VLDL/IDL* particles via the action of *CETP*. The mature particle can also be taken up by the liver through interaction with *SR-B1*. Liver stores of CE can be packaged and resecreted as a component of VLDL or converted to FC and bile acids (*BA*) and excreted in the feces

membrane to the extracellular lipoproteins acceptors is mediated by several different transmembrane proteins, depending on the type of lipoprotein acceptor. Lipid-poor apolipoproteins and pre-β HDL particles largely mediate cholesterol efflux by an ATP-binding cassette transporter A1 (ABCA1)-dependent pathway (Rothblat et al. 2010). The exact mechanism of action for ABCA1 is not known, but it appears to create a specialized lipid domain from which phospholipid and cholesterol are extracted from the plasma membrane. In contrast, larger mature spherical HDL particles appear to mostly promote cholesterol efflux by the ABCG1 transporter or perhaps by other mechanisms, such as aqueous diffusion (Rothblat et al. 2010).

Once onboard an HDL particle, a plasma enzyme called lecithin-cholesterol acyltransferase (LCAT) cleaves a fatty acyl chain from phosphatidylcholine and transesterifies it to the hydroxyl group of a nearby free cholesterol molecule to form cholesteryl esters (Rousset et al. 2011). Hydrophobic cholesteryl ester molecules produced by LCAT then move to the core of the lipoprotein particle where they become

Table 1 Comparison of ApoA-I mimetic peptides

ApoA-I peptide	Sequence	Company	Optimized mechanism of action	Stage of development	Administration route (formulation)	References
ESP24218 Peptide	P-V-L-D-L-F-R-E-L-L-N-E-L-L-E-A-L-K-Q-K-L-K	Esperion	Lipid binding LCAT activation RCT	Phase I Single dose and multiple doses	IV Peptide-lipid HDL particle (SM/DPPC/ESP 24218 = 3.75/3.75/1)	Khan et al. (2003), Miles et al. (2004)
D-4F	Ac-D-W-F-K-A-F-Y-D-K-V-A-E-K-F-K-E-A-F-NH_2	Novartis	Same as L-4F chemical stability	Phase I Single dose	Oral Free peptide	Bloedon et al. (2008)
L-4F	Ac-D-W-F-K-A-F-Y-D-K-V-A-E-K-F-K-E-A-F-NH_2	Novartis	RCT, lipid binding Inflammation reduction	Phase I Single dose and multiple doses	IV and SQ Free peptide	Watson et al. (2011)
Retroinverso peptides	K-L-K-Q-K-L-A-E-L-L-E-N-L-L-E-R-F-L-D-L-V-Inp Ac-F-A-E-K-F-K-E-A-V-K-D-Y-F-A-K-F-W-D-NH_2 (reverse 4F)	Kos pharmaceuticals	Lipid binding cholesterol mobilization in vivo	Preclinical	IV Peptide-lipid particle	Dasseux et al. (2013), Kos Reports on Promising Data Presented at AHA
5A	D-W-L-K-A-F-Y-D-K-V-A-E-K-L-K-E-A-F-P-D-W-A-K-A-A-Y-D-K-A-A-E-K-A-K-E-A-A	KineMed Inc.	ABCA1 activation Low hemolysis Lipid binding	Preclinical	IV Peptide-lipid particle	Amar et al. (2010)
18-A	Ac-EWLEAFYKKVLEKLKELF-NH_2	None	RCT	Preclinical	IV, IP, SQ Free peptide	Wool et al. (2008)
ATI-5261	Ac-E-V-R-S-K-L-E-E-W-F-A-A-F-R-E-F-A-E-E-F-L-A-R-L-K-S-NH_2	Roche	Antioxidant properties Promote ABCA1-dependent cholesterol efflux	Preclinical	SQ Free peptide	Bielicki et al. (2010)

trapped, thus preventing their passive back diffusion to cellular donors. From this point, cholesteryl esters on HDL have two possible fates. The first is that they can be transferred to ApoB-containing lipoproteins in exchange for triglyceride via the cholesteryl ester transfer protein (CETP). Approximately half of cholesterol is thought to return to the liver after the hepatic uptake of ApoB-containing particles (Schwartz et al. 2004). Alternatively, cholesteryl esters can be returned to the liver directly from HDL by a selective lipid uptake process mediated by the scavenger receptor class B member 1 (SR-BI) protein on hepatic cell membranes. Once delivered to the liver, cholesterol can either be stored as a cholesteryl ester, excreted into the bile as either free cholesterol or as a bile salt, or it can be recycled when it is packaged onto a VLDL particle and secreted back into systemic circulation. As shown in Fig. 1, and as will be discussed below, apolipoprotein mimetic peptides are believed to participate in the RCT pathway in much of the same way as full-length ApoA-I.

Apolipoprotein Mimetic Peptides

ESP24218 Peptide

ESP24218 is 22 amino acids in length and was the first apolipoprotein mimetic peptide to reach clinical development (Khan et al. 2003; Miles et al. 2004). The main rationale in the design of ESP24218 was to develop a peptide that would activate LCAT, which mediates a critical step in the RCT pathway (Fig. 1), namely, the esterification of cholesterol. Cholesterol esterification by LCAT is thought to drive net cholesterol efflux from cells and to also promote the eventual uptake of cholesterol by the liver (Rousset et al. 2011). ESP24218 was developed by Dasseux et al. at Esperion Therapeutics, and its sequence optimization is detailed in several patents (Dasseux et al. 2003, 2004, 2006). The original patents were later in-licensed by Esperion Therapeutics where it was formulated into an HDL-like particle by combining it with phospholipid and renamed ETC-642. ETC-642, an rHDL preparation, contains the ESP24218 peptide, 1,2-dipalmitoyl-*sn*-glycero-3-phosphocholine (DPPC), and sphingomyelin (SM) at 1:3.75:3.75 M ratio of peptide/DPPC/SM (Di Bartolo et al. 2011a). The formulation process for producing the rHDL particle involved the co-lyophilization of peptide/phospholipid mixture dissolved in organic solvent following by subsequent hydration with an isotonic neutral buffer (Dasseux 2001).

The ESP24218 peptide sequence was originally derived from an ApoA-I consensus peptide (PVLDEFREKLNEELEALKQKLK), which was constructed by G.M. Anantharamaiah et al. by identifying the most prevalent amino acid residue at each position of the ten amphipathic helices on human ApoA-I (Anantharamaiah et al. 1991; Anantharamaiah et al. 1990). The consensus peptide forms a class A-type amphipathic α-helix that is characterized by a clustering of positively charged amino acid residues, mostly lysine, at the hydrophobic-hydrophilic interface and negatively charged amino acid residues, mostly glutamic acid, at the center of its hydrophilic face (Segrest et al. 1990). The original consensus peptide was

Table 2 Design criteria for ApoA-I peptides for maximum LCAT activation and pre-β HDL formation

Property	Preferred range	Consensus peptide	ESP-24218 peptide $4^{\times}$	Peptide $8^{\times}$
Percent hydrophobic aa	50–60 %	41 %	55 %	55 %
$\langle H_o \rangle$	−0.030 to −0.055	−0.293	−0.013	−0.041
$\langle H_o^{pho} \rangle$	0.94–1.1	0.96	0.99	0.94
$\langle \mu_H \rangle$	0.50–0.60	0.425	0.547	0.521
Pho angle	160–220°	100°	200°	200°
Number of positively charged aa	4	5	4	4
Number of negatively charged aa	4	6	4	4
Net charge	0	−1	0	0
Hydrophobic cluster	3, 6, 9, and 10 are hydrophobic	No	Yes	Yes
Acidic cluster	At least 1 acidic per turn in turns 1–4	Yes	Yes	Yes
Basic cluster	C-terminal	Yes	Yes	Yes
LCAT activity	>70 %	10 %	93 %	83 %
% Helix in solution	N/A	18 %	80 %	20 %
% Helix bound to lipids	N/A	23 %	97 %	61 %

determined to be a relatively poor LCAT activator, with only 10 % activity compared to full-length ApoA-I protein (Dasseux et al. 2003, 2004, 2006). Table 2 compares the properties of the starting ApoA-I consensus peptide with ETC-642 and another comparator peptide called peptide 8 (PVLDLFRELLNEGLEALKQKLK). With the use of the design criteria described in Table 2, a number of peptides besides ETC-642 have been developed with LCAT activation ability nearly approaching 100 % of the activity observed with ApoA-I (Dasseux et al. 2003, 2004, 2006).

EPS24218 readily binds to phospholipids and forms pre-β HDL-like particles, which have similar activity as rHDL particles made with ApoA-I in activating LCAT and in promoting cholesterol efflux when tested in NZW rabbits (Dasseux et al. 2003, 2004, 2006). Multiple administrations of ETC-642 were found to reduce the progression aortic of plaque burden in Watanabe-heritable hyperlipidemic rabbits (WHHR), as measured by IVUS (Iwata et al. 2011). In this study, WHHR rabbits were administered twice weekly either high (50 mg/kg) or low (15 mg/g) doses of ETC-642 or placebo. ETC-642 infusions were also shown to be effective in reducing chronic collar-induced vascular inflammation in NZW rabbits similar to rHDL made with full-length human ApoA-I (Di Bartolo et al. 2011a, b).

A phase I clinical study of ETC-642 was performed in 2002 (Khan et al. 2003; Miles et al. 2004). It was a single-dose intravenous infusion study of 28 patients with stable coronary artery disease and was designed to determine the safety and tolerability of 0.1, 0.3, 1, 3, and 10 mg/kg dose levels of ETC-642 (Khan et al. 2003). After a 4-week observation period, ETC-642 was considered to be safe and well tolerated at all dose levels tested (Khan et al. 2003). Modest increases in HDL-C were observed shortly after the infusion due to presumably increase cholesterol mobilization, and the changes in HDL-C were similar to what has been described for the clinical trials involving the infusion of rHDL made with either purified or recombinant ApoA-I (Krause et al. 2013). A second phase I trial was conducted to test safety of ETC-642 at higher doses of 10, 20, and 30 mg/mg. At the highest dose, evidence of asymptomatic liver function test abnormalities were observed in a single patient, suggesting that a maximum tolerated dose may have been identified (Miles et al. 2004). ETC-642 was also tested in a multiple dose study, involving four weekly infusions (Esperion, Press release 2003), but the results of multiple dose studies have not been publically disclosed. The development of ETC-642 was shortly thereafter terminated in 2006 following the failure of the torcetrapib program when Pfizer decided to "exit" the field of cardiovascular disease drug development (Pfizer 2008).

D-4F Peptide

D-4F is an 18-amino-acid-long amphipathic peptide synthesized with all D-amino acids. It is very similar to the 18A peptide in primary amino acid sequence but contains two additional phenylalanine residues in its hydrophobic face besides the ones already present in the 18-A peptide (Navab et al. 2005a, b) and hence the origin of its name D-4F. The amphipathic helical structure of D-4F is further stabilized by caps at its N- and C-terminus with acetyl and amino groups, respectively. Unlike most of the other peptides discussed in this chapter, D-4F was not specifically designed based on its cholesterol efflux properties, although it does promote cholesterol efflux (Xie et al. 2010). D-4F is primarily believed to protect vascular function by binding pro-inflammatory lipids, particularly oxidized phospholipids (Navab et al. 2004). It was found that the four phenylalanine residues in the hydrophobic face of this peptide are critical for its high affinity for binding to oxidized phospholipids (Van Lenten et al. 2008). Adding D-4F to normal human plasma causes the formation of pre-β HDL, reduces lipoprotein lipid hydroperoxide content, and increases paraoxonase activity, which also likely contributes to its antiatherogenic properties (Navab et al. 2005a, b).

One of the advantages of D-4F is that it can be potentially orally administrated due to its small size and the fact that it is composed of D-amino acids, which are resistant to proteolysis. In one study, oral administration of D-4F in either ApoE-null mice or LDL receptor-null mice showed that compared to its enantiomer peptide made with L-amino acids (L-4F), D-4F showed extended circulation time in plasma and an enhanced ability to protect against LDL oxidation. It also caused a marked reduction in atherosclerotic lesions without causing major changes in total plasma lipids or HDL-C (Navab 2002). Another study showed that a combination of low-dose oral D-4F with pravastatin was also able to reduce atherosclerosis and promote lesion regression (Navab et al. 2005a, b). Numerous animal studies in a wide variety of different disease models have now established D-4F to be effective in decreasing atherosclerosis and inflammation (Navab et al. 2005a, b).

D-4F was licensed by Novartis and advanced into phase I clinical trials in 2008 (Bloedon et al. 2008). A single oral dose of D-4F up to 500 mg was found to be well tolerated. The time to reach maximum D-4F plasma concentration was very short and dose dependent, although peak plasma doses of 2–10 ng/mL were relatively low. Administration of D-4F together with food further reduced the plasma C_{max} and the AUC for the peptide. Despite the low plasma, a significant improvement in the HDL inflammatory index, a functional assay of the antioxidant properties of HDL, was observed after 4 h of administration, with no change in plasma lipid or lipoprotein levels. Although no toxicity was observed in this study, no further clinical trials have been reported possibly because of the low oral availability of the peptide and because of concerns about possible long-term tissue accumulation of the protease-resistant peptide.

L-4F Peptide

L-4F, the enantiomer of D-4F, made with L-amino acids has also been investigated in numerous preclinical animal models (Getz et al. 2010; Ying et al. 2013; Vecoli et al. 2011; Meriwether et al. 2011) and has been tested in one phase I clinical trial (Buga et al. 2010). It appears to mediate most of the same functions as D-4F, such as cholesterol efflux (Wool et al. 2008) indicating the most of the antiatherogenic functions of apolipoprotein mimetic peptides do not depend on a stereoselective process. Interest in L-4F as a therapeutic is mostly in regard to its use as an acute intravenous agent for ACS. A phase I clinical trial of either subcutaneous (SC) or intravenous (IV) administration of L-4F has been performed (Buga et al. 2010). L-4F was well tolerated when administered IV for seven daily doses with the dose range of 3–100 mg and SC for 28 daily dose of 10 and 30 mg. The mean maximal plasma concentration after IV infusion and SC injection was 2,970 ng/ml and 395 ng/ml, respectively, which should be an effective plasma concentration level based on the phase I D-4F study and on animal studies. However, there was no improvement of the HDL inflammatory index, paraoxonase activity, or other lipid measures or inflammatory markers, such as CRP. Subsequent animal studies with both D-4F and L-4F indicate that the main site of action of these peptides may be in the gut in blocking the absorption and/or production of oxidized lipids (Remaley 2013), which could possibly explain the lack of an effect observed after IV administration in the phase I clinical trial.

Retroinverso Peptides

Retroinverso peptides are peptides that are synthesized in reverse order so that the C-terminal amino acid becomes the N-terminus and the rest of the amino acids follow in reverse order (Chorev 2005). They are also synthesized with D-amino acids instead of the L-amino acids. It has been shown that retroinverso peptides maintain the configuration of their side chains in the same spatial orientation as their non-reverse analogue peptide made with L-amino acids (Chorev 2005). The advantage of retroinverso peptides is that they are stable to degradation because they are made with D-amino acids but maintain their stereoselective interactions unlike non-reverse peptides made with D-amino acids.

Two retroinverso peptides being investigated for drug development have been described (Table 1). The first is the retroinverso variant of ESP24218 developed by Cerenis Therapeutics. Only limited information is available on this peptide in the patent literature (Dasseux et al. 2013), but presumably this peptide like ESP24218 is able to activate LCAT through a stereoselective interaction but unlike ESP24218 should be relatively resistant to degradation and thus should show better pharmacokinetic properties. This retroinverso analogue of ESP24218 contains an artificial amino acid isonipecotic (Inp) acid instead of proline, which is believed to provide additional stability against proteolytic degradation. The retroinverso variant of ESP24218 was found to form pre-β HDL particles in the presence of phospholipids and exhibit dose-dependent cholesterol mobilization following administration in NZW rabbits. The pharmacokinetics and dose-dependent mobilization of cholesterol following intravenous administration in rats and monkeys at doses of 15, 30, and 60 mg/kg were also reported.

The other retroinverso peptide is based on 4F and is being investigated by Kos Pharmaceuticals (Table 1) (Murase et al. 2014). It is not clear, however, the advantage of this peptide over D-4F, in regard to cholesterol efflux, because the cholesterol efflux process has already been shown to occur by a non-stereoselective mechanism (Remaley et al. 2003). A stereoselective interaction between apolipoprotein mimetic peptides and the ABCA1 transporter is not necessary for cholesterol efflux, but instead these peptides interact directly with lipids in the plasma membrane, during the cholesterol efflux process. It may be, however, that the retroinverso analogue of 4F preserves some other stereoselective interaction that is necessary for its antiatherogenic function. Retroinverso 4F has been shown to promote cholesterol efflux from cells similar to L-4F and D-4F and like other apolipoprotein mimetic peptides has been shown to have antiatherogenic properties in animal models (Qin et al. 2012; Kos Reports 2005; Du et al. 2013). To date, no clinical trials on the retroinverso peptides have been reported.

5A Peptide

The 5A peptide is a 37-amino-acid bi-helical amphipathic peptide with one high lipid affinity binding helix linked via a proline to a low lipid affinity binding helix. The rationale for containing two helices is that it has been shown that apolipoprotein mimetic peptides containing two or more helices were more potent in lipid binding and in promoting cholesterol efflux by the ABCA1 transporter (Sethi et al. 2008; Zhao et al. 2013; Nion et al. 1998). The first helix is identical to the 18A helix (Table 1). The second helix is also similar to 18A, but five residues in its hydrophobic face were replaced with Ala, hence its name 5A. Alanine is only slightly hydrophobic and thus this substitution decreases the lipid binding affinity of

Table 3 Relationship between physical properties of bi-helical apolipoprotein mimetic peptides and cholesterol efflux

Parameter	Effect on cholesterol efflux
Charge	Charged peptides (+ or –) tend to have lower efflux capacity compared to neutral peptides
Hydrophobicity	A mean hydrophobicity of about –0.5 appears to be optimal
Size of hydrophobic face	Increase in hydrophobic face up to at least half of the helix improves cholesterol efflux
Type of helix	Type of helix (A, G, or Y) had minimal effect on cholesterol efflux
Inter-helical turn	Residues that promote inter-helical turn favor cholesterol efflux
Phospholipid complexation	Increases cholesterol efflux capacity but favors non-ABCA1-dependent pathways

the second helix. This was done because it was observed that a dimer of the 18A helix linked with proline, which is referred to as 37pA, was cytotoxic and also readily lysed red blood cells. It was hypothesized that the high lipid affinity of these bi-helical peptide was promoting the cytotoxicity of cells by a detergent-like process. Similarly, the 37pA peptide was found to promote some cholesterol efflux by the ABCA1 transporter, but the majority of cholesterol efflux that occurred by this peptide was the result of a nonspecific cholesterol extraction from cells most likely because of its strong detergent-like property (Sethi et al. 2008). In contrast, the 5A peptide containing five alanine substitutions in its second helix was noncytotoxic and specifically effluxed cholesterol by the ABCA1 transporter. It was proposed that the 5A peptide possibly mimics the full-length ApoA-I protein, which contains a mixture of low and high lipid affinity binding helices. Two exposed hydrophobic residues in the hinge region of the 5A peptide between the two helices, namely, tryptophan and phenylalanine, were found to be critical in the initial attachment of this peptide to lipid membranes, during the cholesterol efflux process (Sviridov et al. 2013). Detailed examination of structure versus function relationships has revealed several other critical factors in the ability of bi-helical apolipoprotein mimetic peptides to promote cholesterol efflux from macrophages (D'Souza et al. 2010), a summary of which is shown in Table 3.

Reconstitution of the 5A peptide with phosphatidylcholine resulted in the formation of discoidal particles similar to pre-β HDL (Amar et al. 2010). These 5A-PC particles showed enhanced cholesterol efflux by the ABCA1 transporter compared to the free peptide and also showed better pharmacokinetic properties than the free peptide in mice. Reconstitution of the peptide with phospholipid also enabled the peptide to promote cholesterol efflux by the ABCG1 transporter and by aqueous diffusion. In a rabbit collar injury model, the 5A was comparable to full-length ApoA-I in preventing the expression of adhesion proteins on endothelial cells and in blocking leukocyte infiltration (Tabet et al. 2010). Like other apolipoprotein mimetic peptides or reconstituted HDL preparations, IV infusions of 5A-PC were found to block the progression of atherosclerosis in a mouse model (Amar et al. 2010). Although the 5A peptide was developed for promoting cholesterol efflux, it also has potent anti-inflammatory effects. It was shown to be superior to steroids in preventing inflammation in a house dust mice model of asthma (Yao et al. 2011). Currently, the 5A peptide is being developed as potential acute therapy for ACS by KineMed Inc., and phase I trials are planned for 2015.

ATI-5261 Peptide

ATI-5261 is a 26-residue-long peptide based on the last helix of ApoE. Although based on relative abundance, ApoA-I is likely the most important apolipoprotein for mediating cholesterol efflux by the ABCA1 transporter, other apolipoproteins may also participate in this process. In fact, it has been shown that all of the exchangeable-type apolipoproteins can mediate cholesterol efflux from cells transfected with the ABCA1 transporter (Remaley et al. 2001). Based on synthesizing peptides with a mixture of D- and L-amino acids, which disrupt helix stabilization by hydrogen bonding, it appears that the presence of an amphipathic helix is the main structural motif that is necessary for cholesterol efflux (Remaley et al. 2003). ApoE, in particular, may play an important role in cholesterol efflux, because unlike ApoA-I, it is produced by a wide variety of cells like macrophages, and thus there may be high enough local concentrations of ApoE in atherosclerotic plaques for promoting cholesterol efflux.

Previous studies have established that the C-terminal helix of ApoE forms a high lipid affinity binding helix and can promote cholesterol efflux (Vedhachalam et al. 2007). ATI-5261 was modeled after amino acid residues from 238 to 266 in this helix (Bielicki et al. 2010). ATI-5261 differs, however, from the native sequence in ten amino acids. Most of the substitutions were made to increase the hydrophobicity of nonpolar face of the helix and to increase its helicity by adding more salt bridges on the polar face. The presence of several negative charged glutamic acids on the polar face were also found to increase cholesterol efflux of this peptide, although this feature has not been found to be generally important in cholesterol efflux for other apolipoprotein mimetic peptides (Smith et al. 2013). Compared to the native ApoE sequence, ATI-5261 shows much greater helicity even in the absence of bound lipid. Most likely because of its improved helicity, ATI-5261 was found to be very potent in stimulating cholesterol efflux by the ABCA1 transporter and had a molar Km and Vmax comparable to the full-length ApoA-I protein (Vedhachalam et al. 2007). Like other apolipoprotein mimetic peptides, ATI-5261 was found when given interperitoneally as a free peptide to prevent progression of atherosclerosis in both ApoE and LDL-r KO mice (Vedhachalam et al. 2007).

The ATI-5261 peptide was licensed by Roche for drug development, but it was halted when toxicity from skeletal muscle damage was observed in preclinical animal models. The mechanism behind the toxicity is not known at this time, but other nontoxic peptides based on ApoE are now being explored. ApoE-based peptides are also being developed for the treatment of Alzheimer's disease (Laskowitz et al. 2006) and for promoting the hepatic uptake of ApoB-containing lipoproteins (Handattu et al. 2013).

Summary

The field of apolipoprotein mimetic peptides has revealed many new insights into the structure and function of lipoproteins. These peptides are now also being investigated as possible therapeutic agents for cardiovascular disease. Future progress in this area will depend on better understanding the antiatherogenic functions of HDL, which will enable more rational drug design. For example, a better mechanistic into the cholesterol efflux process will also likely lead to future advances in apolipoprotein mimetic peptide design, but it is still not clear whether this process is the most important antiatherogenic property of these peptides. Advances in the use of amino acid analogues in the production of peptides and improvements in their formulation to increase oral availability and their other pharmacokinetic properties will also likely be needed to produce apolipoprotein mimetic peptides that can be safely used for the chronic treatment of cardiovascular disease.

Acknowledgments A.S. and D.L. were supported in part by AHA 13SDG17230049. Research by A.R. and S.G. were supported by intramural research funds from the National Heart, Lung, and Blood Institute.

References

Amar MJ et al (2010) 5A apolipoprotein mimetic peptide promotes cholesterol efflux and reduces atherosclerosis in mice. J Pharmacol Exp Ther 334(2):634–641

Anantharamaiah GM et al (1985) Studies of synthetic peptide analogs of the amphipathic helix. Structure of complexes with dimyristoyl phosphatidylcholine. J Biol Chem 260(18): 10248–10255

Anantharamaiah GM et al (1990) Use of synthetic peptide analogues to localize lecithin: cholesterol acyltransferase activating domain in apolipoprotein A-I. Arterioscler Thromb Vasc Biol 10(1):95–105

Anantharamaiah GM et al (1991) Role of Amphipathic helixes in hdl structure-function. hypercholesterolemia, hypocholesterolemia, hypertriglyceridemia. Invivo Kinetics 285:131–140

Bielicki JK et al (2010) A new HDL mimetic peptide that stimulates cellular cholesterol efflux with high efficiency greatly reduces atherosclerosis in mice. J Lipid Res 51(6):1496–1503

Bloedon LT et al (2008) Safety, pharmacokinetics, and pharmacodynamics of oral apoA-I mimetic peptide D-4F in high-risk cardiovascular patients. J Lipid Res 49(6):1344–1352

Buga GM et al (2010) L-4F alters hyperlipidemic (but not healthy) mouse plasma to reduce platelet aggregation. Arterioscler Thromb Vasc Biol 30(2):283–289

Chorev M (2005) The partial retro-inverso modification: a road traveled together. Biopolymers 80(2–3):67–84

D'Souza W et al (2010) Structure/function relationships of apolipoprotein a-I mimetic peptides: implications for antiatherogenic activities of high-density lipoprotein. Circ Res 107(2): 217–227

Dasseux J-L (2001) Peptide/lipid complex formation by co-lyophilization. US6287590 B1

Dasseux J-L et al (2003) Apolipoprotein A-I agonists and their use to treat dyslipidemic disorders. US20030008827 A1

Dasseux J-L et al (2004) Multimeric Apoa-I agonist compounds. US6753313 B1

Dasseux J-L et al (2006) Apolipoprotein A-I agonists and their use to treat dyslipidemic disorders. US 20060252694 A1

Dasseux J-L et al (2013) Apolipoprotein A-I mimics. US8378068 B2
Di Bartolo BA et al (2011a) The apolipoprotein A-I mimetic peptide ETC-642 exhibits anti-inflammatory properties that are comparable to high density lipoproteins. Atherosclerosis 217(2):395–400
Di Bartolo BA et al (2011b) The apolipoprotein A-I mimetic peptide, ETC-642, reduces chronic vascular inflammation in the rabbit. Lipids Health Dis 10:224
Du L et al (2013) Reverse apolipoprotein A-I mimetic peptide R-D4F inhibits neointimal formation following carotid artery ligation in mice. Am J Pathol 182(5):1932–1939
Esperion begins multiple-dose study of ETC-642 (RLT peptide) in patients with stable atherosclerosis (2003). Available from: http://www.prnewswire.co.uk/news-releases/esperion-begins-multiple-dose-study-of-etc-642-rlt-peptide-in-patients-with-stable-atherosclerosis-154589805.html
Getz GS et al (2010) Biological properties of apolipoprotein a-I mimetic peptides. Curr Atheroscler Rep 12(2):96–104
Handattu SP et al (2013) Two apolipoprotein E mimetic peptides with similar cholesterol reducing properties exhibit differential atheroprotective effects in LDL-R null mice. Atherosclerosis 227(1):58–64
Iwata A et al (2011) Antiatherogenic effects of newly developed apolipoprotein A-I mimetic peptide/phospholipid complexes against aortic plaque burden in Watanabe-heritable hyperlipidemic rabbits. Atherosclerosis 218(2):300–307
Khan M et al (2003) Single-dose intravenous infusion of ETC-642, a 22-Mer ApoA-I analogue and phospholipids complex, elevates HDL-C in atherosclerosis patients. Circulation 108(17): 563–564
Kos reports on promising data presented at AHA: new compound reverse-D4F, a novel Apo A-I mimetic peptide, may reduce the progression of atherosclerosis (2005). Available from: http://www.businesswire.com/news/home/20051114005406/en/Kos-Reports-Promising-Data-Presented-AHA-Compound#.VF0-H_nF9HV
Krause BR et al (2013) Reconstituted HDL for the acute treatment of acute coronary syndrome. Curr Opin Lipidol 24(6):480–486
Laskowitz DT et al (2006) Apolipoprotein E-derived peptides reduce CNS inflammation: implications for therapy of neurological disease. Acta Neurol Scand Suppl 185:15–20
Meriwether D et al (2011) Enhancement by LDL of transfer of L-4F and oxidized lipids to HDL in C57BL/6J mice and human plasma. J Lipid Res 52(10):1795–1809
Miles JM et al (2004) Single-dose tolerability, pharmacokinetics, and cholesterol mobilization in HDL-C fraction following intravenous administration of ETC-642, a 22-mer ApoA-I analogue and phospholipids complex, in atherosclerosis patients. Proceedings of ATVB
Murase K et al (2014) Apo A-I mimetic peptides and methods of treatment. US8748394 B2
Navab M (2002) Oral administration of an Apo A-I mimetic peptide synthesized from D-amino acids dramatically reduces atherosclerosis in mice independent of plasma cholesterol. Circulation 105(3):290–292
Navab M et al (2004) Oral D-4F causes formation of pre-beta high-density lipoprotein and improves high-density lipoprotein-mediated cholesterol efflux and reverse cholesterol transport from macrophages in apolipoprotein E-null mice. Circulation 109(25):3215–3220
Navab M et al (2005a) Apolipoprotein A-I mimetic peptides. Arterioscler Thromb Vasc Biol 25(7):1325–1331
Navab M et al (2005b) D-4F and statins synergize to render HDL antiinflammatory in mice and monkeys and cause lesion regression in old apolipoprotein E-null mice. Arterioscler Thromb Vasc Biol 25(7):1426–1432
Nion S et al (1998) Branched synthetic peptide constructs mimic cellular binding and efflux of apolipoprotein AI in reconstituted high density lipoproteins. Atherosclerosis 141(2):227–235
Pfizer to drop development of drugs for hyperlipidemia, atherosclerosis, and heart failure. (2008). Available from: http://www.medscape.com/viewarticle/581528
Qin S et al (2012) Reverse D4F, an apolipoprotein-AI mimetic peptide, inhibits atherosclerosis in ApoE-null mice. J Cardiovasc Pharmacol Ther 17(3):334–343

Remaley AT (2013) Tomatoes, lysophosphatidic acid, and the small intestine: new pieces in the puzzle of apolipoprotein mimetic peptides? J Lipid Res 54(12):3223–3226
Remaley AT et al (2001) Apolipoprotein specificity for lipid efflux by the human ABCAI transporter. Biochem Biophys Res Commun 280(3):818–823
Remaley AT et al (2003) Synthetic amphipathic helical peptides promote lipid efflux from cells by an ABCA1-dependent and an ABCA1-independent pathway. J Lipid Res 44(4):828–836
Rosenson RS et al (2012) Cholesterol efflux and atheroprotection: advancing the concept of reverse cholesterol transport. Circulation 125(15):1905–1919
Rothblat GH et al (2010) High-density lipoprotein heterogeneity and function in reverse cholesterol transport. Curr Opin Lipidol 21(3):229–238
Rousset X et al (2011) Lecithin cholesterol acyltransferase: an anti- or pro-atherogenic factor? Curr Atheroscler Rep 13(3):249–256
Schwartz CC et al (2004) Lipoprotein cholesteryl ester production, transfer, and output in vivo in humans. J Lipid Res 45(9):1594–1607
Segrest JP et al (1990) Amphipathic helix motif: classes and properties. Proteins Struct Funct Bioinforma 8(2):103–117
Sethi AA et al (2007) Apolipoprotein AI mimetic peptides: possible new agents for the treatment of atherosclerosis. Curr Opin Investig Drugs 8(3):201–212
Sethi AA et al (2008) Asymmetry in the lipid affinity of bihelical amphipathic peptides. A structural determinant for the specificity of ABCA1-dependent cholesterol efflux by peptides. J Biol Chem 283(47):32273–32282
Shah PK et al (2005) Apolipoprotein A-I mimetic peptides: potential role in atherosclerosis management. Trends Cardiovasc Med 15(8):291–296
Smith LE et al (2013) Helical domains that mediate lipid solubilization and ABCA1-specific cholesterol efflux in apolipoproteins C-I and A-II. J Lipid Res 54(7):1939–1948
Sviridov DO et al (2013) Hydrophobic amino acids in the hinge region of the 5A apolipoprotein mimetic peptide are essential for promoting cholesterol efflux by the ABCA1 transporter. J Pharmacol Exp Ther 344(1):50–58
Tabet F et al (2010) The 5A apolipoprotein A-I mimetic peptide displays antiinflammatory and antioxidant properties in vivo and in vitro. Arterioscler Thromb Vasc Biol 30(2):246–252
Van Lenten BJ et al (2008) Anti-inflammatory apoA-I-mimetic peptides bind oxidized lipids with much higher affinity than human apoA-I. J Lipid Res 49(11):2302–2311
Vecoli C et al (2011) Apolipoprotein A-I mimetic peptide L-4F prevents myocardial and coronary dysfunction in diabetic mice. J Cell Biochem 112(9):2616–2626
Vedhachalam C et al (2007) The C-terminal lipid-binding domain of apolipoprotein E is a highly efficient mediator of ABCA1-dependent cholesterol efflux that promotes the assembly of high-density lipoproteins. Biochemistry 46(10):2583–2593
Watson CE et al (2011) Treatment of patients with cardiovascular disease with L-4F, an apo-A1 mimetic, did not improve select biomarkers of HDL function. J Lipid Res 52(2):361–373
Wool GD et al (2008) Apolipoprotein A-I mimetic peptide helix number and helix linker influence potentially anti-atherogenic properties. J Lipid Res 49(6):1268–1283
Xie Q et al (2010) D-4F, an apolipoprotein A-I mimetic peptide, promotes cholesterol efflux from macrophages via ATP-binding cassette transporter A1. Tohoku J Exp Med 220(3):223–228
Yao X et al (2011) 5A, an apolipoprotein A-I mimetic peptide, attenuates the induction of house dust mite-induced asthma. J Immunol 186(1):576–583
Ying R et al (2013) The combination of L-4F and simvastatin stimulate cholesterol efflux and related proteins expressions to reduce atherosclerotic lesions in apoE knockout mice. Lipids Health Dis 12:180
Zhao Y et al (2013) Mimicry of high-density lipoprotein: functional peptide-lipid nanoparticles based on multivalent peptide constructs. J Am Chem Soc 135(36):13414–13424

ApoA-I Mimetic Peptides and Diabetes

Max Benson, Stephen J. Peterson, Parag Mehta, and Nader G. Abraham

Abstract There has been a resurgence of interest in the use of apolipoprotein mimetic peptides in the last decade. Much of the initial scientific application was in the field of cardiovascular disease. This has resulted in a much better understanding of the complex nature and function of HDL. The best understood mechanism is its role in reverse cholesterol transport (RCT), but there is now a much better understanding that HDL reduction does not directly correlate with its anti-inflammatory and antioxidant effects. The use of apoA-I mimetic peptides in diabetes, obesity, and metabolic syndrome has resulted in decreased insulin resistance, weight loss, and increased adiponectin levels. This occurred without major changes in HDL and LDL levels. Visceral abdominal obesity has been recognized as a chronic inflammatory state, especially in the setting of diabetes and metabolic syndrome. The anti-inflammatory and antioxidant response to these mimetic peptides is independent of the effects on HDL levels. There is compelling evidence that these mimetic peptides upregulate heme oxygenase (HO-1), the body's first line of defense against oxidant injury. This upregulation of HO-1 is accompanied by an improvement in the anti-inflammatory index of HDL without a change in the HDL level. This remains to be further elucidated in clinical trials.

M. Benson • S.J. Peterson (✉) • P. Mehta
Department of Medicine, New York Methodist Hospital/Weill Cornell Medical College, New York, NY, USA
e-mail: sjpmunger@icloud.com

N.G. Abraham
Joan C. Edwards School of Medicine, Marshall University, Huntington, UK

G.M. Anantharamaiah, D. Goldberg (eds.), *Apolipoprotein Mimetics in the Management of Human Disease*, DOI 10.1007/978-3-319-17350-4_4

Introduction

We are now facing an epidemic of obesity and obesity-related diabetes of alarming proportion. Obesity and diabetes have long been known to induce oxidative stress, which has been shown to downregulate heme oxygenase (HO-1), the body's first line of defense against oxidative stress. Heme, which is itself pro-oxidant, is broken down by heme oxygenase 1 (HO-1) into bilirubin, carbon monoxide, and iron. Bilirubin and carbon monoxide both have antioxidant properties. We will review in this chapter results of the studies using the apolipoprotein A-I (Apo A-I) mimetic peptide, 4F, to reduce oxidative stress, at least in part, by possible upregulation of heme oxygenase. The 4F peptide shows great promise in its ability to address the redox state, resulting in increased antioxidant, anti-inflammatory, and antiplatelet activity.

ApoA-I is the major protein of HDL, accounting for approximately 70 % of the protein content. ApoA-II accounts for approximately 20 %. The remaining 10 % consists of a multitude of proteins that we are only now beginning to appreciate, but they are becoming increasingly important in comprehending the structure and function of HDL. ApoA-I is a 243-amino acid sequence that is only available in parenteral form, and its use is complicated by both expense and potential endotoxin contamination due to its high lipid affinity. For these reasons, there has been a resurgence of interest in apoA-I mimetics in recent years. In this chapter, we will review the evidence for the use of apoA-I mimetics in the field of diabetes. Visceral adiposity is increasingly recognized as a chronic inflammatory state especially in the setting of diabetes, obesity, and metabolic syndrome. These mimetics have had potent anti-inflammatory and antioxidant effects that were not accompanied by changes in HDL levels.

4F Background

4F, available in both D and L forms, is an analog of 18A which possesses an amphipathic alpha helical structure. This structure is required for the mimetic peptide/ABCA1 interaction. This type A helical structure results in a 1:1 hydrophobic/hydrophilic face (Segrest et al. 1992). The 18-amino acid sequence has four strategically placed phenylalanine residues, rendering the name, 4F. Phenylalanine has the largest hydrophobic surface area of all amino acids, improving lipid affinity. Much of the work on apoA-I mimetic peptides has been done with D-4F. D proteins are not natural to the body, are not easily metabolized, and are resistant to proteolysis when given in the oral form (Navab et al. 2002). GI peptidases recognize and break down L amino acids. Since D bonds are not broken down, there is some concern that this can eventually lead to toxicity. Navab et al. have shown that D-4F increased the antioxidant ability of HDL, which resulted in decreased atherosclerosis, without significant change in HDL levels (Navab et al. 2002).

4F and Diabetes

Oxidative stress has been implicated in the pathogenesis of insulin resistance and its consequent vascular injury (Robertson 2004; Wellen and Hotamisligil 2005). Dr. Nader Abraham's group showed that endothelial injury results from the generation of reactive oxygen species (ROS) with endothelial cell sloughing and increased apoptosis (Kruger et al. 2005). Lin et al. emphasized the role of reactive oxygen species in adipocytes that result in decreased adiponectin levels, increased inflammation, and insulin resistance (Lin et al. 2005; Kruger et al. 2005). Administration of L-4F intraperitoneally to obese mice increased high-molecular-weight serum adiponectin, reduced adiposity, decreased adipogenesis in the bone marrow, improved insulin sensitivity, and improved glucose tolerance. More importantly, IL-1β, IL-6, and superoxides were all reduced (Peterson et al. 2008) (Figs. 1 and 2).

L-4F treatment increased both the levels of HO-1 protein as well as HO-1 activity, which was significantly greater than age-matched lean controls. The levels of high-molecular-weight adiponectin paralleled those of the HO-1 protein. Inducers of HO-1 have been reported to increase serum adiponectin levels in diabetic rats (Lin et al. 2007; Abraham et al. 2008; Abraham and Kappas 2008). The weight loss was remarkable. When L-4F was discontinued at week 10, the mice gained weight to the level of obese mice by week 12. Reintroduction of L-4F returned weight to baseline by week 14 (Fig. 3).

L-4F has also been shown to decrease hepatic lipid content and increase the numbers of adipocytes of small size, which are more insulin sensitive. Adipocytes of large cell size are more insulin resistant (Figs. 4 and 5) (Peterson et al. 2009).

MRI showed reduction in both visceral and subcutaneous fat in obese mice. L-4F resulted in improved vascular function with increased levels of pAMPK, pAKT, and phosphorylation of insulin receptors, with improved insulin sensitivity and blood glucose levels. L-4F has been shown to improve metabolic syndrome in obese female mice independent of body weight (Marino et al. 2012). The metabolic syndrome is characterized by visceral adiposity, insulin resistance, elevated blood pressure, and cholesterol levels. This is a low-grade chronic inflammatory state. L-4F increased serum adiponectin and decreased inflammatory cytokines TNF-α, IL-1β, and IL-6 while restoring insulin sensitivity. Interestingly, male mice lost weight while female mice did not. However, the female mice had improvement in all the same parameters on L-4F, independent of body weight. HO-1 activity was increased by L-4F and was subsequently

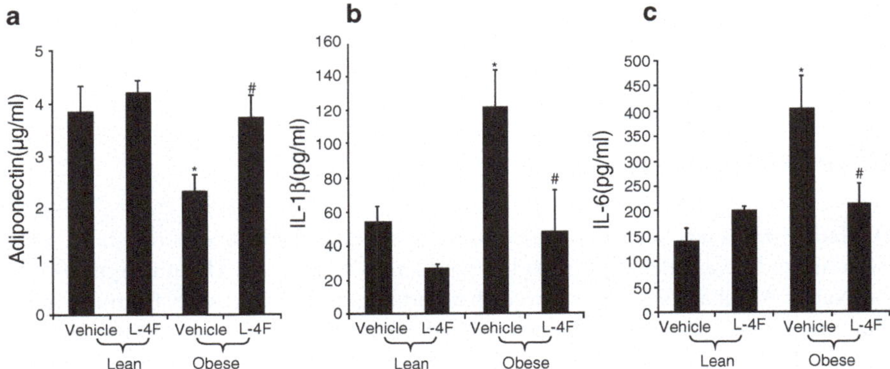

Fig. 1 (**a**) Adiponectin levels in lean and obese mice. Vehicle or vehicle-containing L-4F was administered daily for 6 weeks (as described in Materials and Methods), and serum samples were obtained immediately prior to euthanization. The results are expressed as mg/ml serum. *P, 0.027 vehicle-treated lean versus vehicle-treated obese mice; #P, 0.04L-4F-treated obese versus vehicle-treated obese mice. (**b**, **c**) Serum IL-1b and IL-6 levels in lean and obese mice. Vehicle or vehicle-containing L-4F was administered as described in Materials and Methods. Serum samples were obtained immediately prior to euthanization. (**b**) The results for lean vehicle-treated or obese L-4F-treated versus obese vehicle-treated mice for IL-1b; *P, 0.02 vehicle-treated obese versus vehicle-treated lean mice; #P, 0.05L-4F-treated obese versus vehicle-treated obese mice. (**c**) The results for lean vehicle-treated or obese L-4 F-treated versus obese vehicle-treated mice for IL-6; *P, 0.05 vehicle-treated obese versus vehicle-treated lean mice; #P, 0.05L-4F-treated obese versus vehicle-treated obese mice. Results are shown as the mean 6 SEM (Peterson et al. 2008)

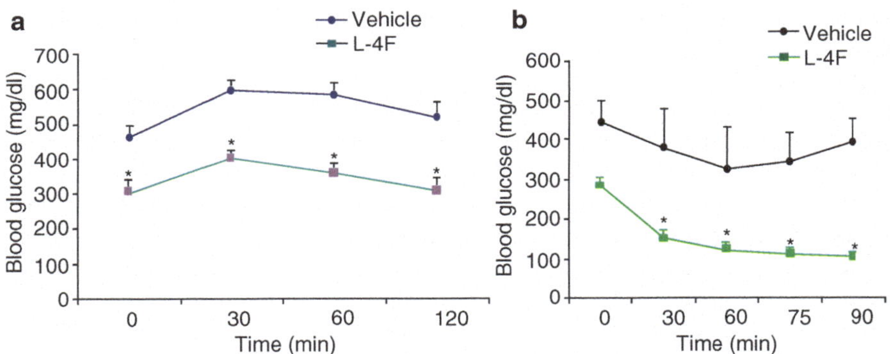

Fig. 2 (**a**) Glucose tolerance and insulin sensitivity after treatment with vehicle or vehicle containing L-4F. After 6 weeks of treatment with vehicle or vehicle containing L-4F, obese mice were injected intraperitoneally with 2 g/kg of glucose, and plasma glucose levels were determined as described in Materials and Methods for the intraperitoneal glucose tolerance test. *$P < 0.05$ versus vehicle-treated obese mice. (**b**) After 6 weeks of treatment with vehicle or vehicle containing L-4F, obese mice were injected intraperitoneally with 2.0 U/kg of insulin, and plasma glucose levels were determined as described in Materials and Methods for the intraperitoneal insulin tolerance test. *$P < 0.001$ versus L-4F-treated obese mice, 0 min. The results are expressed as mean ± SEM; n = 4 (Peterson et al. 2008)

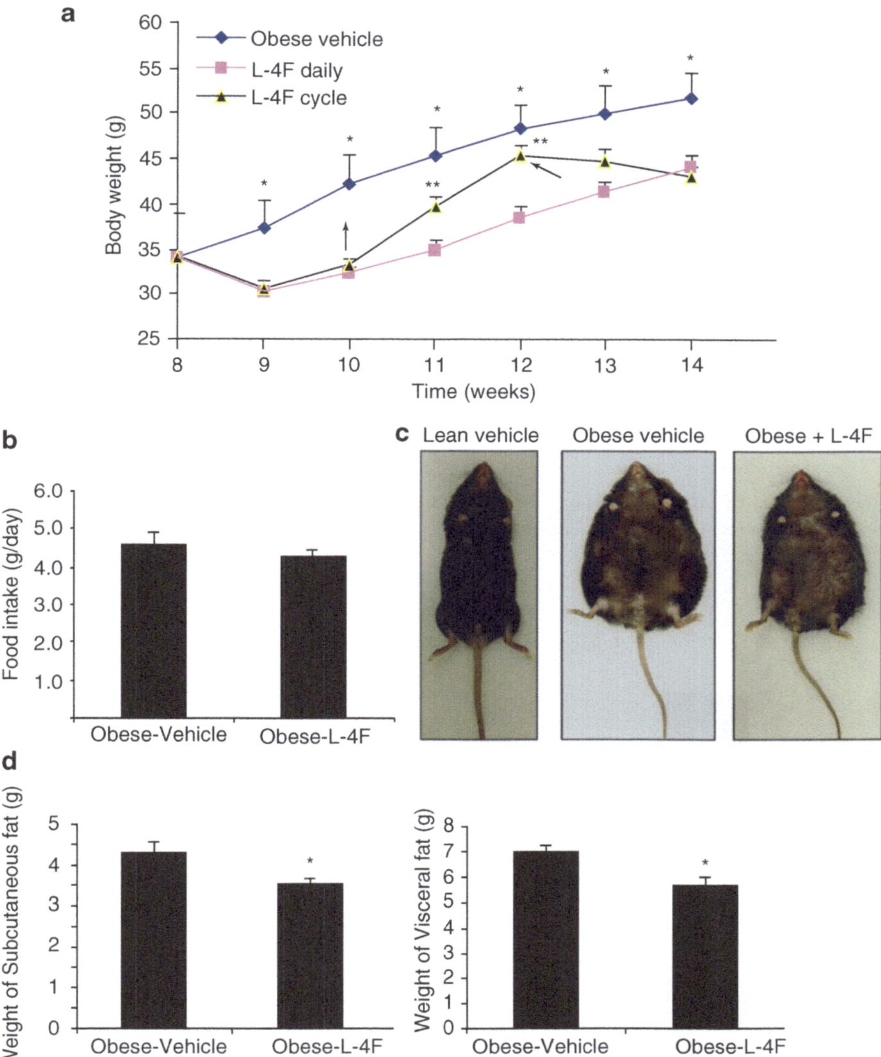

Fig. 3 (**a**) Body weight of vehicle-treated or L-4F-treated obese mice. The mice were weighed at the times shown on the X-axis given as the age of the mice in weeks. The data are the weights in grams as mean ± SEM (average of two independent experiments); n = 8 for vehicle-treated and n = 10 for L-4F-treated, L-4F discontinued, L-4F recommended. *$P < 0.05$ obese vehicle-treated versus obese L-4Ftreated mice. **$P < 0.05$ compared to continuous administration of L-4F. (**b**) Food intake in vehicle-treated or L-4F-treated obese mice during the first 2 weeks of treatment. (**c**) Representative photographs of mice after 6 weeks of treatment. (**d**) Weight of subcutaneous and visceral fat after L-4F treatment; *$P < 0.05$ versus vehicle-treated obese animals (Peterson et al. 2008)

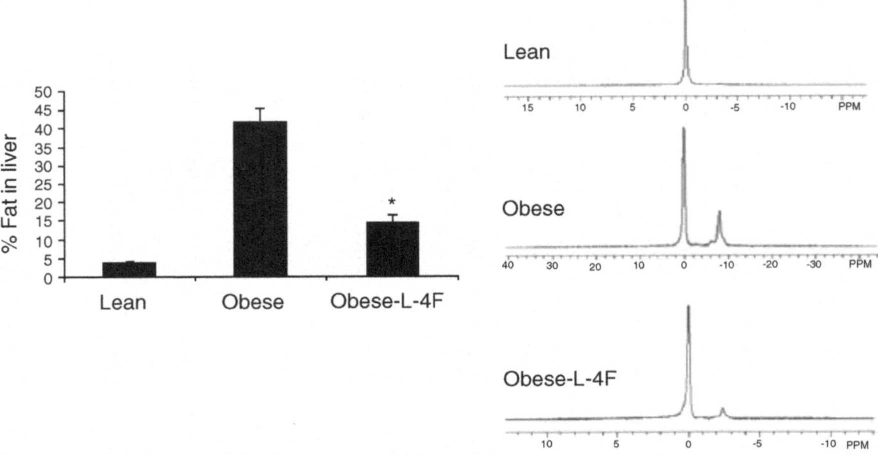

Fig. 4 Effect of L-4F on percentage of fat in the liver of ob mice measured by MRS. Analysis of lipid content percentage of fat was calculated as described earlier by us (*P, 0.01 vs. obese, n 5 3) (Segrest et al. 1992)

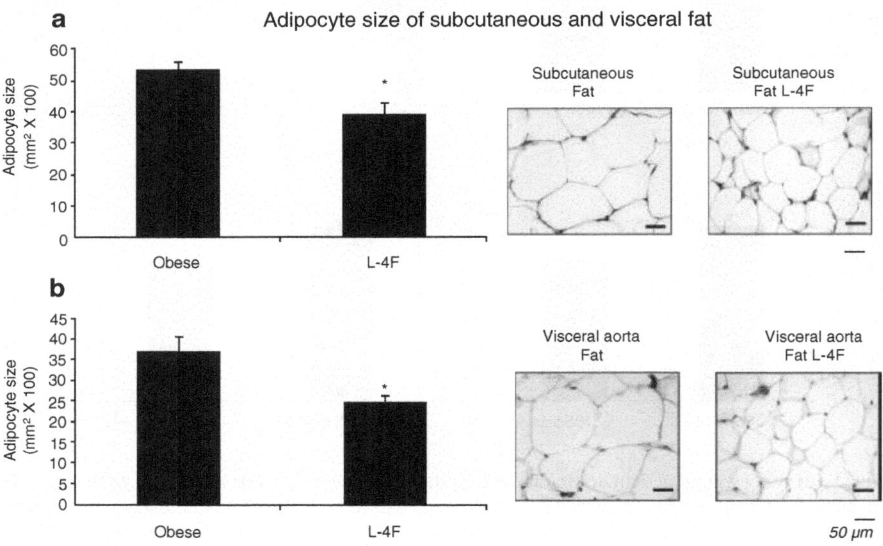

Fig. 5 Effect of L-4F on subcutaneous (**a**) and visceral (**b**) fat in ob mice. Hematoxylin-eosin staining of subcutaneous (**a**) and visceral (**b**) fat in ob and L-4F-treated ob mice. Bars = 50 mm. Quantitative analysis of adipocyte size in subcutaneous fat and visceral fat surrounding the aorta of ob or L-4F-treated ob mice is displayed. Data are expressed as means 6 SD (* *P*, 0.05 vs. ob) (Peterson et al. 2009)

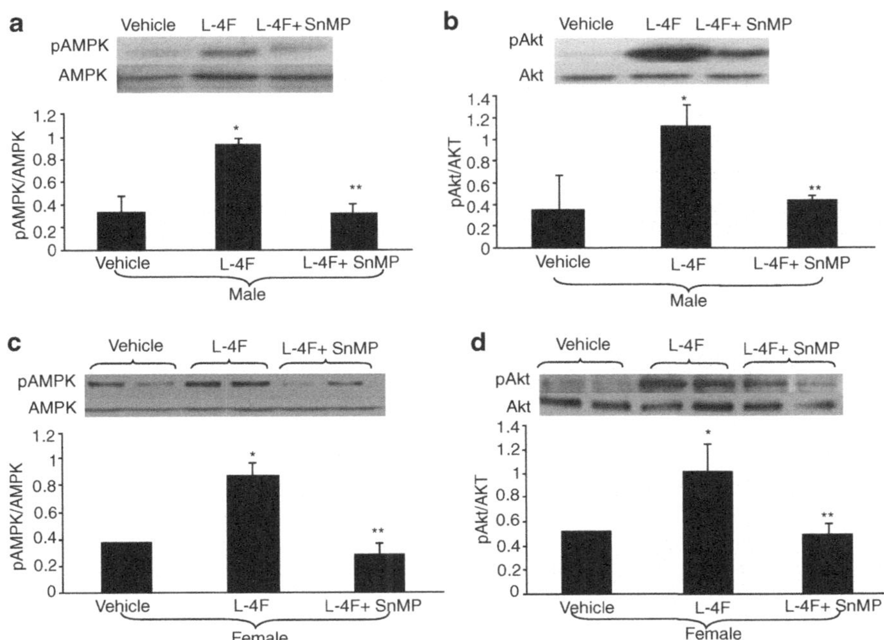

Fig. 6 (**a**–**d**) Effect of L-4F and SnMP inhibition of HO activity on pAMPK, pAKT, and a-actin in the kidneys of control and L-4F-treated ob males and females. All data are represented as phosphorylated/total. (**a**) Western blot and densitometry analysis of renal pAMPK protein in ob males. Results are means ± s.e., n¼4. *P=0.01 vs. ob male and **P=0.001 vs. ob maleþL-4F. (**b**) Representative Western blot and densitometry analysis of pAKT protein in ob male mice. Results are means ± s.e., n¼4. *P=0.05 vs. ob male and **P=0.05 vs. ob maleþL-4F. (**c**) Representative Western blot and densitometry analysis of pAMPK protein in ob females. Results are means ± s.e., n¼4. *P=0.05 vs. ob female and **P=0.05 vs. ob femaleþL-4F. (**d**) Representative Western blot and densitometry analysis of pAMPK protein in ob females. Results are means ± s.e., n¼4. *P=0.05 vs. ob female and **P=0.01 vs. ob femaleþL-4F (Marino et al. 2012)

blocked by stannous mesoporphyrin (SnMP), a known antagonist of heme oxygenase. Marino et al. showed that this mimetic peptide improved cardiovascular risk factors, improved insulin sensitivity, and vascular health. L-4F was shown to increase pAKT and pAMPK in an HO-dependent manner (Fig. 6) (Marino et al. 2012).

Morgantini et al. (2011) have shown that type 2 diabetics have impaired anti-inflammatory and antioxidant properties. Impaired or dysfunctional HDL is incapable of preventing the oxidation of LDL. He further illustrated that D-4F could prevent the development of atherosclerosis in mice with diabetes as a preexisting condition (Morgantini et al. 2010; Morgantini et al. 2011).

Kruger et al. (2005) used streptozotocin to induce diabetes in Sprague Dawley rats. This resulted in endothelial cell sloughing, the first step in endothelial cell dysfunction. There was reduction in HO-1 as well as superoxide dismutase, leading to marked increases in superoxides. D-4F administration via injection increased HO-1 and superoxide dismutase. It also decreased the number of sloughed, circulating endothelial cells and decreased superoxide levels.

Peterson et al. (2007) used D-4F in type 1 diabetic rats resulting in upregulation of heme oxygenase, endothelial cell marker (CD31+), and thrombomodulin (TM) expression with an increase in the number of endothelial progenitor cells (EPCs). D-4F prevented increases in oxidized LDL and reversed the increases in reactive oxygen species (ROS) and superoxide production. It also increased endothelial nitric oxide synthetase (eNOS).

Cao et al. have shown that L-4F was able to induce HO-1 expression and decrease oxidative stress and obesity in HO-2 knockout mice via HO-1-induced increase in adiponectin, PAMPK, and LKB1 (Cao et al. 2012). LKB1 is a kinase that controls the phosphorylation of AMPK (Shackelford and Shaw 2009). pAMPK is responsible for the metabolism in adipose tissue. Vanella et al. have demonstrated that L-4F was able to reverse adipocyte dysfunction in vivo and in vitro (Vanella et al. 2012). The hypothesis was that adiponectin came from mesenchymal stem cell (MSC)-derived adipocytes and that these levels were decreased in diabetes. L-4F reduced IL-1β and Il-6 and blood glucose levels while simultaneously increasing adiponectin and improving insulin sensitivity. Treatment of these MSCs with L-4F increased MSC-derived adipocytes by 50 % in S phase. L-4F was used to treat these MSC-derived adipocytes, which increase Wnt10B and decreased peg1/MEST. This study was very important because it showed that HO-1 was involved with adipogenic markers. The increased Wnt10b and decreased Peg1/MEST was accompanied by improved insulin sensitivity. Wnt10B is a protein encoded by the Wnt10B gene. While this gene has been implicated in oncogenesis, it was studied here for its role as a molecular "switch" that governs adipogenesis (Isakson et al. 2009; Aslanidi et al. 2007; Wright et al. 2007). Peg1/MEST is an imprinted gene from the father. Paternally expressed (Peg1)/mesoderm-specific transcript/Peg1/MEST is markedly elevated in obese adipose tissue (Takahashi et al. 2005). The L-4F-induced HO-1 increase was accompanied by increases in Wnt10B and decreases in Peg1/MEST. It also was accompanied by reduction in PPAR-γ. PPAR-γ is mainly present in adipose tissue. PPAR-γ stimulates the genes that stimulate lipid uptake and increase adipogenesis (Wright et al. 2014). Reducing PPAR-γ, as in this case, has exactly the opposite effect, reducing adipogenesis. This was a dramatic effect of L-4F in vivo in animals as well as on mesenchymal stem cells. L-4F increased Wnt10B signaling in adipose tissue while decreasing signaling of Peg1/MEST. Since these effects were blocked by SnMP, a known blocker of HO-1 (Cao et al. 2009), the effect appeared to be upregulation of HO-1 by L-4F with dramatic effects on adipose tissue directly (Figs. 7, 8, and 9).

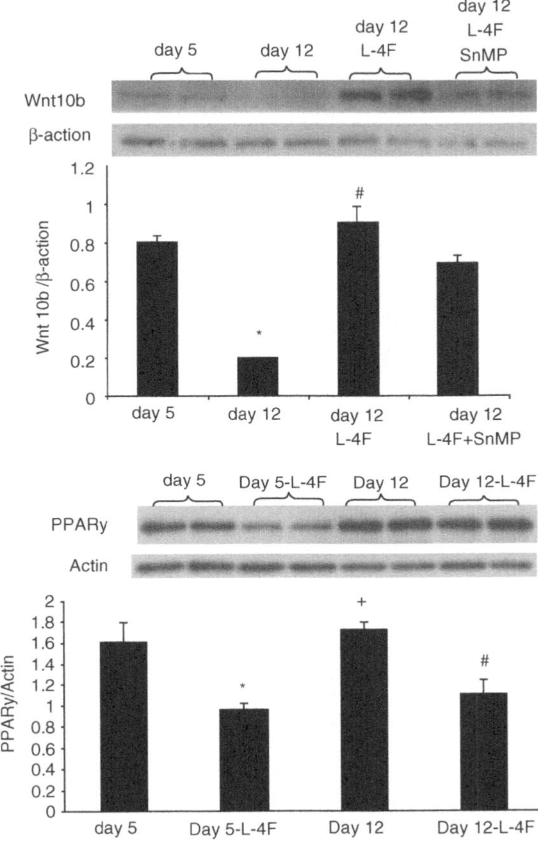

Fig. 7 Effect of L-4F on Wnt10b, β-catenin, and PPARγ levels. Western blot of Wnt10b, β-catenin, PPARγ, and actin proteins in MSC-derived adipocytes treated with L-4F alone or in combination with SnMP. Representative immunoblots are shown ($n=4$). Quantitative densitometry evaluation of Wnt10b β-catenin and actin proteins ratio was determined. Data are expressed as means ± SD (*$p<0.05$ vs. day 5, #$p<0.05$ vs. day 12, +$p<0.05$ vs. day5 + L-4F) (Vanella et al. 2012)

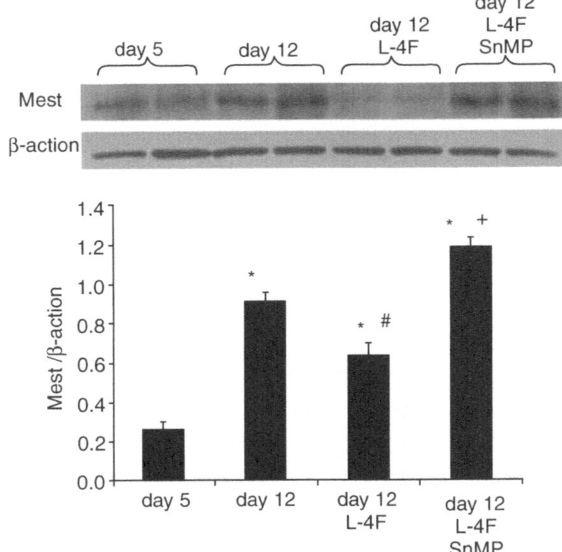

Fig. 8 Effect of L-4F on MEST and IRP-Tyr1146. Western blot of MEST, IRP-Tyr1146, and actin proteins in MSC-derived adipocytes treated with L-4F alone or in combination with SnMP. Representative immunoblots are shown ($n=4$). Quantitative densitometry evaluation of MEST, IRP-Tyr1146, and actin proteins ratio was determined. Data are expressed as means ± SD (*$p<0.05$ vs. day 5, #$p<0.05$ vs. day 12, +$p<0.05$ vs. day 5 + L-4F) (Vanella et al. 2012)

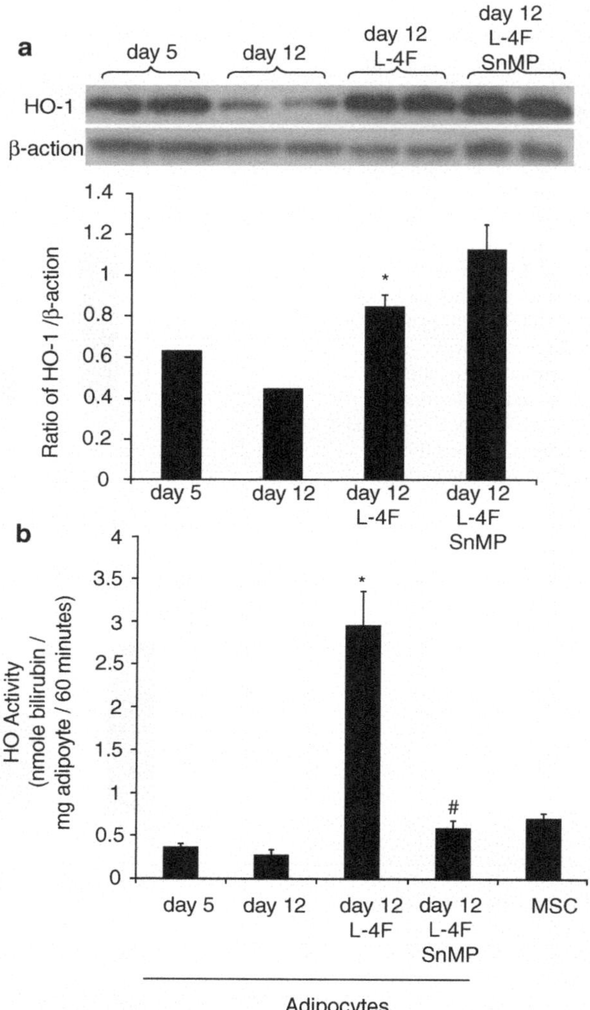

Fig. 9 Effect of L-4F on HO-1 expression and activity. (**a**) Western blot of HO-1 proteins in MSC-derived adipocytes treated with L-4F and SnMP. Representative immunoblots are shown ($n=4$). MSCs were cultured in adipogenic differentiation media, and L-4F was added every 3 days. Quantitative densitometry evaluation of HO-1 and actin proteins ratio was determined. Data are expressed as means ± SD ($^*p<0.05$ vs. day 12). (**b**) Effect of L-4F on HO activity as measured by bilirubin generation. Bilirubin formed in cellular homogenates in the presence of heme and NADPH was measured ($^*p<0.001$ vs. day 12). Combination of L-4F with SnMP reduces HO activity ($\#p<0.001$ vs. day 12 + L-4F) (Vanella et al. 2012)

Conclusion

ApoA-1 comprises 70 % of the total protein of HDL and is largely responsible for the beneficial effects of HDL. It would be prohibitively expensive to manufacture this 243 amino acid protein. ApoA-1 mimetic proteins, such as D-4F and L-4F are 18A amphipathic alpha helical peptides, are relatively cheap and easy to produce and offer an enhanced ability to form lipid complexes while retaining the ability to promote cholesterol efflux.

D-4F is an oral peptide made with D-amino acids that is resistant to proteolysis. Since D bonds are not broken down, there is some concern that D-4F will eventually lead to toxicity. GI peptidases recognize and break down L amino acids. L-4F may have more utility in the future with a better safety profile if it can be made into an oral delivery system that would be resistant to proteolysis.

4F has been shown to have tremendous beneficial effects in diabetes, obesity, and metabolic syndrome. It appears to do this independent of cholesterol levels and weight loss. The results are anti-inflammatory, antioxidant, and antiplatelet.

It also appears to upregulate HO-1, thereby increasing adiponectin, improving blood glucose levels, reducing insulin resistance, and reducing visceral and subcutaneous adiposity. More work needs to be done to determine the future of this class of drugs, but it certainly shows promise in this area. Future possibilities include combination with metformin, as they both reduce insulin levels and insulin resistance, but have very different mechanisms of action. Since diabetics have increased cardiovascular risk, the conversion of proinflammatory HDL to anti-inflammatory HDL (bad HDL to good HDL), with its enhanced ability to promote cholesterol efflux independent of HDL levels is a very important aspect of 4F. The epidemic of obesity, diabetes, and metabolic syndrome may offer the perfect setting for clinical trials for this indication.

References

Abraham NG, Kappas A (2008) Pharmacological and clinical aspects of heme oxygenase. Pharmacol Rev 60:79–127

Abraham N, Tsenovoy P, McClung J, Drummond G (2008) Heme oxygenase: a target gene for anti-diabetic and obesity. Curr Pharm Des 14:412–421

Aslanidi G, Kroutov V, Philipsberg G, Lamb K, Campbell-Thompson M, Walter GA, Kurenov S, Ignacio Aguirre J, Keller P, Hankenson K, Macdougald OA, Zolotukhin S (2007) Ectopic expression of Wnt10b decreases adiposity and improves glucose homeostasis in obese rats. Am J Physiol Endocrinol Metab 293(3):E726–E736, Epub 2007 Jun 19

Cao J, Sodhi K, Puri N, Monu SR, Rezzani R, Abraham NG (2011) High fat diet enhances cardiac abnormalities in SHR rats: protective role of heme oxygenase-adiponectin axis. Diabetol Metab Syndr 3(1):37. doi:10.1186/1758-5996-3-37, Nat Rev Cancer. 2009;9(8):563–575. doi: 10.1038/nrc2676

Cao J, Puri N, Sodhi K, Bellner L, Abraham NG, Kappas A (2012) Apo A1 mimetic rescues the diabetic phenotype of HO-2 knockout mice via an increase in HO-1 adiponectin and LKBI signaling pathway. Int J Hypertens 2012:628147. doi:10.1155/2012/628147, Epub 2012 Apr 4

Isakson P, Hammarstedt A, Gustafson B, Smith U (2009) Impaired preadipocyte differentiation in human abdominal obesity: role of Wnt, tumor necrosis factor-alpha, and inflammation. Diabetes 58(7):1550–1557. doi:10.2337/db08-1770, Epub 2009 Apr 7

Kruger AL, Peterson S, Turkseven S, Kaminski PM, Zhang FF, Quan S, Wolin MS, Abraham NG (2005) D-4F induces heme oxygenase-1 and extracellular superoxide dismutase, decreases endothelial cell sloughing, and improves vascular reactivity in rat model of diabetes. Circulation 111(23):3126–3134, Epub 2005 Jun 6

Lin Y, Berg AH, Iyengar P, Lam TK, Giacca A, Combs TP, Rajala MW, Du X, Rollman B, Li W, Hawkins M, Barzilai N, Rhodes CJ, Fantus IG, Brownlee M, Scherer PE (2005) The hyperglycemia-induced inflammatory response in adipocytes: the role of reactive oxygen species. J Biol Chem 280(6):4617–4626, Epub 2004 Nov 9

Lin HV, Kim JY, Pocai A, Rossetti L, Shapiro L, Scherer PE, Accili D (2007) Adiponectin resistance exacerbates insulin resistance in insulin receptor transgenic/knockout mice. Diabetes 56(8):1969–1976, Epub 2007 May 2

Marino JS, Peterson SJ, Li M, Vanella L, Sodhi K, Hikll JW, Abraham NG (2012) ApoA-1 mimetic restores adiponectin expression and insulin sensitivity independent of changes in body weight in female obese mice. Nutr Diabetes 2:e33. doi:10.1038/nutd.2012.4

Morgantini C, Imaizumi S, Grijalva V, Navab M, Fogelman AM, Reddy ST (2010) Apolipoprotein A-I mimetic peptides prevent atherosclerosis development and reduce plaque inflammation in a murine model of diabetes. Diabetes 59(12):3223–3228. doi:10.2337/db10-0844, Epub 2010 Sep 8

Morgantini C, Natali A, Boldrini B, Imaizumi S, Navab M, Fogelman AM, Ferrannini E, Reddy ST (2011) Anti-inflammatory and antioxidant properties of HDLs are impaired in type 2 diabetes. Diabetes 60(10):2617–2623. doi:10.2337/db11-0378, Epub 2011 Aug 18

Navab M, Anantharamaiah GM, Hama S, Garber DW, Chaddha M, Hough G, Lallone R, Fogelman AM (2002) Oral administration of an Apo A-I mimetic peptide synthesized from D-amino acids dramatically reduces atherosclerosis in mice independent of plasma cholesterol. Circulation 105(3):290–292

Peterson SJ, Husney D, Kruger AL, Olszanecki R, Ricci F, Rodella LF, Stacchiotti A, Rezzani R, McClung JA, Aronow WS, Ikehara S, Abraham NG (2007) Long-term treatment with the apolipoprotein A1 mimetic peptide increases antioxidants and vascular repair in type I diabetic rats. J Pharmacol Exp Ther 322(2):514–520, Epub 2007 May 8

Peterson SJ, Drummond G, Kim DH, Li M, Kruger AL, Ikehara S, Abraham NG (2008) L-4F treatment reduces adiposity, increases adiponectin levels, and improves insulin sensitivity in obese mice. J Lipid Res 49(8):1658–1669. doi:10.1194/jlr.M800046-JLR200, Epub 2008 Apr 19

Peterson SJ, Kim DH, Li M, Positano V, Vanella L, Rodella LF, Piccolomini F, Puri N, Gastaldelli A, Kusmic C, L'Abbate A, Abraham NG (2009) The L-4F mimetic peptide prevents insulin resistance through increased levels of HO-1, pAMPK, and pAKT in obese mice. J Lipid Res 50(7):1293–1304. doi:10.1194/jlr.M800610-JLR200, Epub 2009 Feb 17

Robertson RP (2004) Chronic oxidative stress as a central mechanism for glucose toxicity in pancreatic islet beta cells in diabetes. J Biol Chem 279(41):42351–42354, Epub 2004 Jul 16. Review

Segrest JP, Jones MK, De Loof H, Brouillette CG, Venkatachalapathi YV, Anantharamaiah GM (1992) The amphipathic helix in the exchangeable apolipoproteins: a review of secondary structure and function. J Lipid Res 33(2):141–166, Review

Shackelford DB, Shaw RJ (2009) The LKB1-AMPK pathway: metabolism and growth control in tumour suppression. Nat Rev Cancer 9(8):563–575. doi:10.1038/nrc2676

Takahashi M, Kamei Y, Ezaki O (2005) Mest/Peg1 imprinted gene enlarges adipocytes and is a marker of adipocyte size. Am J Physiol Endocrinol Metab 288(1):E117–E124, Epub 2004 Sep 7

Vanella L, Li M, Kim D, Malfa G, Bellner L, Kawakami T, Abraham NG (2012) ApoA1: mimetic peptide reverses adipocyte dysfunction in vivo and in vitro via an increase in heme oxygenase (HO-1) and Wnt10b. Cell Cycle 11(4):706–714. doi:10.4161/cc.11.4.19125, Epub 2012 Feb 15

Wellen KE, Hotamisligil GS (2005) Inflammation, stress, and diabetes. J Clin Invest 115(5):1111–1119, Review

Wright WS, Longo KA, Dolinsky VW, Gerin I, Kang S, Bennett CN, Chiang SH, Prestwich TC, Gress C, Burant CF, Susulic VS, MacDougald OA (2007) Wnt10b inhibits obesity in ob/ob and agouti mice. Diabetes 56(2):295–303

Wright MB, Bortolini M, Tadayyon M, Bopst M (2014) Minireview: challenges and opportunities in development of PPAR agonists. Mol Endocrinol 28:1756, Aug 22:me20131427. [Epub ahead of print]

Apolipoprotein A-I Mimetic Peptides in Mouse Models of Cancer

Robin Farias-Eisner, Feng Su, G.M. Anantharamahiah, Mohamad Navab, Alan M. Fogelman, and Srinivasa T. Reddy

Abstract Novel therapeutic approaches, free of secondary side effects, are desperately needed for the treatment of cancers especially recurrent, chemotherapy-resistant cancers. It is now established that inflammation and lipoprotein metabolism play an important role in cancer development and progression. The serendipitous discovery that plasma/serum levels of HDL-associated proteins, apolipoprotein A-I (ApoA-I), transthyretin, and transferrin, are markers for the detection of early-stage ovarian cancer led to the hypothesis that HDL may play a critical role in the development and progression of cancer. Studies in mouse models established that apoA-I has antitumorigenic properties. ApoA-I mimetic peptides administered orally or subcutaneously reduce tumor growth and tumor burden in mouse models of ovarian

R. Farias-Eisner • F. Su
Department of Obstetrics and Gynecology, David Geffen School of Medicine at UCLA, Los Angeles, CA, USA

G.M. Anantharamahiah, PhD
Department of Medicine, University of Alabama at Birmingham, Birmingham, AL, USA
e-mail: ganantha@uabmc.edu

M. Navab • A.M. Fogelman
Division of Cardiology, Department of Medicine, David Geffen School of Medicine at UCLA, Los Angeles, CA, USA

S.T. Reddy, PhD (✉)
Department of Obstetrics and Gynecology, David Geffen School of Medicine at UCLA, Los Angeles, CA, USA

Division of Cardiology, Department of Medicine, David Geffen School of Medicine at UCLA, Los Angeles, CA, USA

Department of Molecular and Medical Pharmacology, David Geffen School of Medicine at UCLA, Los Angeles, CA, USA

Division of Cardiology, Department of Medicine, David Geffen School of Medicine at UCLA, 10833 Le Conte Avenue, Los Angeles, CA 90095-1679, USA
e-mail: sreddy@mednet.ucla.edu

G.M. Anantharamaiah, D. Goldberg (eds.), *Apolipoprotein Mimetics in the Management of Human Disease*, DOI 10.1007/978-3-319-17350-4_5

cancer and colon cancer by suppressing angiogenesis and proliferation. Antioxidant, lipid-binding, and anti-inflammatory properties of apoA-I mimetic peptides appear to be their primary mechanism of action. In vivo and in vitro studies implicate multiple pathways including VEGF, MnSOD, and HIF1-α in mediating the antiangiogenic and antiproliferative properties of apoA-I mimetic peptides. The antiproliferative effects of apoA-I mimetic peptides on the viability of human papillary serous adenocarcinoma cell lines resistant to cis-platinum suggest that apoA-I mimetic peptides may be efficacious for the treatment of at least some of the chemotherapy-resistant types of cancer.

Introduction

One of the greatest clinical challenges we face in the twenty-first century is the treatment of recurrent and chemotherapy-resistant cancer. More than 75 % of these patients will succumb to the disease. The 5-year survival rate is exceedingly low (e.g., 28 % for metastatic ovarian cancer) and has not improved in spite of more than three decades of clinical trials using conventional radiation and chemotherapeutic agents. The lack of effective therapeutic strategies has led to the inevitable emergence of chemotherapy (e.g., cis-platinum)-resistant cancer, and the associated incapacitating toxicity has led to the current clinical crisis in cancer treatment. Thus, what is desperately needed is a novel therapeutic approach that is free of secondary side effects for the treatment of recurrent and chemotherapy-resistant cancer.

Inflammation and Lipoproteins in Cancer

Although a link was established between inflammation and cancer in the nineteenth century, the molecular mechanisms and pathways underlying cancer-related inflammation have only been examined in the last two decades (Mantovani et al. 2008). There is now evidence suggesting that inflammation promotes all aspects of tumorigenesis including angiogenesis, tumor growth, and invasion (Mantovani et al. 2008). Mitochondrial reactive oxygen species (ROS) derived as a result of activation of Ras, Myc, and p53 contribute to inflammation-associated cancers (Kamp et al. 2011). Moreover, it is now well established that macrophages, the hallmark of inflammation, play an important role in the progression and metastasis of cancers (Qian and Pollard 2010). Lipoproteins participate in the integral network of lipid transport to and from all cells and tissues. Lipoprotein levels and metabolism play a critical role in inflammation and are recognized as key components of inflammatory diseases including cancer (Barter 2005; Navab et al. 2005). Indeed, epidemiological studies showed that risk for endometrial cancer (Cust et al. 2007) and colon cancer (van Duijnhoven et al. 2011) is inversely correlated with HDL-cholesterol levels.

ApoA-I and Ovarian Cancer

Ovarian cancer has the highest mortality rate among all gynecologic malignancies (Edwards et al. 2010). At the time of diagnosis, over 85 % of patients with ovarian cancer present with advanced stage III or IV disease characterized by intraperitoneal, lymphatic, and/or distant spread of disease; the poor prognosis associated with ovarian cancer is attributed to a lack of as yet undetectable symptoms at early stages of the disease as well as a lack of known biomarkers for the detection of early-stage disease. Moreover, despite appropriate surgery and receiving frequently or largely effective first-line chemotherapy, approximately 20–30 % of patients with advanced stage disease continue to have evidence of residual disease during the treatment and never have a complete clinical response. There is therefore an immediate need for both biomarkers and therapeutic targets for treating ovarian cancer (Nossov et al. 2008).

Kozak et al. utilized mass spectrometry and demonstrated that three proteins associated with high-density lipoprotein (HDL) are lower in the serum of patients with early-stage ovarian neoplasia compared to normal individuals (Kozak et al. 2003). The three ovarian cancer biomarkers, apolipoprotein A-I (apoA-I), transthyretin (TTR), and transferrin (TF) (Kozak et al. 2003, 2005; Nossov et al. 2008, 2009), when used as a panel were better predictors of early-stage ovarian cancer, compared to serum CA125 levels. More recently (09/12/2009), the US Food and Drug Administration (FDA) cleared the first laboratory test that can indicate the likelihood of ovarian cancer, OVA1™ test, which utilizes apoA-I, TTR, TF, CA125, and beta2-microglobulin (Fung 2010). Since lipid transport, inflammation, and oxidative stress are associated with the development and progression of cancer, Su et al. hypothesized that the reduced levels of apoA-I in ovarian cancer patients may have been causal in disease progression and further hypothesized that apoA-I plays an antitumorigenic role in ovarian cancer (Su et al. 2010). Su et al. demonstrated, for the first time, that overexpression of human apoA-I in transgenic mice inhibits tumor growth and improves survival in a mouse model of ovarian cancer (Su et al. 2010). Subsequently, Zamanian-Daryoush et al. (2013) reported that apoA-I potently suppressed tumor growth and metastasis in multiple animal tumor models through both innate and adaptive immune processes.

ApoA-I Mimetic Peptides as Cancer Therapeutics

ApoA-I is recognized as a key functional entity of HDL that confers many of the antiatherogenic, antioxidant, and anti-inflammatory properties assigned to HDL. Based on this rationale, peptides that contained lipid-binding properties similar to apoA-I were developed as candidate therapeutic agents for the treatment of inflammatory diseases, primarily atherosclerosis. In preclinical studies, apoA-I mimetic peptides have proven to be excellent agents for the treatment of a number of inflammatory diseases (Van Lenten et al. 2008a). Following the tumor studies on apoA-I protein, Su et al. tested whether apoA-I mimetic peptides can prevent tumorigenesis (Su et al. 2010). In a series of experiments, Su et al. demonstrated, for the first time, that L-4F (an apoA-I mimetic peptide with four phenylalanines) and 5F (an apoA-I mimetic peptide with five phenylalanines) reduced the viability and proliferation of ID8 cells (a mouse epithelial ovarian cancer cell line) and cis-platinum-resistant human ovarian cancer cells and decreased ID-8 cell-mediated tumor burden in C57BL/6J mice when administered subcutaneously or orally (Su et al. 2010).

Su et al. further demonstrated that the apoA-I mimetic peptides 4F and 5F decreased the levels of lysophosphatidic acid (LPA), a known tumor growth promoter, in vitro and in vivo (Su et al. 2010). Since apoA-I mimetic peptides bind oxidized lipids including LPA with high affinity (Van Lenten et al. 2008b), these results suggest that binding and removal of LPA might be a potential mechanism for the inhibition of tumor development by apoA-I mimetic peptides. In support of this, the inhibition of cell growth is the dominant mechanism of apoA-I mimetic peptides as there were no differences in apoptosis but did see significant differences in BrdU incorporation in cells following peptide treatment. In vitro, the apoA-I mimetic peptide L-4F reduced the viability of human papillary serous adenocarcinoma cell lines resistant to cis-platinum, namely, SKOV3, OV2008, and A2780 (Su et al. 2010). These results have important clinical implications because the majority of patients treated for advanced stage ovarian cancer will succumb to their disease secondary to the development of cis-platinum-resistant recurrent disease (Cannistra 2004).

Besides the binding and removal of oxidized phospholipids and/or LPA, a number of other mechanisms have also been examined and identified for the antitumorigenic effects of apoA-I mimetic peptides. Gao and colleagues demonstrated that inhibition of angiogenesis is one of the mechanisms (Gao et al. 2011). The apoA-I mimetic peptide, L-5F, inhibited both vascular endothelial growth factor (VEGF)- and basic fibroblast growth factor (bFGF)-induced proliferation, cell viability, migration, invasion, and tube formation in HUVECs by altering Akt and ERK1/2 signaling pathways (Gao et al. 2011). Gao et al. also demonstrated that daily injection of L-5F (10 mg kg^{-1}) decreased both the quantity and size of tumor vessels in mice, suggesting a critical role in neo-angiogenesis for the apoA-I mimetic peptide.

Expression and activity of hypoxia-inducible factor-1 alpha (HIF-1α) play an important role in the production of angiogenic factors and angiogenesis. Gao et al. demonstrated that L-4F treatment dramatically decreased HIF-1α expression in mouse ovarian tumor tissues (Gao et al. 2012). L-4F inhibited the expression and activity of HIF-1α induced by low oxygen concentration, lysophosphatidic acid, and insulin in two human ovarian cancer cell lines, OV2008 and CAOV-3 (Gao et al. 2012). Gao et al. further showed that the inhibitory effect of L-4F on HIF-1α expression is mediated by the reactive oxygen species (ROS) scavenging effect of L-4F, suggesting the inhibition of HIF-1α may be a critical mechanism responsible for the suppression of tumor progression by apoA-I mimetic peptides (Gao et al. 2012).

The ROS scavenging effect of apoA-I mimetic peptides fits with the antioxidant properties associated with these peptides. Ganapathy and coworkers demonstrated that D-4F (the D amino acid analogue of 4F) induces MnSOD (but not Cu/Zn SOD) mRNA, protein, and activity (Ganapathy et al. 2012). D-4F treatment significantly reduced the viability and proliferation of ID8 cells and improved the antioxidant status of ID8 cells measured by lipid peroxidation, protein carbonyl, superoxide anion, and hydrogen peroxide levels (Ganapathy et al. 2012). Ganapathy et al. suggested that induction of MnSOD is a part of the mechanism of action of the apoA-I mimetic peptides (Ganapathy et al. 2012).

ApoA-I Mimetic Peptides and Colon Cancer

Colon cancer is the third most common cancer worldwide and the third leading cause of cancer death in both men and women in the USA, with approximately 150,000 new cases diagnosed and 50,000 disease-related deaths every year (Jemal et al. 2010). Like most cancers, early diagnosis and surgery significantly improve the chances of cure for colon cancer. HDL levels are inversely related to colon cancer risk (van Duijnhoven et al. 2011). Su et al. examined whether apoA-I mimetic peptides affect tumor growth and development in mouse models of colon cancer (Su et al. 2012). ApoA-I mimetics reduced the viability and proliferation of CT26 cells, a mouse colon adenocarcinoma cell line, and decreased CT26 cell-mediated tumor burden in BALB/c mice when administered subcutaneously or orally. Plasma levels of LPA, a serum biomarker for colon cancer, were significantly reduced in mice that received apoA-I mimetic peptides, suggesting that pro-inflammatory lipid scavenging is a potential mechanism for the inhibition of tumor development. L-4F significantly reduced size and number of polyps in $APC^{min/+}$ mice, a mouse model for human familial adenomatous polyposis, suggesting that apoA-I mimetic peptides are effective in inhibiting the development of both induced and spontaneous cancers of the colon (Su et al. 2012).

Conclusions

Inflammation and oxidative stress mediated by lipoprotein metabolism are now recognized to be important contributors to cancer development, progression, and metastases. Recent studies have suggested that apoA-I and apoA-I mimetic peptides may provide novel therapeutic strategies in the treatment of a number of malignancies (Su et al. 2010, 2012; Zamanian-Daryoush et al. 2013; Gao et al. 2011, 2012; Ganapathy et al. 2012). In mouse models of ovarian cancer and of colon cancer in which the mice have a normal immune system, it was found that transgenic expression of human apoA-I, or administration of apoA-I mimetic peptides, significantly decreased tumor burden (Su et al. 2010, 2012; Zamanian-Daryoush et al. 2013; Gao et al. 2011, 2012; Ganapathy et al. 2012). A common mechanism of action for these agents appears to be the reduction of pro-inflammatory lipids including LPA, a well-studied tumor promoter. Interestingly, LPA has been reported to increase the expression of scavenger receptor A (SR-A) on macrophages (Chang et al. 2008). SR-A expression on macrophages has been shown to be necessary and sufficient to promote tumor invasiveness (Neyen et al. 2013a). The 4F peptide was reported to be a potent inhibitor of SR-A (Neyen et al. 2009), and administration of the 4F peptide inhibited tumor invasiveness (Neyen et al. 2013b). Although 4F (at low doses tested – dose of 0.43 mg/kg) did not improve inflammatory markers in a recent clinical trial (Watson et al. 2011), Chattopadhyay et al. developed a novel strategy by overexpressing apoA-I mimetic peptide 6F (an apoA-I mimetic peptide with six phenylalanines) in tomato plants and demonstrated that transgenic tomatoes prevented atherosclerosis in mice (Chattopadhyay et al. 2013). Interestingly, these novel therapies also carry antitumorigenic activities. In conclusion, apoA-I mimetic peptides will be free of secondary side effects and have the potential for the treatment of cancers especially recurrent, chemotherapy-resistant cancer.

Disclosures M.N., S.T.R, G.M.A, and A.M.F. are principals in Bruin Pharma, and A.M.F. is an officer in Bruin Pharma.

Acknowledgments This work was supported in part by US Public Health Service Research Grants HL-30568, a Network grant from the Leducq Foundation, the Laubisch, Castera, and M.K. Grey Funds at UCLA, the Women's Endowment, the Carl and Roberta Deutsch Family Foundation, the Joan English Fund for Women's Cancer Research, Kelly Day, the OVARIAN CANCER Coalition, the Helen Beller Foundation, Wendy Stark Foundation, and Sue and Mel Geliebter Family Foundation.

References

Barter P (2005) The inflammation: lipoprotein cycle. Atheroscler Suppl 6:15–20

Cannistra SA (2004) Cancer of the ovary. N Engl J Med 351:2519–2529

Chang C-L, Hsu H-Y, Lin H-Y, Chiang W, Lee H (2008) Lysophosphatidic acid-induced oxidized low-density lipoprotein uptake is class A scavenger receptor-dependent in macrophages. Prostaglandins Other Lipid Mediat 87:20–25

Chattopadhyay A, Navab M, Hough G, Gao F, Meriwether D, Grijalva V, Springstead JR, Palgunachari MN, Namiri-Kalantari R, Su F, Van Lenten BJ, Wagner AC, Anantharamaiah GM, Farias-Eisener R, Reddy ST, Fogelman AM (2013) A novel approach to oral apoA-I mimetic therapy. J Lipid Res 54:995–1010

Cust AE, Kaaks R, Friedenreich C, Bonnet F, Laville M, Tjonneland A, Olsen A, Overvad K, Jakobsen MU, Chajes V, Clavel-Chapelon F, Boutron-Ruault MC, Linseisen J, Lukanova A, Boeing H, Pischon T, Trichopoulou A, Christina B, Trichopoulos D, Palli D, Berrino F, Pnico S, Tumino R, Sacerdote C, Gram IT, Lund E, Quiros JR, Travier N, Martinez-Garcia C, Larranga N, Chiriaque MD, Ardanaz E, Berglund G, Lundin E, Bueno-de-Mesquita HB, van Duijnhoven FJ, Peeters PH, Bingham S, Khaw KT, Allen N, Key T, Ferrari P, Rinaldi S, Slimani N, Riboli E (2007) Metabolic syndrome, plasma lipid, lipoprotein and glucose levels, and endometrial cancer risk in the European Prospective Investigation into Cancer and Nutrition (EPIC). Endocr Relat Cancer 14:755–767

Edwards BK et al (2010) Annual report to the nation on the status of cancer, 1975–2006, featuring colorectal cancer trends and impact of interventions (risk factors, screening, and treatment) to reduce future rates. Cancer 116:544–573

Fung ET (2010) A recipe for proteomics diagnostic test development: the OVA1 test, from biomarker discovery to FDA clearance. Clin Chem 56:327–329

Ganapathy E, Su F, Meriwhether D, Devarajan A, Grijalva V, Gao F, Chattopadhyay A, Anantharamaiah GM, Navab M, Fogelman AM, Reddy ST, Farias-Eisner R (2012) D-4F, an apoA-I mimetic peptide, inhibits proliferation and tumorigenicity of epithelial ovarian cancer cells by upregulating the antioxidant enzyme MnSOD. Int J Cancer 130:1071–1081

Gao F, Vasquez SX, Su F, Roberts S, Shah N, Grijalva V, Imaizumi S, Chattopadhyay A, Ganapathy E, Meriwhether D, Johnston B, Anantharamaiah GM, Navab M, Fogelman AM, Reddy ST, Farias-Eisner R (2011) L-5F, an apolipoprotein A-I mimetic, inhibits tumor angiogenesis by suppressing VEGF/basic FGF signaling pathways. Integr Biol 3:479–489

Gao F, Chattopadhyay A, Navab M, Grijalva V, Su F, Fogelman AM, Reddy ST, Farias-Eisner R (2012) Apolipoprotein A-I mimetic peptides inhibit expression and activity of hypoxia-inducible factor-1α in human ovarian cancer cell lines and a mouse ovarian cancer model. J Pharmacol Exp Ther 342:255–262

Jemal A, Siegel R, Xu J, Ward E (2010) Cancer statistics 2010. CA Cancer J Clin 60:277–300

Kamp DW, Shacter E, Weitzman SA (2011) Chronic inflammation and cancer: the role of the mitochondria. Oncology 25:400–410

Kozak KR, Amneus MW, Puseyu SM, Su F, Luong MN, Luong SA, Reddy ST, Farias-Eisner R (2003) Identification of biomarkers for ovarian cancer using strong anion-exchange ProteinChips: potential use in diagnosis and prognosis. Proc Natl Acad Sci U S A 100:12343–12348

Kozak KR, Su F, Whitelegge JP, Faull K, Reddy S, Farias-Eisner R (2005) Characterization of serum biomarkers for detection of early stage ovarian cancer. Proteomics 5:4589–4596

Mantovani A, Allavena P, Sica A, Balkwill F (2008) Cancer-related inflammation. Nature 454: 436–444

Navab M, Anantharamaiah GM, Fogelman AM (2005) The role of high-density lipoprotein in inflammation. Trends Cardiovasc Med 15:158–161

Neyen C, Pluddemann A, Roversi P, Thomas B, Cai L, van derWesthuyzen DR, Sim RB, Gordon S (2009) Macrophage scavenger receptor A mediates adhesion to apolipoproteins A-I and E. Biochemistry 48:11858–11871

Neyen C, Pluddemann A, Mukhopadhyay S, Maniati E, Bossard M, Gordon S, Hagemann T (2013a) Macrophage scavenger receptor A promotes tumor progression in murine models of ovarian and pancreatic cancer. J Immunol 190:3798–3805

Neyen C, Mukhopadhyay S, Gordon S, Hagemann T (2013b) An apolipoprotein A-I mimetic targets scavenger receptor A on tumor-associated macrophages. A prospective treatment? Oncoimmunology 2:e24461

Nossov V et al (2008) The early detection of ovarian cancer: from traditional methods to proteomics. Can we really do better than serum CA-125? Am J Obstet Gynecol 199:215–223

Nossov V, Su F, Amneus M, Birrer M, Robbins T, Kotlerman J, Reddy S, Farias-Eisner R (2009) Validation of serum biomarkers for detection of early-stage ovarian cancer. Am J Obstet Gynecol 200:639.e1–639.e5

Qian B-Z, Pollard JW (2010) Macrophage diversity enhances tumor progression and metastasis. Cell 141:39–51

Su F, Kozak KR, Imaizumi S, Gao F, Amneus MW, Grijalva V, Ng C, Wagner A, Hough G, Farias-Eisner G, Anantharamaiah GM, Van Lenten BJ, Navab M, Fogelman AM, Reddy ST, Farias-Eisner R (2010) Apolipoprotein A-I (apoA-I) and apoA-I mimetic peptides inhibit tumor development in a mouse model of ovarian cancer. Proc Natl Acad Sci U S A 107:19997–20002

Su F, Grijalva V, Navab K, Ganapathy E, Meriwether D, Imaizumi S, Navab M, Fogelman AM, Reddy ST, Farias-Eisner R (2012) HDL mimetics inhibit tumor development in both induced and spontaneous mouse models of colon cancer. Mol Cancer Ther 11:1311–1319

van Duijnhoven FJ, Bueno-De-Mesquita HB, Calligaro M, Jenab M, Pischon T, Jansen EH, Frohlich J, Ayyobi A, Overvad K, Toft-Petersen AP, Tjonneland A, Hansen L, Boutron-Ruault MC, Clavel-Chapelon F, Cottet V, Palli D, Tagliabue G, Panico S, Tumino R, Vineis P, Kaaks R, Teucher B, Boeing H, Drogan D, Trichopoulou A, Lagiou P, Dilis V, Peeters PH, Siersema PD, Rodriguez L, Gonzalez CA, Molina-Montes E, Dorronsoro M, Tormo MJ, Barricarte A, Palmqvist R, Hallmans G, Khaw KT, Tsilidis KK, Crowe FL, Chajes V, Fedirko V, Rinaldi S, Norat T, Riboli E (2011) Blood lipid and lipoprotein concentrations and colorectal cancer risk in the European Prospective Investigation into Cancer and Nutrition. Gut 60:1094–1102

Van Lenten BJ, Navab M, Anantharamaiah GM, Buga GM, Reddy ST, Fogelman AM (2008a) Multiple indications for anti-inflammatory apolipoprotein mimetic peptides. Curr Opin Investig Drugs 9:1157–1162

Van Lenten BJ et al (2008b) Anti-inflammatory apoA-I-mimetic peptides bind oxidized lipids with much higher affinity than human apoA-I. J Lipid Res 49:2302–2311

Watson CE, Weissbach N, Kjems L, Ayalasomayajula S, Zhang Y, Chang I, Navab M, Hama S, Hough G, Reddy ST, Soffer D, Rader DJ, Fogelman AM, Schecter A (2011) Treatment of patients with cardiovascular disease with L-4F, an apo-A1 mimetic, did not improve select biomarkers of HDL function. J Lipid Res 52:361–373

Zamanian-Daryoush M, Linder D, Tallant TC, Wang Z, Buffa J, Klipfell E, Parker Y, Hatala D, Parsons-Wingerter P, Rayman P, Yusufishaq MSS, Fisher EA, Smith JD, Finke J, DiDonato JA, Hazen SL (2013) The cardioprotective protein apolipoprotein A1 promotes potent anti-tumorigenic effects. J Biol Chem 288:21237–21252

Effects of ApoA-I Mimetic Peptide L-4F in LPS-Mediated Inflammation

Oleg F. Sharifov, G.M. Anantharamaiah, and Himanshu Gupta

Abstract Despite recent advances in antimicrobial and anti-inflammatory therapy, sepsis continues to be a major cause of death in hospitalized patients. To date few interventions have been successful in treating sepsis. Microbes, via their unique molecular patterns, activate a cascade of events that leads to the clinical manifestation of sepsis. Lipopolysaccharide (LPS), a component of the outer membrane of gram-negative bacteria, mediates many of the toxic effects associated with sepsis. The innate immune response is activated during sepsis to protect the host. Circulating lipoproteins especially high-density lipoproteins (HDL) are important components of this immune response. Low concentrations of cholesterol and HDL are associated with oxidative stress and elevated inflammatory mediators in response to LPS. This is associated with poorer outcomes in septic patients. Apolipoprotein (apo) A-I is the principle protein component of HDL that is responsible for many of the anti-inflammatory properties of HDL. Results of studies indicate that HDL/apoA-I administration may be effective in treating sepsis. However obtaining therapeutic quantities of the HDL/apoA-I is impractical. Peptide 18A and its structural variant 4F are only 18 amino acid residues in length (compared to 243 amino acids

O.F. Sharifov, MD, PhD
Department of Medicine, University of Alabama at Birmingham,
ZRB-334, 703 19th Street South, Birmingham, AL 35294, USA
e-mail: sharifov@uab.edu

G.M. Anantharamaiah, PhD
Department of Medicine, University of Alabama at Birmingham,
Department of Biochemistry and Molecular Genetics, University of Alabama at Birmingham,
BDB-668, 1808 7th Avenue South, Birmingham, AL 35294, USA
e-mail: ananth@uab.edu

H. Gupta, MD, FACC (✉)
Department of Medicine, University of Alabama at Birmingham,
Birmingham Veterans Affairs Medical Center,
BDB-101, 1808 7th Avenue South, Birmingham, AL 35294, USA
e-mail: hgutpa@uab.edu

G.M. Anantharamaiah, D. Goldberg (eds.), *Apolipoprotein Mimetics in the Management of Human Disease*, DOI 10.1007/978-3-319-17350-4_6

present in human apoA-I). They have no sequence similarity with apoA-I, but they mimic the class A amphipathic helixes contained in apoA-I with lipid-binding properties. Recent in vitro and in vivo studies indicate that 4F efficiently inhibits LPS-mediated inflammatory responses and could be considered as an effective alternative to HDL/apoA-I therapy in conditions mediated by gram-negative infection. Major mechanisms of anti-inflammatory properties of 4F might include a direct binding and neutralization of LPS, strong antioxidant properties, effects on HDL function, and effects on cell membranes.

Abbreviations

apoA-I	Apolipoprotein A-I
apoB	Apolipoprotein B
apoE	Apolipoprotein E
CD14	Membrane (m) or soluble (s) pattern recognition receptor (cluster of differentiation 14)
HDL	High-density lipoproteins
IL	Interleukin
LAL	Limulus amebocyte lysate
LBP	Lipopolysaccharide-binding protein
LDL	Low-density lipoproteins
LPS	Lipopolysaccharide
NF-κB	Nuclear factor kappa-light-chain-enhancer of activated B cells
PON 1	Paraoxonase 1
rHDL	Reconstituted HDL
TNF-α	Tumor necrosis factor alpha
TLR	Toll-like receptor
VCAM-1	Vascular cell adhesion protein 1
VLDL	Very low-density lipoproteins

Introduction

Despite recent advances in antimicrobial and anti-inflammatory therapy, sepsis continues to be a major cause of death in hospitalized patients. An observational cohort study provides estimates of 751,000 cases of severe sepsis in hospitals in the United States in 1995 (Angus et al. 2001). Approximately 50 % of patients in intensive care units develop severe sepsis and the overall mortality rate of all affected patients is 29 % (Angus et al. 2001). Circulating high-density lipoprotein (HDL) and apolipoprotein (apo) A-I have important anti-inflammatory effects and may be potential therapeutic adjunct for the treatment of sepsis. ApoA-I mimetic peptides, including L-4F peptide, could represent a potential therapeutic approach for HDL/ApoA-I replacement in gram-negative sepsis.

LPS and Sepsis

Mortality in sepsis caused by gram-negative bacteria is due, in large part, to the cytotoxic actions of lipopolysaccharide (LPS, endotoxin), a component of the outer membrane of the gram-negative bacteria. Even low concentrations of LPS (<500 pg/ml) are able to cause endotoxemia and septic shock in patients (Opal and Gluck 2003). LPS is composed of a core oligosaccharide, a repeating polysaccharide side chain, and the glycolipid moiety lipid A (Opal and Gluck 2003). Pro-inflammatory and cytotoxic effects of LPS are mainly mediated by lipid A (David 2001). LPS is released from bacterial membranes into the circulation where it interacts with lipopolysaccharide-binding protein (LBP), a member of the superfamily of phospholipid-binding proteins. LBP binds to lipid A and mediates the disaggregation of LPS to form an LBP-LPS complex (Tobias et al. 1999). LBP directs LPS to membrane-associated CD14 receptors (mCD14) on myeloid cells including monocytes and neutrophils (Guha and Mackman 2001; Zhou et al. 2005). mCD14 is a cell surface-anchored protein that facilitates the binding of LPS and activation of Toll-like receptor 4 (TLR4) which acts as the cellular transducer of LPS action (Opal and Gluck 2003; Zhou et al. 2005). Plasma LPS-LBP may also interact with soluble CD14 (sCD14) to form a complex that activates TLRs on endothelial, epithelial, Kupffer, and other cells (Tobias et al. 1999). By activating NF-κB-dependent signaling mechanisms, LPS stimulates the synthesis/release of inflammatory cytokines that play an important role in the innate immune response (Guha and Mackman 2001). Dysregulation of this response leads to the development of endothelial dysfunction, intravascular coagulation, pulmonary injury, multiple organ failure, and death (Munford 2006; Cohen 2002).

It is now realized that lipid A from different bacterial strains have different efficacies in causing upregulation of inflammatory cascade (Netea et al. 2002; Miller et al. 2005). One postulated mechanism is based on the cross-sectional differences in the structure of lipid A (Netea et al. 2002). Lipid A that has conical cross section can interact with TLR4 to produce septic effects. However if the lipid A is cylindrical in shape, it may not even interact with TLR4 (Netea et al. 2002).

HDL and LPS

Plasma lipoproteins play an important role in LPS neutralization by binding to circulating LPS and transporting it to the liver where it gets metabolized and excreted in the bile (Read et al. 1993; Kitchens et al. 2003; Feingold et al. 1995). HDL possesses the highest binding capacity for LPS compared to other lipoproteins (Levels et al. 2001; Kitchens et al. 2003). In normal situation, of the various lipoproteins, HDL is most abundant in terms of particle number and surface area (Kitchens et al. 2003). HDL appears to be an important component of innate immune response to sepsis (Shiflett et al. 2005). Acute endotoxemia causes decrease in LDL, HDL, apo B, apo A-I, phospholipids, and total cholesterol (Hudgins et al. 2003). There may be associated increase in triglycerides and VLDL. Septic patients have decreased plasma HDL levels (van Leeuwen et al. 2003). In sepsis, HDL undergoes remodeling and is converted to an acute-phase lipoprotein with pro-inflammatory and pro-oxidant properties (Van Lenten et al. 1995, 2003; Fogelman 2004). Many of these structural and functional changes occur in the apo A-I present in HDL (Fogelman 2004). Clinical data suggests that reduced HDL is strongly associated with increased mortality in septic patients (Opal and Gluck 2003). Several factors might lead to HDL and apo A-I reduction in sepsis. First, it may be due to increased utilization of these particles for clearance of toxic substances (Levels et al. 2001). Second, LPS induces acute inflammation/injury in the liver which is the major site for apoA-I biosynthesis (Haddad et al. 1986). Reduction of apoA-I synthesis in the liver likely occurs through LPS-mediated NF-kB activation and cytokine production (Morishima et al. 2003; Cohen 2002; Ettinger et al. 1994). Third, the liver actively synthesizes acute-phase proteins in response to infection; incorporation of these proteins in the HDL particle has been linked to an increase in the catabolism of HDL and its apolipoproteins (Tietge et al. 2002; Cabana et al. 1989). Increasing plasma HDL concentration reduces complications associated with endotoxemia in mice. In this respect, it was shown that a twofold increase in plasma HDL enhances binding of intraperitoneally administered LPS to HDL, reduces plasma cytokine levels, and improves survival in transgenic mice (Levine et al. 1993). Intravenous infusion of reconstituted HDL (rHDL) or apo A-I also confers protection against LPS in wild-type mice (Levine et al. 1993). Similar effects of rHDL in preventing the LPS-dependent induction of pro-inflammatory mediators and organ injury have been demonstrated in rat model of endotoxic shock (McDonald et al. 2003). In vitro, rHDL inhibited VCAM-1 expression in endothelial cells stimulated by LPS (Calabresi et al. 1997). While these results suggest that HDL administration may be effective in treating sepsis, obtaining therapeutic quantities of the lipoprotein is impractical. Other pharmacological approaches to raise plasma HDL have yielded variable results (Shah et al. 2001a).

One mechanism by which HDL neutralizes LPS is thought to occur by masking of the lipid A domain into the phospholipids on the surface of HDL (Parker et al. 1995; Levine et al. 1993). Phospholipids may therefore play an important role in attenuating the toxic effects of LPS. It has been demonstrated that pretreatment with phospholipid emulsion of septic porcine model results in improved survival as compared to the controls (Goldfarb et al. 2003). Similarly, pretreatment of healthy volunteers with phospholipid emulsion before a sublethal dose of LPS results in attenuation of toxic effects of LPS as compared to the placebo controls (Gordon et al. 2005). The mechanism of action of these phospholipids emulsions may be related to the increased endotoxin neutralizing action of various lipoproteins as phospholipids quickly distribute across them. However their effectiveness in human trials is still untested. Furthermore phospholipids may not be as effective in ongoing sepsis as they provide no efficient means of mobilizing bound LPS from monocyte and endothelial surfaces.

ApoA-I and Sepsis

Apo A-I is 243 amino acid residue protein and represents the major protein component of HDL. It has multiple putative class A helical domains that have the ability to associate with lipids (Brouillette et al. 2001). Apo A-I is known to inhibit inflammatory processes such as those associated with atherosclerosis and sepsis (Shah et al. 2001b). Low apo A-I levels are associated with increased mortality in septic patients (Chien et al. 2005). This was demonstrated in an observational study where initial apo A-I levels below 100 mg/dl had 83 % sensitivity, 73 % specificity, and 76 % accuracy in predicting 30-day mortality due to sepsis (Chien et al. 2005). The mechanism of action of apo A-I in attenuating effects of LPS may be related to the direct actions of apo A-I in inactivating LPS (Ma et al. 2004; Flegel et al. 1993; Emancipator et al. 1992). The helical domains of apo A-I have a wedge-shaped cross-sectional structure (Tytler et al. 1993; Mishra et al. 1998; Brouillette et al. 2001). It has been noticed that this shape is complementary to the cross-sectional shape of lipid A of LPS and therefore makes it highly probable that apo A-I can directly interact with lipid A. Interaction of lipid A and apo A-I may prevent activation of TLR4 receptor which is critical to upregulate inflammatory mediators in response to LPS. There may be other mechanisms also that may be responsible for the protective effects of apo A-I against LPS. These include competitive binding of the LPS-LBP-CD14 complex to apo A-I (Parker et al. 1995; Massamiri et al. 1997; Kitchens and Thompson 2003). It is also suggested that apo A-I displaces and clears LPS bound to surface receptors on monocytes (Kitchens and Thompson 2003).

ApoA-I Mimetic Peptides 18A and 4F

One of first effective apolipoprotein A-I mimetic peptides is the class A amphipathic helix peptide 18A, which was synthesized by Dr. Anantharamaiah (1986; Anantharamaiah et al. 1985). Peptide 18A is only 18 amino acid residues in length (compared to 243 amino acids present in human apoA-I) (Anantharamaiah 1986; Anantharamaiah et al. 1985). It has no sequence similarity with apoA-I, but it mimics the class A amphipathic helixes contained in apoA-I and some apoA-I lipid-binding and anti-inflammatory properties (Mendez et al. 1994; Anantharamaiah et al. 1985). Indeed, this peptide was designed to provide a strong support for the theory of the amphipathic helix as the binding motif present in exchangeable apolipoproteins such as apoA-I and is responsible for associating to lipids present in lipoproteins. It has been reported that administration of the apoA-I mimetic peptide 18A prolongs survival in LPS-injected mice (Levine et al. 1993). Original peptide 18A contains 2 phenylalanine residues (2F) on the hydrophobic face. A family of apoA-I mimetic peptides that were structural variants of 18A (2F) was subsequently developed. It was found that sequential substitution of aliphatic amino acids (Leu, Val) on the nonpolar face of 18A with phenylalanine (F) resulted in the formation of class A peptides 3F, 4F, 5F, 6F, and 7F with increased hydrophobicity and lipid-binding affinity (Datta et al. 2001). Two of these peptides, 4F and 5F, revealed the greatest phospholipid-binding capacity; both peptides formed discoidal HDL-like structures with phospholipids (Datta et al. 2001). However, 4F was superior to 5F in inhibiting LDL-induced monocyte chemotaxis and in solubility properties (Datta et al. 2001). Due to its superior antioxidative effects, peptide 4F has been extensively studied in several laboratories (White et al. 2014; Van Lenten et al. 2008; Navab et al. 2005). In vitro and in vivo studies demonstrate that 4F peptide mimics apoA-I anti-atherogenic and anti-inflammatory properties (White et al. 2014; Van Lenten et al. 2008; Navab et al. 2005).

ApoA-I Mimetic Peptide L-4F and LPS

Table 1 summarizes results of multiple in vitro and in vivo experiments that provide strong support for effects of L-4F against LPS. Beneficial effects of L-4F in inhibiting LPS-mediated inflammatory responses are due to several mechanisms. Table 2 presents evidence supporting the hypothesis that L-4F directly binds to LPS with high affinity and neutralizes LPS endotoxin activity. Binding and neutralizing LPS properties of L-4F seem to be superior to that of human apoA-I (Fig. 1). It is hypothesized that strong 4F binding to LPS could be due to complementary shapes of 4F peptide and lipid A of LPS. However, this needs further experimental testing. By interacting with LPS, L-4F inhibits LPS binding to plasma components responsible for transferring LPS to cells (e.g., LBP, sCD14), also to endothelial cells and leukocytes (Fig. 2), and likely to other LPS-sensitive cells in LPS-targeted tissues. L-4F might also facilitate LPS binding to HDL (Fig. 3), in part likely due to direct L-4F association with HDL (Fig. 4).

Table 3 summarizes additional anti-inflammatory mechanisms that play an important role in efficient inhibition of LPS/septic inflammation and organ injury. L-4F has strong antioxidant properties (Fig. 5). It also improves HDL function and maintains HDL quantitative levels (Fig. 5). L-4F, similar to apoA-I, produces direct effects on cells by altering the assembly of TLR-ligand complexes in cell membranes and inhibiting pro-inflammatory gene expression in monocyte-derived macrophages. Figure 6 provides a schematic description of multiple mechanisms of 4F against LPS-induced inflammation. Likely due to such multiple mechanisms of anti-inflammatory activity of 4F, it was effective in reducing LPS-mediated organ injury and overall mortality in animal experiments with delayed administration of L-4F (Table 1). In addition to anti-LPS effects of L-4F, several laboratories have demonstrated potent anti-atherogenic, antiviral, anticancer, antihypertensive, anti-asthmatic, and other effects of 4F in different in vitro, animal, and human studies (Gao et al. 2012; Van Lenten et al. 2002, 2004; Kelesidis et al. 2011; Sharma et al. 2014; Nandedkar et al. 2011; Ou et al. 2012; Navab et al. 2005; White et al. 2014). The mechanisms responsible for the effects of L-4F in these models might be also in part involved in anti-inflammatory effects of L-4F in LPS studies.

ApoA-I Mimetic Peptide L-4F in Polymicrobial Septic Models

Two independent groups tested L-4F in rat model of polymicrobial sepsis using cecal ligation and puncture (Zhang et al. 2009; Moreira et al. 2014). In the research work published by Zhang et al. (2009), L-4F, 10 mg/kg, administered i.p. 6 h post CLP procedure, effectively improved survival rate by reducing inflammatory cytokines level, preventing a drop in cardiac function, and maintaining a proper plasma total cholesterol level and HDL protein composition. In a similar model, L-4F attenuated kidney injury, heart injury, and endothelial dysfunction in HDL-dependent manner (Moreira et al. 2014).

Table 1 Evidence of inhibition of LPS-induced inflammatory responses by L-4F

Effect/target	Study	LPS	L-4F	Time after LPS	Measurement indices
In cell media					
Inhibits inflammatory response in HUVEC monolayer	Gupta et al. (2005)	1 μg/ml *E. coli* (O26:B6)	Up to 50 μg/ml concurrently	6 h post LPS	IL-6, IL-8, IFN-γ, TNF-α, MCP-1, E-selectin, ICAM-1, VCAM-1, VCAM-1 mRNA
Inhibits inflammatory response in human monocyte THP-1 cells	Gupta et al. (2005)	1 μg/ml *E. coli* (O26:B6)	Up to 50 μg/ml concurrently	6 h post LPS	Binding to HUVEC monolayer
	Sharifov et al. (2014a)	0.5 μg/ml *E. coli* (O55:B5, O26:B6, and O11:B4) and *P. aeruginosa*	10 μg/ml seconds after LPS	22 h	TNF-α and IL-6 levels in media
Inhibits inflammatory response in isolated human neutrophils	Sharifov et al. (2013)	Incubated in endotoxemic plasma of ARDS patients	40 μg/ml	1 h	Plasma MPO level, cellular cd11b expression
	Sharifov et al. (2014b)	1 μg/ml (*E. coli* 026:B6) in 50 % human plasma	40 μg/ml seconds after LPS	By 3 h post LPS	Plasma TNF-α, IL-6, MPO; flow cytometry: cd11b expression, lipid raft abundance
Inhibits inflammatory response in isolated human leukocytes	Sharifov et al. (2013)	Incubated in endotoxemic plasma of ARDS patients	40 μg/ml	1 h	Superoxide formation measured with lucigenin-amplified chemiluminescence
	Sharifov et al. (2014b)	1 μg/ml (*E. coli* 026:B6) in human plasma	40 μg/ml seconds after LPS	By 3 h post LPS	Superoxide formation measured with lucigenin-amplified chemiluminescence
In human blood/plasma ex vivo					
Inhibits inflammatory response in human blood	Sharifov et al. (2013)	1 μg/ml (*E. coli* 026:B6)	40 μg/ml concurrently	By 12 h post LPS	Plasma level of IL-6
	Sharifov et al. (2014b)	1 μg/ml (*E. coli* 026:B6)	40 μg/ml concurrently	By 3 h post LPS	Plasma levels of TNF-α, IL-6 (compared to human apoA-I)
Inhibits alterations in HDL/Apo A-I/PON1 functionality	Sharifov et al. (2013)	1 μg/ml (*E. coli* 026:B6) in human blood	40 μg/ml concurrently	By 12 h post LPS	Size exclusion chromatography, HDL-C, HDL-PON1 activity
	Sharifov et al. (2013)	Endotoxemic plasma of ARDS patients	40 μg/ml concurrently	By 1 h	Plasma activity of HDL PON1

(continued)

Table 1 (continued)

Effect/target	Study	LPS	L-4F	Time after LPS	Measurement indices
In vivo					
Inhibits VCAM-1 expression in aorta	Gupta et al. (2005) (rats)	10 mg/kg i.p. *E. coli* (026:B6)	25 mg/kg concurrently	6 h post LPS	VCAM-1 expression by WB
Prevents vascular defects (NOS2 and NO formation)	Dai et al. (2010) (rats)	10 mg/kg i.v. (*E. coli* 026:B6)	10 mg/kg i.v. min after LPS	By 6 h post LPS	Systemic blood pressure; contractile response to PE in isolated aortic ring segments; gel electrophoresis and WB; plasma NO metabolite level
Preserves cardiac function	Datta et al. (2011) (rats)	10 mg/kg i.p. (*E. coli* 026:B6)	10 mg/kg i.p. concurrently	By 24 h post LPS	Systemic blood pressure, cardiac pressure by catheterization, cardiac volumes by echocardiography
Inhibits HDL/ Apo A-I alterations	Datta et al. (2011) (rats)	10 mg/kg i.p. (*E. coli* 026:B6)	10 mg/kg i.p. concurrently	By 24 h post LPS	HDL-associated apoA-I, apoA-IV
	Sharifov et al. (2013) (rats)	30 mg/kg i.p. (*E. coli* 026:B6)	10 mg/kg i.v. 1 h after LPS	By 6 h post LPS	Plasma levels of apoA-I and HDL-C, activity of HDL PON1
	Kwon et al. (2012) (rats)	10 mg/kg i.v. (*E. coli* 026:B6)	10 mg/kg i.p. 10 min after LPS	By 6 h post LPS	Plasma HDL-C
Inhibits systemic inflammation and lipid oxidation	Dai et al. (2010) (rats)	30 mg/kg i.v. (*E. coli* 026:B6)	10 mg/kg i.v. min after LPS	By 2 h post LPS	Plasma TNF-α level
	Datta et al. (2011) (rats)	10 mg/kg i.p. (*E. coli* 026:B6)	10 mg/kg i.p. concurrently	By 24 h post LPS	Plasma levels of TNF-α, IL-6, CINC-2α
	Sharifov et al. (2013) (rats)	30 mg/kg i.p. (*E. coli* 026:B6)	10 mg/kg i.v. 1 h after LPS	By 6 h post LPS	Plasma activity of MPO, plasma levels of IL-6 and reactive oxygen species
	Sharifov et al. (2014a) (mice)	50 μg i.v. (*E. coli* 026:B6 and 055:B6)	100 μg i.v. 5 min post LPS	By 3 h post LPS	Plasma levels of IL-6, reactive oxygen species, SAA, INF-γ
Inhibits recruitment of PMN and macrophages to inflamed lungs	Madenspacher et al. (2012) (mice)	300 μg/ml, 20 min aerosol (*E. coli* is not specified)	20 mg/kg i.v. 2 h before LPS	By 4 h and 24 h	PMN and macrophages concentration in bronchoalveolar lavage fluid

Table 1 (continued)

Effect/target	Study	LPS	L-4F	Time after LPS	Measurement indices
Inhibits acute lung injury	Sharifov et al. (2013) (rats)	30 mg/kg i.p. (*E. coli* 026:B6)	10 mg/kg i.v. 1 h after LPS	By 6 h post LPS	Rat lung histological analysis, BALF levels of TNF-α, IL-6, MPO
	Kwon et al. (2012) (rats)	10 mg/kg i.v. (*E. coli* 026:B6)	10 mg/kg i.p. 10 min after LPS	By 6 h post LPS	Lung histological analysis, $S1P_1$, P-Akt/Akt ratio, cytoplasmic P-IkB-α/IkB-α ratio, NF-κB p65 DNA activity, E-selection, ICAM-1, MPO
Inhibits acute liver injury	Sharifov et al. (2013) (rats)	30 mg/kg i.p. (*E. coli* 026:B6)	10 mg/kg i.v. 1 h after LPS	By 6 h post LPS	Rat liver histological analysis, plasma levels of ALT, AST, ALP, TB, TRG
Improves survival rate	Dai et al. (2010) (rats)	30 mg/kg i.p. (*E. coli* 026:B6)	10 mg/kg i.v. 1 min after LPS	By 24 h post LPS	Rat survival rate
	Sharifov et al. (2013) (rats)	30 mg/kg i.p. (*E. coli* 026:B6)	10 mg/kg. concurrently or i.v. 1 h after LPS	By 24 h post LPS	Rat survival rate
	Kwon et al. (2012) (rats)	10 mg/kg i.v. (*E. coli* 026:B6)	10 mg/kg i.p. 10 min after LPS	By 72 h post LPS	Rat survival rate

LPS lipopolysaccharide, *PMN* polymorphonuclear leukocytes, *ARDS* acute respiratory distress syndrome, *PE* phenylephrine, *WB* Western blotting, *MPO* myeloperoxidase, *HUVEC* human umbilical vein endothelial cells, *ALT* alanine transaminase, *AST* aspartate transaminase, *ALP* alkaline phosphatase, *TB* total bilirubin, *TRG* triglycerides, *VCAM-1* vascular cell adhesion molecule 1, *MCP-1* monocyte chemoattractant protein-1, *IL-6 and IL-8* interleukins, *IFN-γ* interferon gamma, *TNF-α* tumor necrosis factor alpha, *Akt* protein kinase B (PKB), *IκB-α* nuclear factor of kappa-light polypeptide gene enhancer in B-cell inhibitor, alpha, *NF-κB* nuclear factor kappa-light-chain-enhancer of activated B cells

Efficacy of L-4F in Different Models of Atherosclerosis and Metabolic Syndrome (Diabetes) Could Be in Part Accounted for by Its Anti-endotoxin Property

Multiple experimental and clinical studies suggest that LPS-mediated endotoxemia promotes atherosclerosis (Feng et al. 2010; Wiesner et al. 2010; Szeto et al. 2008; Wiedermann et al. 1999; Seitz et al. 1996; Pasterkamp et al. 2004; Vikatmaa et al. 2010; Lakio et al. 2006; Lalla et al. 2003; Kallio et al. 2008; Rufail et al. 2007). TLR4, the major cellular target for LPS in humans, may play a role in the initiation and

Table 2 Evidence supporting direct interaction of L-4F with LPS

Effect	Study	LPS	L-4F	Time after LPS	Measurement
In aqueous solution					
Formation of L-4F-LPS complex	Gupta et al. (2005)	10 μg BODIPY-LPS (*E. coli* 055:B5)	3.4 μg ^{125}I-L-4F		Size exclusion chromatography
	Sharifov et al. (2013)	1 mg/kg (*E. coli* 026:B6)	100 μg/kg seconds after LPS	By 1 min post LPS	Circular dichroism spectroscopy (change in mean residue ellipticity)
	Sharifov et al. (2014a)	1, 5, 10 μg/ml *E. coli* (O55:B5)	1 μg	By 1 min post LPS	Agarose gel (change in polarity)
Disaggregation of LPS aggregates	Sharifov et al. (2014a)	5 μg/ml BODIPY-LPS (*E. coli* O55:B5)	100 μg/ml co-incubation for 15 min	By 15–30 min	Size exclusion chromatography
Binding kinetics to LPS	Sharifov et al. (2014b)	0–0.4 mg/ml (*E. coli* 026:B6) over CM5 chip	L-4F on CM5 chip	By 2.5 min post LPS	Surface plasmon resonance (compared to human apoA-I)
Inhibits endotoxin activity	Sharifov et al. (2013)	1 μg/ml (*E. coli* 026:B6)	1, 10, 100 μg/kg seconds after LPS	By 1 min post LPS	LAL assay
	Sharifov et al. (2014b)	1 μg/ml (*E. coli* 026:B6)	1, 10, 100 μg/kg seconds after LPS	By 1 min post LPS	LAL assay (compared to human apoA-I)
	Sharifov et al. (2014a)	0.5 μg/ml *E. coli* (O55:B5, O26:B6) and *P. aeruginosa*	1, 10, 100 μg/kg seconds after LPS	By 1 min post LPS	LAL assay
In cell media					
Inhibits binding of LPS to HUVEC monolayer	Gupta et al. (2005)	1 μg/ml *E. coli* (^{125}I-LPS-ASD))	Up to 50 μg/ml concurrently	6 h post LPS	VCAM-1 expression by RT-PCR
Inhibits binding of LPS to LBP	Gupta et al. (2005)	1 μg/ml biotinylated LPS	Up to 50 μg/ml concurrently	6 h post LPS	ELISA

In human blood/plasma ex vivo					
Inhibits endotoxin activity	Sharifov et al. (2013)	1 μg/ml (*E. coli* 026:B6)	40 μg/kg seconds after LPS	By 12 h post LPS	LAL assay
	Sharifov et al. (2013)	Endotoxemic plasma of ARDS patients	40 μg/kg	By 12 h post LPS	LAL assay
	Sharifov et al. (2014a)	1 μg/ml (*E. coli* 026:B6)	40 μg/kg seconds after LPS	By 6 h post LPS	LAL assay
Inhibits binding of LPS to leukocytes	Sharifov et al. (2013)	1 μg/ml (BODIPY-LPS *E. coli* 055:B5)	40 μg/kg seconds after LPS	By 30 min post LPS	Flow cytometry
In vivo					
Facilitates binding of LPS to HDL	Dai et al. (2010)	10 mg/kg i.v. (BODIPY-LPS *E. coli* 055:B5)	^{14}C-L-4 F 10 mg/kg i.v. min after LPS	By 10 min post LPS	Size exclusion chromatography, plasma kinetic of BODIPY-LPS and ^{14}C-L-4 F
Neutralization of LPS charge	Datta et al. (2011) (rats)	10 mg/kg i.p. (*E. coli* 026:B6)	10 mg/kg i.p. concurrently	By 24 h post LPS	Plasma gel electrophoresis and WB for apoA-I
Inhibits endotoxin activity in plasma	Dai et al. (2010) (rats)	30 mg/kg i.v. (*E. coli* 026:B6)	10 mg/kg i.v. min after LPS	By 2 h post LPS	LAL assay
	Sharifov et al. (2013) (rats)	30 mg/kg i.p. (*E. coli* 026:B6)	10 mg/kg i.v. 1 h after LPS	By 6 h post LPS	LAL assay
	Sharifov et al. (2014a) (mice)	50 μg i.v. (*E. coli* 026:B6 and 055:B6)	100 μg i.v. 5 min post LPS	By 3 h post LPS	LAL assay

LPS lipopolysaccharide, *HDL* high-density lipoprotein, *LAL* limulus amebocyte lysate, *WB* Western blotting, *HUVEC* human umbilical vein endothelial cells, *VCAM-1* vascular cell adhesion molecule 1, *ELISA* enzyme-linked immunosorbent assay, *RT-PCR* reverse transcription polymerase chain reaction

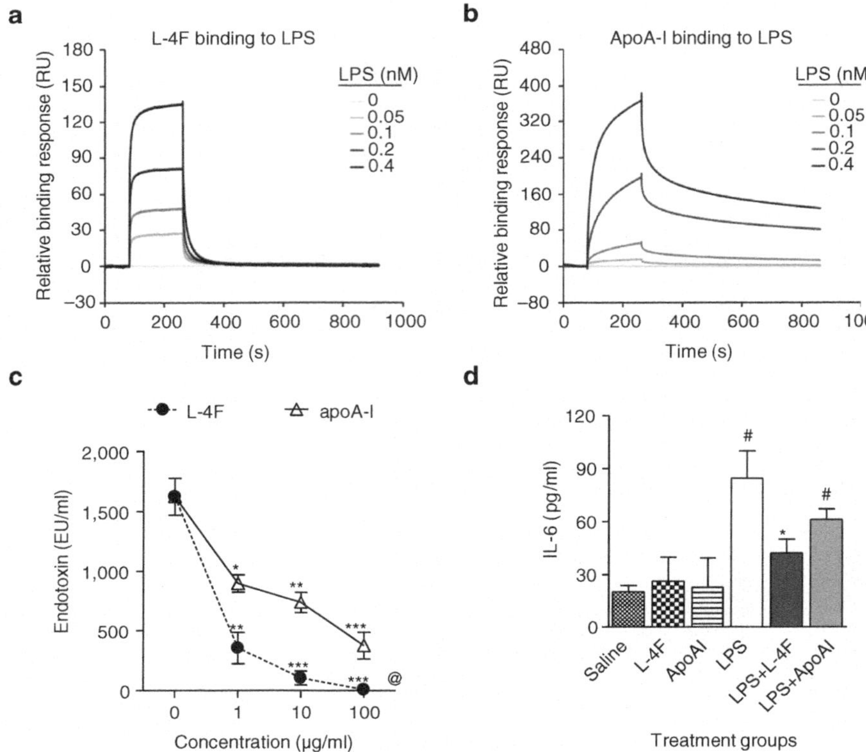

Fig. 1 L-4F and apoA-I bind LPS, neutralize entotoxin activity, and inhibit LPS-mediated inflammatory response. (**a**, **b**) Representative sensograms of L-4F (**a**) and apoA-I (**b**) binding to LPS obtained in surface plasmon resonance (SPR) studies. LPS binding was measured by observing the change in the SPR angle of the L-4F or apoA-I immobilized to the CM5 chip when LPS flowed over the chip. Compared to apoA-I, L-4F has a faster binding kinetics with a higher calculated steady-state affinity (KD (M) = $3.727E^{-7}$ for L-4F vs. KD (M) = $2.073E^{-6}$ for apoA-I). (**c**) L-4F and apoA-I inhibit LAL endotoxin activity in aqueous solution. LPS (1 μg/ml) was mixed with L-4F or apoA-I in saline and endotoxin activity was immediately measured with LAL assay. L-4F and apoA-I neutralized endotoxin activity in a dose-dependent manner ($P<0.001$, $n=4$); L-4F inhibited endotoxin activity more effectively than apoA-I. (**d**) L-4F and apoA-I inhibit LPS-mediated production of IL-6 by isolated human neutrophils. Isolated human neutrophils were incubated in donor plasma with saline, L-4F or apoA-I (40 μg/ml), LPS (1 μg/ml), and LPS plus L-4F or apoA-I for 3 h ($n=3$). In all experiments, LPS from *E. coli* 026:B6 was used. *$P<0.05$, **$P<0.01$, ***$P<0.001$ vs. LPS; @$P<0.05$ vs. apoA-I; #$P<0.05$ vs. control groups (Modified from Sharifov et al. (2014b)

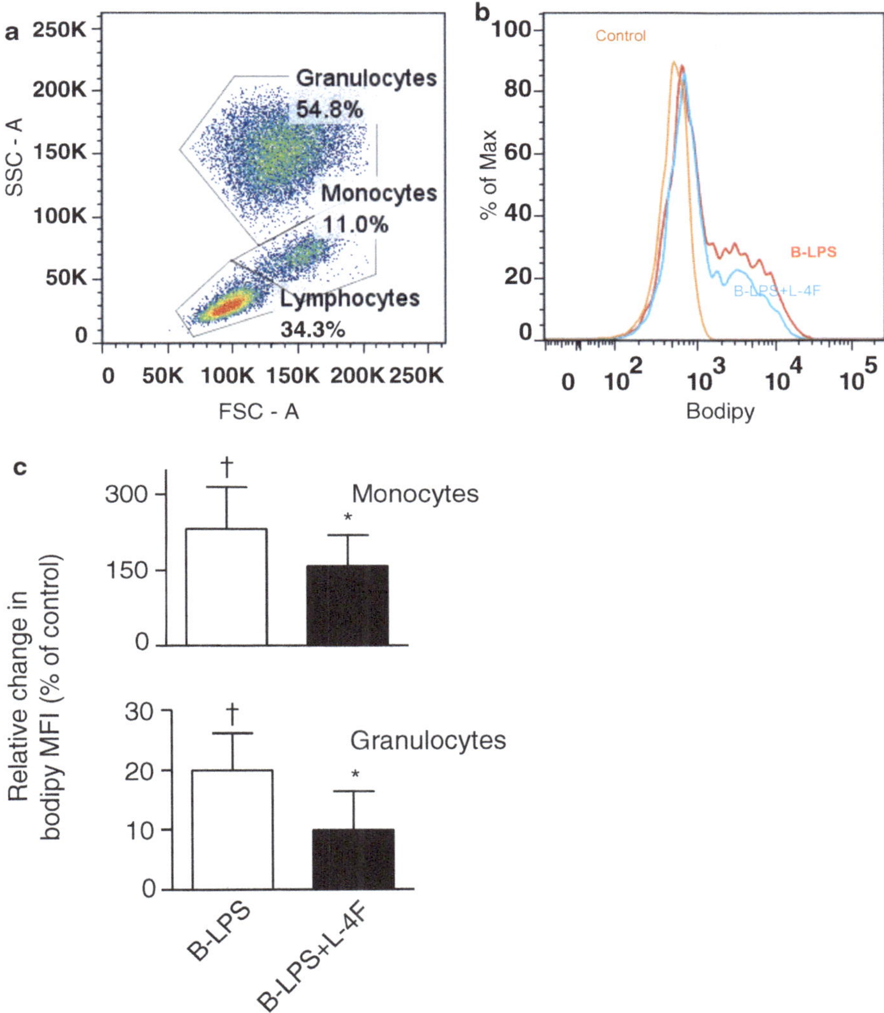

Fig. 2 L-4F inhibits LPS binding to leukocytes. Following incubation of BODIPY-LPS (B-LPS, from *E. coli* 055:B5) for 30 min in human whole blood ex vivo ($n=5$), fluorescence due to binding of B-LPS to leukocytes was measured using flow cytometry. (**a**) A representative example of side scatter and forward scatter characteristics of leukocytes with major populations of lymphocytes, monocytes, and granulocytes isolated after incubation with either control (saline or L-4F), B-LPS (1 μg/ml), or B-LPS and L-4F (40 μg/ml). (**b**) Cells selected as monocytes in (**a**) are plotted depending on intensity of BODIPY signal. (**c**) Relative changes of BODIPY mean fluorescence intensity (*MFI*) compared to control MFI for monocytes and granulocytes are shown. *$P<0.05$ vs. LPS or B-LPS, †$P<0.05$ vs. saline and L-4F alone (Modified from Sharifov et al. (2013))

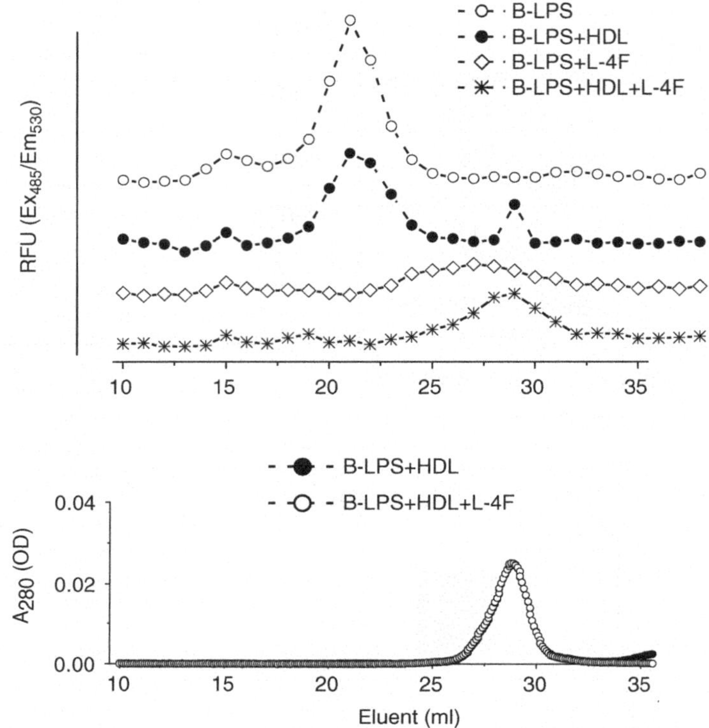

Fig. 3 L-4F binds and disaggregates large LPS micelles (aggregates) to form complexes in the range of HDL size. *Top panel*: Disaggregation and binding of LPS to HDL and L-4F. In fast protein liquid chromatography (FPLC) eluent, BODIPY-LPS (B-LPS from *E. coli* 055:B5, 5 μg/ml) aggregates are seen as large single fluorescent peak. When incubated with HDL (2.6 mg/ml), some B-LPS binds to HDL that results in another smaller peak. In the presence of L-4F, only single but broader peak in the HDL region was noted suggesting that L-4F disaggregates LPS to smaller particles that coelute in HDL region ($n = 3$). In the presence of both L-4F and HDL, B-LPS fluorescent peak narrows in HDL region. *Bottom panel*: Identification of HDL in FPLC eluent by absorbance at 280 nm

progression of inflammation and atherosclerosis (Pasterkamp et al. 2004). In a rodent model, increased adhesion of monocytes and T cells to aortic endothelium is found in response to endotoxin (Seitz et al. 1996). It has also been demonstrated that LPS promotes the binding of oxidized LDL to activated human macrophages resulting in foam cell formation (Feng et al. 2010). Pro-atherogenic activation of macrophages via TLR4 can occur cooperatively by low subclinical concentrations of endotoxin and minimally oxidized LDL (Wiesner et al. 2010). Increased carotid atherosclerosis has been shown to be associated with higher levels of LPS in plasma and/or in arterial wall (Wiedermann et al. 1999; Vikatmaa et al. 2010; Szeto et al. 2008). A link has been demonstrated between periodontal disease-associated endotoxemia and atherosclerosis (Rufail et al. 2007; Lalla et al. 2003; Lakio et al. 2006; Kallio et al. 2008). In addition, LPS-mediated inflammation may contribute to metabolic disorders in humans

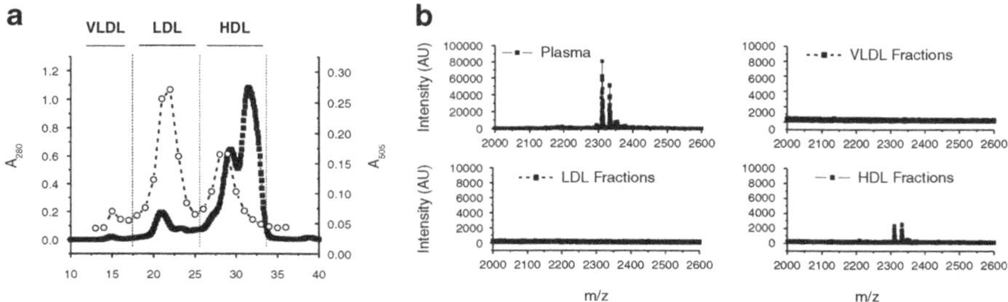

Fig. 4 L-4F presents in FPLC eluents associated with HDL in human blood in the absence and presence of LPS. In this experiment, L-4F (40 μg/ml) was incubated in healthy human whole blood for 30 min at 37 °C and 5 %CO2/95 % air in the presence or absence of LPS (1 μg/ml, from *E. coli* 026:B6) . Plasma was collected and fractionated by FPLC. (**a**) Superimposed profiles of total cholesterol (A_{505}) and protein (A_{280}) for plasma FPLC fractions are shown. (**b**) VLDL, LDL, and HDL fractions were pooled and L-4F was detected using MALDI-TOF mass spectroscopy. The presence of L-4F is evident as a peak at 2,310 (m/z) that is accompanied by a second peak at 2,332 (m/z) due to high sodium concentration. Measurements of L-4F are shown in plasma and for VLDL, LDL, and HDL pools. Among pooled lipoproteins, L-4F was identified only in HDL pool in both L-4F alone and LPS+L-4F (not shown) conditions. Similar result was obtained for L-4F incubation in human blood with and without LPS for 12 h (not shown)

(Nakarai et al. 2012; Lajunen et al. 2008). Humans are persistently exposed to LPS during their entire life span. In both animal and human studies, endotoxin levels in blood increase significantly with the increased consumption of food (Pendyala et al. 2012; Cani et al. 2007). Chronic endotoxemia, and therefore systemic inflammation, especially owing to the Western diet, might be an important pathogenic factor in the development of metabolic syndrome and atherosclerosis (Pendyala et al. 2012; Nakarai et al. 2012; Lajunen et al. 2008; Cani et al. 2007).

It has been shown that apoE-null mice are highly susceptible to endotoxemia, likely due to a decreased LPS-neutralizing capacity of apoE-deficient plasma (de Bont et al. 1999). Reconstitution of hepatic apoE expression in the liver of apoE-deficient mice normalizes the inflammatory response to low doses of LPS (Ali et al. 2005). The apoE-deficient mouse and/or the Western diet is extensively used to study atherosclerosis. It therefore can be suggested that a high-fat-diet-induced endotoxemia, especially in the absence of endogenous apoE, may contribute to systemic inflammation. This might be an important factor that contributes to atherosclerosis along with hyperlipidemia in apoE-deficient mice. Therefore, anti-atherogenic effects of the apoA-I mimetic peptide 4F (which has no effect on cholesterol levels) in apoE-null mice and in LDL-receptor null mice on the Western diet (Navab et al. 2002) could, in part, be due to its strong anti-endotoxin activity. Recent studies in female apoE-null mice with already existing lesions have found that Ac-hE18A-NH_2 (apoE mimetic peptide) is more effective in inhibiting lesions than 4F (Nayyar et al. 2012a). As our recent work indicates that the anti-endotoxin activity of Ac-hE18A-NH_2 is superior to 4F (Sharifov et al. 2014a), such activity may also contribute to the superior effect of Ac-hE18A-NH_2 in apoE-null mice (Nayyar et al. 2012a). However, the relative role of endogenous endotoxemia in atherosclerosis

Table 3 Indirect anti-inflammatory effects of L-4F

Effect	Study	Baseline condition	L-4F	Time after L-4F	Measurement indices
In solution					
Binds oxidized lipids with higher affinity than human apoA-I	Van Lenten et al. (2008)	Different oxidized lipids in HBS-EP buffer over CM5 chip	L-4F on CM5 chip	3 min	Surface plasmon resonance (compared to human apoA-I)
Transfers oxidized LDL to HDL	Meriwether et al. (2011)	0.5 mg human LDL loaded with 15HETE-d_8 and 0.5 mg human HDL	25 μg	1 h	LC/MS/MS
In complex with lipid serves as a platform for PON1	Mishra et al. (2013)	rPON1	L-4F:POPC complex	3 h	ELISA, gel electrophoresis, paraoxonase activity, PON1 stability to trypsin digestion
Binds and neutralizes with MPO-derived hypochlorous acid	White et al. (2012a)	Various concentrations of HOCl	Various concentrations of L-4F	15 min	Fluorescent measurement of HOCl-dependent oxidation of APF
In cell media					
Inhibition of LDL-induced monocyte migration to human artery wall cells	Datta et al. (2001)	Human LDL (250 μg/ml) in co-culture of HAEC and HASMC cells, with human monocytes	20 μg/ml	8 h	MCP-1, M-CSF
Changing differentiation of human monocyte THP-1 cells	Smythies et al. (2010)	RPMI treated with saline	50 μg/10^6 cells	7 days	Decreased: HLA-DR, CD86, CD11b, CD11c, TLR-4, CD14, CD32, lipid raft abundance Increased: cholesterol efflux; IL-10 mRNA Decreased response to LPS: MCP-1, MIP-1, RANTES, IL-6, TNF-α, adhesion to HUVECs

Changing differentiation of monocyte-derived macrophages (from human peripheral blood)	Smythies et al. (2010)	RPMI treated with saline	50 μg/10^6 cells	7 days	Decreased: HLA-DR, CD86, CD11b, CD11c, TLR-4, CD14, CD32, lipid raft abundance Increased: cholesterol efflux; IL-10 mRNA Decreased response to LPS: MCP-1, MIP-1, RANTES, IL-6, TNF-α, adhesion to HUVECs
	White et al. (2012b)	RPMI treated with saline	50 μg/10^6 cells	7 days	Decreased: TLR4,5,6, IkBα, caveolin (lipid raft component) Decreased response to LPS: genes encoding TLR1,2,6, MyD88-dependent and MyD88-independent pathways; TLR4 recycling, p-IkBα, NF-kB, IL-6 and TNF-α Decreased response to LTA: IL-6 and TNF-α
Chemoattraction of human PMN and monocytes	Madenspacher et al. (2012)	10^6/ml human PMN or monocytes in RPMI	Up to 50 μg/ml in RPMI	60–90 min	Microchemotaxis chamber technique
In human blood/plasma ex vivo					
HDL/Apo A-I improvement	Sharifov et al. (2013)	Whole blood	40 μg/ml	12 h incubation	Plasma activity of HDL PON1
Association with HDL and formation of pre-β HDL	Nayyar et al. (2012b)	Plasma	^{14}C-L-4F	Overnight incubation	Size exclusion chromatography, gel electrophoresis
	Sharifov and Gupta (unpublished)	Whole blood	40 μg/ml	1 h or 12 h	Size exclusion chromatography, gel electrophoresis, MALDI-TOF MS

(continued)

Table 3 (continued)

Effect	Study	Baseline condition	L-4F	Time after L-4F	Measurement indices
In vivo					
Formation of pre-β HDL enriched in apoA-I and PON1 activity	Navab et al. (2004) (mice)	apoE-null mice	0.5 mg (D-4F)	20 min after D-4F	Gel electrophoresis, size exclusion chromatography, paraoxonase activity
Improvement of anti-inflammatory index of HDL	Van Lenten et al. (2007) (rabbits)	HDL from high-fat-diet rabbits treated with L-4F in HAEC culture for 8 h	10 mg/kg/day s.q.	1 month treatment	MCP-1 level in supernatant
HDL/Apo A-I improvement	Sharifov et al. (2013) (rats)	Rats treated with saline	10 mg/kg i.v.	By 6 h post L-4F	Tend to raise plasma levels of apoA-I and HDL-C, activity of HDL PON1

LPS lipopolysaccharide, *HDL and LDL* high- and low-density lipoproteins, *THP-1* human monocytic cell line derived from an acute monocytic leukemia patient, *PMN* polymorphonuclear leukocytes, *HUVEC* human umbilical vein endothelial cells, *HAEC and HASMC* human aortic endothelial cells and smooth muscle cells, *HOCl* hypochlorous acid, *HLA* human leukocyte antigen, *VCAM-1* vascular cell adhesion molecule 1, *MCP-1* monocyte chemoattractant protein-1, *RANTES* chemokine CCL5, *IL-6 and IL-8* interleukins, *IFN-γ* interferon gamma, *TNF-α* tumor necrosis factor alpha, *IκB-α* nuclear factor of kappa-light polypeptide gene enhancer in B-cell inhibitor, alpha, *NF-κB* nuclear factor kappa-light-chain-enhancer of activated B cells, *LC/MS* liquid chromatography–mass spectrometry, *MS* mass spectrometry

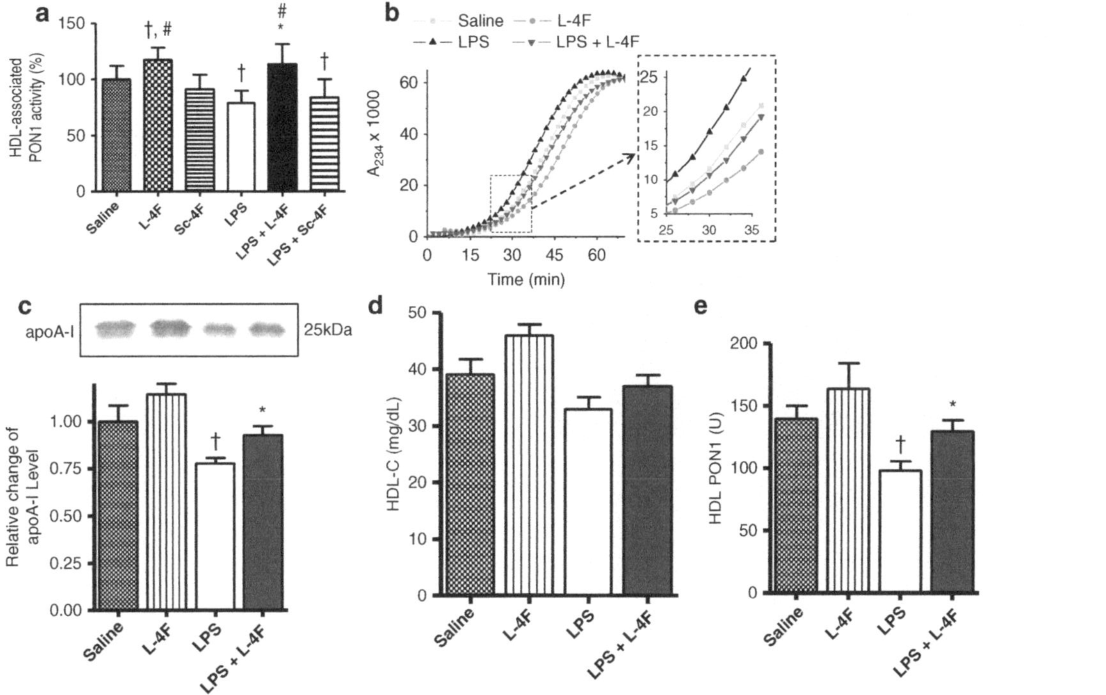

Fig. 5 4F effects on HDL. (**a**, **b**) In vitro effects: (**a**) L-4F (40 μg/ml), but not scramble 4F (Sc-4F), increases HDL-associated PON1 activity in the healthy human whole blood ex vivo and preserves this activity after co-incubation with 1 μg/ml LPS (n=6/group); (**b**) L-4F preserves antioxidant potency of HDL to inhibit $CuSO_4$-induced LDL oxidation at 37 °C. HDL was isolated from human whole blood incubated with saline, L-4F, LPS, and LPS and L-4F (n=8). In a representative example, HDL isolated after LPS incubation resulted in faster rate of $CuSO_4$-induced LDL oxidation (magnified insert) than in saline controls or L-4F-treated groups. (**c–e**) In vivo effects: Plasma measurements taken at 6 h following 10 mg/kg i.p. LPS injection in rats. L-4F was administered i.v. 1 h after LPS. (**c**) Western analysis of relative levels of apoA-I (based on plasma SDS-PAGE gel electrophoresis followed by immunoblotting for apoA-I); (**d**) HDL-cholesterol (HDL-C) levels; (**e**) HDL-associated PON1 activity. *$P<0.05$ vs. LPS, †$P<0.05$ vs. saline, #$P<0.05$ vs. Sc-4F (n=8 for controls, n=12–14 for LPS groups). In all these experiments, LPS from *E. coli* 026:B6 was used (Modified from Sharifov et al. (2013))

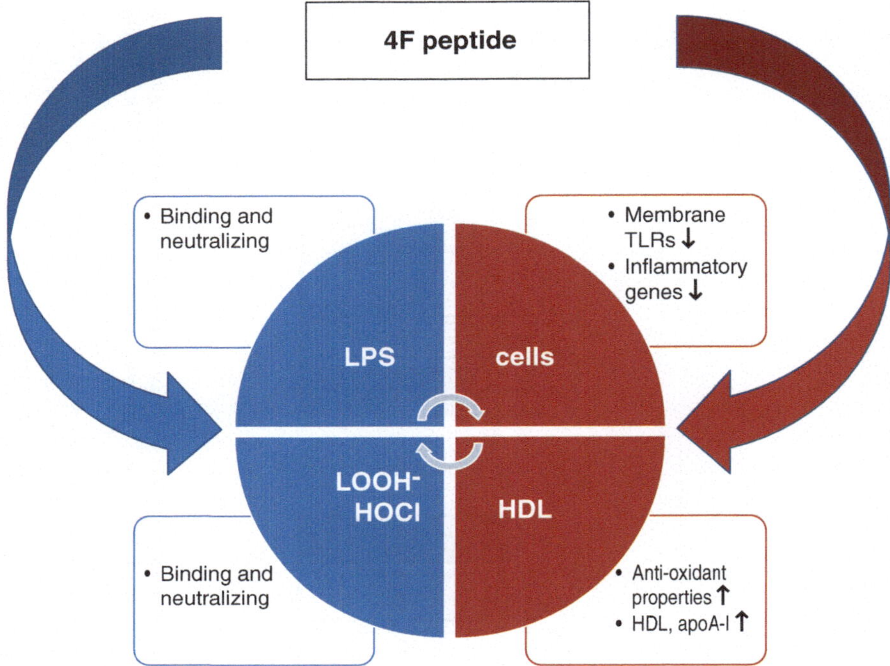

Fig. 6 A schematic representing major anti-inflammatory properties of 4F against LPS-induced inflammation. *LOOH* oxidized lipids, *HOCl* myeloperoxidase-derived hypochlorous acid

development and the protective effects of the peptides need to be better evaluated in future research.

References

Ali K, Middleton M, Pure E, Rader DJ (2005) Apolipoprotein E suppresses the type I inflammatory response in vivo. Circ Res 97(9):922–927. doi:10.1161/01.res.0000187467.67684.43

Anantharamaiah GM (1986) Synthetic peptide analogs of apolipoproteins. Methods Enzymol 128:627–647

Anantharamaiah GM, Jones JL, Brouillette CG, Schmidt CF, Chung BH, Hughes TA, Bhown AS, Segrest JP (1985) Studies of synthetic peptide analogs of the amphipathic helix. Structure of complexes with dimyristoyl phosphatidylcholine. J Biol Chem 260(18):10248–10255

Angus DC, Linde-Zwirble WT, Lidicker J, Clermont G, Carcillo J, Pinsky MR (2001) Epidemiology of severe sepsis in the United States: analysis of incidence, outcome, and associated costs of care. Crit Care Med 29(7):1303–1310

Brouillette CG, Anantharamaiah GM, Engler JA, Borhani DW (2001) Structural models of human apolipoprotein A-I: a critical analysis and review. Biochim Biophys Acta 1531(1–2):4–46

Cabana VG, Siegel JN, Sabesin SM (1989) Effects of the acute phase response on the concentration and density distribution of plasma lipids and apolipoproteins. J Lipid Res 30(1):39–49

Calabresi L, Franceschini G, Sirtori CR, De Palma A, Saresella M, Ferrante P, Taramelli D (1997) Inhibition of VCAM-1 expression in endothelial cells by reconstituted high density lipoproteins. Biochem Biophys Res Commun 238(1):61–65. doi:10.1006/bbrc.1997.7236

Cani PD, Amar J, Iglesias MA, Poggi M, Knauf C, Bastelica D, Neyrinck AM, Fava F, Tuohy KM, Chabo C, Waget A, Delmee E, Cousin B, Sulpice T, Chamontin B, Ferrieres J, Tanti JF, Gibson GR, Casteilla L, Delzenne NM, Alessi MC, Burcelin R (2007) Metabolic endotoxemia initiates obesity and insulin resistance. Diabetes 56(7):1761–1772. doi:10.2337/db06-1491

Chien J-Y, Jerng J-S, Yu C-J, Yang P-C (2005) Low serum level of high-density lipoprotein cholesterol is a poor prognostic factor for severe sepsis. Crit Care Med 33:1688–1693

Cohen J (2002) The immunopathogenesis of sepsis. Nature 420(6917):885–891. doi:10.1038/nature01326

Dai L, Datta G, Zhang Z, Gupta H, Patel R, Honavar J, Modi S, Wyss JM, Palgunachari M, Anantharamaiah GM, White CR (2010) The apolipoprotein A-I mimetic peptide 4F prevents defects in vascular function in endotoxemic rats. J Lipid Res 51:2695–2705. doi:10.1194/jlr.M008086

Datta G, Chaddha M, Hama S, Navab M, Fogelman AM, Garber DW, Mishra VK, Epand RM, Epand RF, Lund-Katz S, Phillips MC, Segrest JP, Anantharamaiah GM (2001) Effects of increasing hydrophobicity on the physical-chemical and biological properties of a class A amphipathic helical peptide. J Lipid Res 42(7):1096–1104

Datta G, Gupta H, Zhang Z, Mayakonda P, Anantharamaiah GM, White CR (2011) HDL mimetic peptide administration improves left ventricular filling and cardiac output in lipopolysaccharide-treated rats. J Clin Exp Cardiol 2:172. doi:10.4172/2155-9880.1000172

David SA (2001) Towards a rational development of anti-endotoxin agents: novel approaches to sequestration of bacterial endotoxins with small molecules. J Mol Recog: JMR 14(6):370–387. doi:10.1002/jmr.549

de Bont N, Netea MG, Demacker PN, Verschueren I, Kullberg BJ, van Dijk KW, van der Meer JW, Stalenhoef AF (1999) Apolipoprotein E knock-out mice are highly susceptible to endotoxemia and Klebsiella pneumoniae infection. J Lipid Res 40(4):680–685

Emancipator K, Csako G, Elin RJ (1992) In vitro inactivation of bacterial endotoxin by human lipoproteins and apolipoproteins. Infect Immun 60(2):596–601

Ettinger WH, Varma VK, Sorci-Thomas M, Parks JS, Sigmon RC, Smith TK, Verdery RB (1994) Cytokines decrease apolipoprotein accumulation in medium from Hep G2 cells. Arterioscler Thromb: J Vasc Biol/Am Heart Assoc 14(1):8–13

Feingold KR, Funk JL, Moser AH, Shigenaga JK, Rapp JH, Grunfeld C (1995) Role for circulating lipoproteins in protection from endotoxin toxicity. Infect Immun 63(5):2041–2046

Feng X, Zhang Y, Xu R, Xie X, Tao L, Gao H, Gao Y, He Z, Wang H (2010) Lipopolysaccharide up-regulates the expression of Fcalpha/mu receptor and promotes the binding of oxidized low-density lipoprotein and its IgM antibody complex to activated human macrophages. Atherosclerosis 208(2):396–405

Flegel WA, Baumstark MW, Weinstock C, Berg A, Northoff H (1993) Prevention of endotoxin-induced monokine release by human low- and high-density lipoproteins and by apolipoprotein A-I. Infect Immun 61(12):5140–5146

Fogelman AM (2004) When good cholesterol goes bad. Nat Med 10(9):902–903. doi:10.1038/nm0904-902

Gao F, Chattopadhyay A, Navab M, Grijalva V, Su F, Fogelman AM, Reddy ST, Farias-Eisner R (2012) Apolipoprotein A-I mimetic peptides inhibit expression and activity of hypoxia-inducible factor-1alpha in human ovarian cancer cell lines and a mouse ovarian cancer model. J Pharmacol Exp Ther 342(2):255–262. doi:10.1124/jpet.112.191544

Goldfarb RD, Parker TS, Levine DM, Glock D, Akhter I, Alkhudari A, McCarthy RJ, David EM, Gordon BR, Saal SD, Rubin AL, Trenholme GM, Parrillo JE (2003) Protein-free phospholipid emulsion treatment improved cardiopulmonary function and survival in porcine sepsis. Am J Physiol Regul Integr Comp Physiol 284(2):R550–R557. doi:10.1152/ajpregu.00285.2002

Gordon BR, Parker TS, Levine DM, Feuerbach F, Saal SD, Sloan BJ, Chu C, Stenzel KH, Parrillo JE, Rubin AL (2005) Neutralization of endotoxin by a phospholipid emulsion in healthy volunteers. J Infect Dis 191(9):1515–1522. doi:10.1086/428908

Guha M, Mackman N (2001) LPS induction of gene expression in human monocytes. Cell Signal 13(2):85–94

Gupta H, Dai L, Datta G, Garber DW, Grenett H, Li Y, Mishra V, Palgunachari MN, Handattu S, Gianturco SH, Bradley WA, Anantharamaiah GM, White CR (2005) Inhibition of lipopolysaccharide-induced inflammatory responses by an apolipoprotein AI mimetic peptide. Circ Res 97:236–243. doi:10.1161/01.RES.0000176530.66400.48

Haddad IA, Ordovas JM, Fitzpatrick T, Karathanasis SK (1986) Linkage, evolution, and expression of the rat apolipoprotein A-I, C-III, and A-IV genes. J Biol Chem 261(28): 13268–13277

Hudgins LC, Parker TS, Levine DM, Gordon BR, Saal SD, Jiang XC, Seidman CE, Tremaroli JD, Lai J, Rubin AL (2003) A single intravenous dose of endotoxin rapidly alters serum lipoproteins and lipid transfer proteins in normal volunteers. J Lipid Res 44(8):1489–1498. doi:10.1194/jlr. M200440-JLR200

Kallio KA, Buhlin K, Jauhiainen M, Keva R, Tuomainen AM, Klinge B, Gustafsson A, Pussinen PJ (2008) Lipopolysaccharide associates with pro-atherogenic lipoproteins in periodontitis patients. Innate Immun 14(4):247–253. doi:10.1177/1753425908095130

Kelesidis T, Yang OO, Currier JS, Navab K, Fogelman AM, Navab M (2011) HIV-1 infected patients with suppressed plasma viremia on treatment have pro-inflammatory HDL. Lipids Health Dis 10:35. doi:10.1186/1476-511x-10-35

Kitchens RL, Thompson PA (2003) Impact of sepsis-induced changes in plasma on LPS interactions with monocytes and plasma lipoproteins: roles of soluble CD14, LBP, and acute phase lipoproteins. J Endotoxin Res 9(2):113–118. doi:10.1179/096805103125001504

Kitchens RL, Thompson PA, Munford RS, O'Keefe GE (2003) Acute inflammation and infection maintain circulating phospholipid levels and enhance lipopolysaccharide binding to plasma lipoproteins. J Lipid Res 44(12):2339–2348

Kwon WY, Suh GJ, Kim KS, Kwak YH, Kim K (2012) 4F, apolipoprotein AI mimetic peptide, attenuates acute lung injury and improves survival in endotoxemic rats. J Trauma Acute Care Surg 72:1576–1583. doi:10.1097/TA.0b013e3182493ab4

Lajunen T, Vikatmaa P, Bloigu A, Ikonen T, Lepantalo M, Pussinen PJ, Saikku P, Leinonen M (2008) Chlamydial LPS and high-sensitivity CRP levels in serum are associated with an elevated body mass index in patients with cardiovascular disease. Innate Immun 14(6):375–382. doi:10.1177/1753425908099172

Lakio L, Lehto M, Tuomainen AM, Jauhiainen M, Malle E, Asikainen S, Pussinen PJ (2006) Proatherogenic properties of lipopolysaccharide from the periodontal pathogen Actinobacillus actinomycetemcomitans. J Endotoxin Res 12(1):57–64. doi:10.1179/096805106x89099

Lalla E, Lamster IB, Hofmann MA, Bucciarelli L, Jerud AP, Tucker S, Lu Y, Papapanou PN, Schmidt AM (2003) Oral infection with a periodontal pathogen accelerates early atherosclerosis in apolipoprotein E-null mice. Arterioscler Thromb Vasc Biol 23(8):1405–1411. doi:10.1161/01.atv.0000082462.26258.fe

Levels JH, Abraham PR, van den Ende A, van Deventer SJ (2001) Distribution and kinetics of lipoprotein-bound endotoxin. Infect Immun 69(5):2821–2828. doi:10.1128/iai. 69.5.2821-2828.2001

Levine DM, Parker TS, Donnelly TM, Walsh A, Rubin AL (1993) In vivo protection against endotoxin by plasma high density lipoprotein. Proc Natl Acad Sci U S A 90(24):12040–12044

Ma J, Liao XL, Lou B, Wu MP (2004) Role of apolipoprotein A-I in protecting against endotoxin toxicity. Acta Biochim Biophys Sin 36(6):419–424

Madenspacher JH, Azzam KM, Gong W, Gowdy KM, Vitek MP, Laskowitz DT, Remaley AT, Wang JM, Fessler MB (2012) Apolipoproteins and apolipoprotein mimetic peptides modulate phagocyte trafficking through chemotactic activity. J Biol Chem 287(52):43730–43740. doi:10.1074/jbc.M112.377192

Massamiri T, Tobias PS, Curtiss LK (1997) Structural determinants for the interaction of lipopolysaccharide binding protein with purified high density lipoproteins: role of apolipoprotein A-I. J Lipid Res 38(3):516–525

McDonald MC, Dhadly P, Cockerill GW, Cuzzocrea S, Mota-Filipe H, Hinds CJ, Miller NE, Thiemermann C (2003) Reconstituted high-density lipoprotein attenuates organ injury and adhesion molecule expression in a rodent model of endotoxic shock. Shock (Augusta, Ga) 20:551–557. doi:10.1097/01.shk.0000097249.97298.a3

Mendez AJ, Anantharamaiah GM, Segrest JP, Oram JF (1994) Synthetic amphipathic helical peptides that mimic apolipoprotein A-I in clearing cellular cholesterol. J Clin Invest 94(4):1698–1705. doi:10.1172/jci117515

Meriwether D, Imaizumi S, Grijalva V, Hough G, Vakili L, Anantharamaiah GM, Farias-Eisner R, Navab M, Fogelman AM, Reddy ST, Shechter I (2011) Enhancement by LDL of transfer of L-4F and oxidized lipids to HDL in C57BL/6J mice and human plasma. J Lipid Res 52:1795–1809. doi:10.1194/jlr.M016741

Miller SI, Ernst RK, Bader MW (2005) LPS, TLR4 and infectious disease diversity. Nat Rev Microbiol 3(1):36–46. doi:10.1038/nrmicro1068

Mishra VK, Palgunachari MN, Datta G, Phillips MC, Lund-Katz S, Adeyeye SO, Segrest JP, Anantharamaiah GM (1998) Studies of synthetic peptides of human apolipoprotein A-I containing tandem amphipathic alpha-helixes. Biochemistry 37(28):10313–10324. doi:10.1021/bi980042o

Mishra VK, Palgunachari MN, McPherson DT, Anantharamaiah GM (2013) Lipid complex of apolipoprotein A-I mimetic peptide 4F is a novel platform for paraoxonase-1 binding and enhancing its activity and stability. Biochem Biophys Res Commun 430(3):975–980. doi:10.1016/j.bbrc.2012.11.128

Moreira RS, Irigoyen M, Sanches TR, Volpini RA, Camara NOS, Malheiros DM, Shimizu MHM, Seguro AC, Andrade L (2014) Apolipoprotein A-I mimetic peptide 4F attenuates kidney injury, heart injury, and endothelial dysfunction in sepsis. Am J Physiol Regul Integr Comp Physiol 307:R514–R524. doi:10.1152/ajpregu.00445.2013

Morishima A, Ohkubo N, Maeda N, Miki T, Mitsuda N (2003) NFkappaB regulates plasma apolipoprotein A-I and high density lipoprotein cholesterol through inhibition of peroxisome proliferator-activated receptor alpha. J Biol Chem 278(40):38188–38193. doi:10.1074/jbc.M306336200

Munford RS (2006) Severe sepsis and septic shock: the role of gram-negative bacteremia. Annu Rev Pathol 1:467–496. doi:10.1146/annurev.pathol.1.110304.100200

Nakarai H, Yamashita A, Nagayasu S, Iwashita M, Kumamoto S, Ohyama H, Hata M, Soga Y, Kushiyama A, Asano T, Abiko Y, Nishimura F (2012) Adipocyte-macrophage interaction may mediate LPS-induced low-grade inflammation: potential link with metabolic complications. Innate Immun 18(1):164–170. doi:10.1177/1753425910393370

Nandedkar SD, Weihrauch D, Xu H, Shi Y, Feroah T, Hutchins W, Rickaby DA, Duzgunes N, Hillery CA, Konduri KS, Pritchard KA Jr (2011) D-4F, an apoA-1 mimetic, decreases airway hyperresponsiveness, inflammation, and oxidative stress in a murine model of asthma. J Lipid Res 52(3):499–508. doi:10.1194/jlr.M012724

Navab M, Anantharamaiah GM, Hama S, Garber DW, Chaddha M, Hough G, Lallone R, Fogelman AM (2002) Oral administration of an Apo A-I mimetic Peptide synthesized from D-amino acids dramatically reduces atherosclerosis in mice independent of plasma cholesterol. Circulation 105(3):290–292

Navab M, Anantharamaiah GM, Reddy ST, Hama S, Hough G, Grijalva VR, Wagner AC, Frank JS, Datta G, Garber D, Fogelman AM (2004) Oral D-4F causes formation of pre-beta high-density lipoprotein and improves high-density lipoprotein-mediated cholesterol efflux and reverse cholesterol transport from macrophages in apolipoprotein E-null mice. Circulation 109(25):3215–3220. doi:10.1161/01.cir.0000134275.90823.87

Navab M, Anantharamaiah GM, Reddy ST, Hama S, Hough G, Grijalva VR, Yu N, Ansell BJ, Datta G, Garber DW, Fogelman AM (2005) Apolipoprotein A-I mimetic peptides. Arterioscler Thromb Vasc Biol 25(7):1325–1331. doi:10.1161/01.atv.0000165694.39518.95

Nayyar G, Garber DW, Palgunachari MN, Monroe CE, Keenum TD, Handattu SP, Mishra VK, Anantharamaiah GM (2012a) Apolipoprotein E mimetic is more effective than apolipoprotein A-I mimetic in reducing lesion formation in older female apo E null mice. Atherosclerosis. doi:10.1016/j.atherosclerosis.2012.05.040

Nayyar G, Mishra VK, Handattu SP, Palgunachari MN, Shin R, McPherson DT, Deivanayagam CC, Garber DW, Segrest JP, Anantharamaiah GM (2012b) Sidedness of interfacial arginine residues and anti-atherogenicity of apolipoprotein A-I mimetic peptides. J Lipid Res 53(5):849–858. doi:10.1194/jlr.M019844

Netea MG, van Deuren M, Kullberg BJ, Cavaillon JM, Van der Meer JW (2002) Does the shape of lipid A determine the interaction of LPS with toll-like receptors? Trends Immunol 23(3):135–139

Opal SM, Gluck T (2003) Endotoxin as a drug target. Crit Care Med 31(1 Suppl):S57–S64. doi:10.1097/01.ccm.0000042472.07935.9c

Ou ZJ, Li L, Liao XL, Wang YM, Hu XX, Zhang QL, Wang ZP, Yu H, Zhang X, Hu P, Xu YQ, Liang QL, Ou JS, Luo G (2012) Apolipoprotein A-I mimetic peptide inhibits atherosclerosis by altering plasma metabolites in hypercholesterolemia. Am J Physiol Endocrinol Metab 303(6):E683–E694. doi:10.1152/ajpendo.00136.2012

Parker TS, Levine DM, Chang JC, Laxer J, Coffin CC, Rubin AL (1995) Reconstituted high-density lipoprotein neutralizes gram-negative bacterial lipopolysaccharides in human whole blood. Infect Immun 63(1):253–258

Pasterkamp G, Van Keulen JK, De Kleijn DP (2004) Role of Toll-like receptor 4 in the initiation and progression of atherosclerotic disease. Eur J Clin Invest 34(5):328–334. doi:10.1111/j.1365-2362.2004.01338.x

Pendyala S, Walker JM, Holt PR (2012) A high-fat diet is associated with endotoxemia that originates from the gut. Gastroenterology 142(5):1100–1101 e1102. doi:10.1053/j.gastro.2012.01.034

Read TE, Harris HW, Grunfeld C, Feingold KR, Calhoun MC, Kane JP, Rapp JH (1993) Chylomicrons enhance endotoxin excretion in bile. Infect Immun 61(8):3496–3502

Rufail ML, Schenkein HA, Koertge TE, Best AM, Barbour SE, Tew JG, van Antwerpen R (2007) Atherogenic lipoprotein parameters in patients with aggressive periodontitis. J Periodontal Res 42(6):495–502. doi:10.1111/j.1600-0765.2007.00973.x

Seitz CS, Kleindienst R, Xu Q, Wick G (1996) Coexpression of heat-shock protein 60 and intercellular-adhesion molecule-1 is related to increased adhesion of monocytes and T cells to aortic endothelium of rats in response to endotoxin. Lab Invest 74(1):241–252

Shah PK, Kaul S, Nilsson J, Cercek B (2001a) Exploiting the vascular protective effects of high-density lipoprotein and its apolipoproteins: an idea whose time for testing is coming, part II. Circulation 104(20):2498–2502

Shah PK, Kaul S, Nilsson J, Cercek B (2001b) Exploiting the vascular protective effects of high-density lipoprotein and its apolipoproteins: an idea whose time for testing is coming, part I. Circulation 104(19):2376–2383

Sharifov OF, Xu X, Gaggar A, Grizzle WE, Mishra VK, Honavar J, Litovsky SH, Palgunachari MN, White CR, Anantharamaiah GM, Gupta H (2013) Anti-inflammatory mechanisms of apolipoprotein A-I mimetic peptide in acute respiratory distress syndrome secondary to sepsis. PLoS ONE 8:e64486. doi:10.1371/journal.pone.0064486

Sharifov OF, Nayyar G, Ternovoy VV, Palgunachari MN, Garber DW, Anantharamaiah G, Gupta H (2014a) Comparison of anti-endotoxin activity of apoE and apoA mimetic derivatives of a model amphipathic peptide 18A. Innate Immun 20(8):867–880. doi:10.1177/1753425913514621

Sharifov OF, Xu X, Gaggar A, Tabengwa EM, White CR, Palgunachari MN, Anantharamaiah GM, Gupta H (2014b) L-4F inhibits lipopolysaccharide-mediated activation of primary human neutrophils. Inflammation 37(5):1401–1412. doi:10.1007/s10753-014-9864-7

Sharma S, Umar S, Potus F, Iorga A, Wong G, Meriwether D, Breuils-Bonnet S, Mai D, Navab K, Ross D, Navab M, Provencher S, Fogelman AM, Bonnet S, Reddy ST, Eghbali M (2014) Apolipoprotein A-I mimetic peptide 4F rescues pulmonary hypertension by inducing microRNA-193-3p. Circulation 130(9):776–785. doi:10.1161/circulationaha.114.007405

Shiflett AM, Bishop JR, Pahwa A, Hajduk SL (2005) Human high density lipoproteins are platforms for the assembly of multi-component innate immune complexes. J Biol Chem 280(38):32578–32585. doi:10.1074/jbc.M503510200

Smythies LE, White CR, Maheshwari A, Palgunachari MN, Anantharamaiah GM, Chaddha M, Kurundkar AR, Datta G (2010) Apolipoprotein A-I mimetic 4F alters the function of human monocyte-derived macrophages. Am J Physiol Cell Physiol 298:C1538–C1548. doi:10.1152/ajpcell.00467.2009

Szeto CC, Kwan BC, Chow KM, Lai KB, Chung KY, Leung CB, Li PK (2008) Endotoxemia is related to systemic inflammation and atherosclerosis in peritoneal dialysis patients. Clin J Am Soc Nephrol 3(2):431–436

Tietge UJ, Maugeais C, Lund-Katz S, Grass D, deBeer FC, Rader DJ (2002) Human secretory phospholipase A2 mediates decreased plasma levels of HDL cholesterol and apoA-I in response to inflammation in human apoA-I transgenic mice. Arterioscler Thromb Vasc Biol 22(7):1213–1218

Tobias PS, Tapping RI, Gegner JA (1999) Endotoxin interactions with lipopolysaccharide-responsive cells. Clin Infect Dis: Off Publ Infect Dis Soc Am 28(3):476–481. doi:10.1086/515163

Tytler EM, Segrest JP, Epand RM, Nie SQ, Epand RF, Mishra VK, Venkatachalapathi YV, Anantharamaiah GM (1993) Reciprocal effects of apolipoprotein and lytic peptide analogs on membranes. Cross-sectional molecular shapes of amphipathic alpha helixes control membrane stability. J Biol Chem 268(29):22112–22118

van Leeuwen HJ, Heezius ECJM, Dallinga GM, van Strijp JAG, Verhoef J, van Kessel KPM (2003) Lipoprotein metabolism in patients with severe sepsis. Crit Care Med 31:1359–1366. doi:10.1097/01.CCM.0000059724.08290.51

Van Lenten BJ, Hama SY, de Beer FC, Stafforini DM, McIntyre TM, Prescott SM, La Du BN, Fogelman AM, Navab M (1995) Anti-inflammatory HDL becomes pro-inflammatory during the acute phase response. Loss of protective effect of HDL against LDL oxidation in aortic wall cell cocultures. J Clin Invest 96(6):2758–2767. doi:10.1172/jci118345

Van Lenten BJ, Wagner AC, Anantharamaiah GM, Garber DW, Fishbein MC, Adhikary L, Nayak DP, Hama S, Navab M, Fogelman AM (2002) Influenza infection promotes macrophage traffic into arteries of mice that is prevented by D-4F, an apolipoprotein A-I mimetic peptide. Circulation 106(9):1127–1132

Van Lenten BJ, Wagner AC, Navab M, Anantharamaiah GM, Hui EK, Nayak DP, Fogelman AM (2004) D-4F, an apolipoprotein A-I mimetic peptide, inhibits the inflammatory response induced by influenza A infection of human type II pneumocytes. Circulation 110(20):3252–3258. doi:10.1161/01.cir.0000147232.75456.b3

Van Lenten BJ, Wagner AC, Navab M, Anantharamaiah GM, Hama S, Reddy ST, Fogelman AM (2007) Lipoprotein inflammatory properties and serum amyloid A levels but not cholesterol levels predict lesion area in cholesterol-fed rabbits. J Lipid Res 48(11):2344–2353. doi:10.1194/jlr. M700138-JLR200

Van Lenten BJ, Wagner AC, Jung CL, Ruchala P, Waring AJ, Lehrer RI, Watson AD, Hama S, Navab M, Anantharamaiah GM, Fogelman AM (2008) Anti-inflammatory apoA-I-mimetic peptides bind oxidized lipids with much higher affinity than human apoA-I. J Lipid Res 49(11):2302–2311

Vikatmaa P, Lajunen T, Ikonen TS, Pussinen PJ, Lepantalo M, Leinonen M, Saikku P (2010) Chlamydial lipopolysaccharide (cLPS) is present in atherosclerotic and aneurysmal arterial wall–cLPS levels depend on disease manifestation. Cardiovasc Pathol 19(1):48–54

White CR, Datta G, Buck AK, Chaddha M, Reddy G, Wilson L, Palgunachari MN, Abbasi M, Anantharamaiah GM (2012a) Preservation of biological function despite oxidative modification of the apolipoprotein A-I mimetic peptide 4F. J Lipid Res 53(8):1576–1587. doi:10.1194/jlr.M026278

White CR, Smythies LE, Crossman DK, Palgunachari MN, Anantharamaiah GM, Datta G (2012b) Regulation of pattern recognition receptors by the apolipoprotein A-I mimetic peptide 4F. Arterioscler Thromb Vasc Biol 32:2631–2639. doi:10.1161/ATVBAHA.112.300167

White CR, Garber DW, Anantharamaiah GM (2014) Anti-inflammatory and cholesterol-reducing properties of apolipoprotein mimetics: a review. J Lipid Res 55:2007–2021. doi:10.1194/jlr. R051367

Wiedermann CJ, Kiechl S, Dunzendorfer S, Schratzberger P, Egger G, Oberhollenzer F, Willeit J (1999) Association of endotoxemia with carotid atherosclerosis and cardiovascular disease: prospective results from the Bruneck Study. J Am Coll Cardiol 34(7):1975–1981

Wiesner P, Choi SH, Almazan F, Benner C, Huang W, Diehl CJ, Gonen A, Butler S, Witztum JL, Glass CK, Miller YI (2010) Low doses of lipopolysaccharide and minimally oxidized low-density lipoprotein cooperatively activate macrophages via nuclear factor kappa B and activator protein-1: possible mechanism for acceleration of atherosclerosis by subclinical endotoxemia. Circ Res 107(1):56–65

Zhang Z, Datta G, Zhang Y, Miller AP, Mochon P, Chen Y-F, Chatham J, Anantharamaiah GM, White CR (2009) Apolipoprotein A-I mimetic peptide treatment inhibits inflammatory responses and improves survival in septic rats. Am J Physiol Heart Circ Physiol 297:H866–H873. doi:10.1152/ajpheart.01232.2008

Zhou X, Gao XP, Fan J, Liu Q, Anwar KN, Frey RS, Malik AB (2005) LPS activation of Toll-like receptor 4 signals CD11b/CD18 expression in neutrophils. Am J Physiol Lung Cell Mol Physiol 288(4):L655–L662. doi:10.1152/ajplung.00327.2004

Apolipoprotein Mimetics in the Amelioration of Respiratory Inflammation

Kirkwood A. Pritchard Jr.

Abstract Asthma induces chronic inflammation, airway hyperresponsiveness, collagen deposition, and airway remodeling. Left unchecked, it can lead to progressive and irreversible lung damage. Oxidative stress and inflammation have been hypothesized to play causal roles in asthma. Interestingly, high-density lipoprotein (HDL) and apolipoprotein A-I, the major anti-inflammatory apolipoprotein of HDL, which are well recognized for protecting against atherosclerosis, have recently been shown to play important roles in reducing inflammation and oxidative stress in the lung. Typically, asthma is treated with inhaled corticosteroids. However, chronic corticosteroid therapy induces side effects that reduce their appeal as a long-term therapeutic. Accordingly, there is a great need for the development of new strategies for inhibiting oxidative stress and inflammation in asthma that does not rely on corticosteroids. In this chapter, we review the cell biology of HDL and apoA-I in the lung and the mechanisms by which apolipoprotein mimetics reduce oxidative stress and inflammation in the asthmatic lung.

Introduction

The relationship between chronic airway inflammation, lipoproteins, atherosclerosis, and asthma has been recognized since 1980 (Jefferys et al. 1980). Asthma induces chronic airway inflammation, which reduces airflow and increases bronchospasm and shortness of breath. In women, adult-onset asthma has been shown to significantly increase the risk of carotid artery atherosclerosis (Onufrak et al. 2007).

K.A. Pritchard Jr., PhD
Department of Surgery, Division of Pediatric Surgery, Medical College of Wisconsin, 8701 Watertown Plank Road, C4420, Milwaukee, WI 53226, USA
e-mail: kpritch@mcw.edu

G.M. Anantharamaiah, D. Goldberg (eds.), *Apolipoprotein Mimetics in the Management of Human Disease*, DOI 10.1007/978-3-319-17350-4_7

Asthma has profound effects on the oxidation status of low-density lipoprotein (LDL) and HDL, resulting, in part, from a decrease in activity of paraoxonase (PON1) associated with HDL. Although corticosteroids are often used to treat inflammation in asthma, they alter plasma lipids in ways that are considered to increase the risk of heart disease (Jefferys et al. 1980). Although asthma and its treatments appear to increase the atherogenic nature of lipoprotein profiles, there is growing evidence that lipoprotein profiles credited with increasing atherosclerosis also contribute to airway inflammation and asthma. Of particular note are studies in children that suggest that these changes take root in early childhood (Gidding et al. 2004) and can be influenced by diet (Schafer et al. 2003).

Strong interactions exist between general health, diet, and airway inflammation. As asthma increases the pro-atherogenic properties of lipoproteins, it also has become credited with increasing the risk of atherosclerosis. To better understand how HDL impacts on the lung, our laboratory investigated the effects of genetic deletion of apolipoprotein A-I (apoA-I) on lung physiology, inflammation, and oxidative stress in mice. Although apoA-1 knockout (*ApoA-I*$^{-/-}$) mice are not more susceptible to atherosclerosis (Plump et al. 1997), deletion of apoA-I in murine models of atherosclerosis greatly enhances the atherogenic mechanisms driving vascular disease (Ou et al. 2005). If apoA-I is important for protecting against atherosclerotic lesion formation, it should also be important for protecting vascular function in other organs. Accordingly, genetic deletion of apoA-I could adversely affect vascular function in vascular beds subjected to oxidative stress. The one vascular bed that is known to experience chronic states of oxidative stress is the lung.

Genetic Deletion of ApoA-I

Previously, we showed that *ApoA-I*$^{-/-}$ mice had reduced total and HDL cholesterol (Wang et al. 2010) confirming findings by Plump et al. (1997). However, additional analysis revealed that HDL in *apoA-I*$^{-/-}$ mice had higher levels of proinflammatory HDL (p-HDL) than C57BL/6J mice (Wang et al. 2010). While the exact cause for an increase in p-HDL in these mice remains unknown, we observed that paraoxonase 1 (PON1) activity in *apoA-I*$^{-/-}$ mice was decreased in spite of the fact that total PON1 protein was increased. The cell biology of PON1 indicates that apoA-I binds PON1 which is expressed in the liver and promotes its entry into the circulation (Sorenson et al. 1999). Possibly, in the absence of apoA-I, PON1 binds to alternative partners and is therefore more susceptible to inactivation. It has been shown that among HDL subspecies, HDL particles that contain only A-I exhibits enhanced PON-1 activity compared to HDL particles that contain A-I/A-II. While the exact reason for why apolipoprotein composition in HDL particles alters PON1 activity is unknown, it is possible that apoA-I in the smaller HDL particle directly activates PON1 which apoA-I and apoA-II in larger HDL particles are less effective. Additional studies will be required to sort out such a possibility (Davidson et al. 2009; Kontush et al. 2003).

One of the common effects of dyslipoproteinemia on endothelial cell function is a shift in the balance of nitric oxide and superoxide generation by endothelial nitric oxide synthase (eNOS) (Ou et al. 2003b; Pritchard et al. 1995, 2002). To determine the effects of apoA-I deficiency on eNOS, we measured total plasma nitrite and nitrate and 3-nitrotyrosine. As anticipated, *apoA-I*$^{-/-}$ mice had lower nitrite and nitrate but increased 3-nitrotyrosine than wild-type mice. These data are consistent with the idea that the apoA-I in HDL stimulates eNOS activity (Mineo et al. 2003) and that dysfunctional HDL uncouples eNOS (Chang et al. 2014).

With evidence supporting the idea that the loss of apoA-I adversely impacts eNOS activity, we next determined whether the vascular physiology in these mice was altered. Vasodilation studies revealed that in *apoA-I*$^{-/-}$ mice, the *facialis* artery was unaffected, but the pulmonary artery contracted at higher doses of vasodilators compared to the responses in control mice. These data were one of the first clues that apoA-I and HDL played an important role in lung physiology (Wang 2010 #13191). To better understand the impact of apoA-I on lung physiology, we examined airway responsiveness in C57Bl/6J and *apoA-I*$^{-/-}$ mice.

Although no differences in airway resistance were observed in large airways, tissue dampening and elastance were both increased in the *apoA-I*$^{-/-}$ mice in response to methacholine challenge and to positive end-expired pressures (Wang et al. 2010). These observations indicate that the small airways are stiffer and less elastic in *apoA-I*$^{-/-}$ mice. Such changes are important for inspiration and expiration. Stiffer airways means that the lung has to work harder during inspiration. Reductions in elasticity mean that the lungs contain less stored-up energy for pushing the air out of the lung during expiration. These data indicate that ventilation is more difficult in *apoA-I*$^{-/-}$ mice all around and that the *apoA-I*$^{-/-}$ mice work harder during inspiration and expiration than C57BL/6J mice.

With such fundamental differences in vascular and airway physiology, it was not surprising that *apoA-I*$^{-/-}$ mice also had more pulmonary inflammation than C57BL/6J mice. Histology studies revealed that the lungs of *apoA-I*$^{-/-}$ mice contained more eosinophils and lymphocytes and expressed higher levels of collagen than the lungs of C57BL/6J mice. Examination of the lungs for evidence of oxidative stress and inflammation revealed that apoA-I deficiency increased the formation of 3-nitrotyrosine and 4-hydroxynonenal, which co-localized with increased expression of TGF-β, one of the primary mechanisms for increasing collagen expression and making a stiffer lung. To understand the impact of apoA-I deficiency on oxidative stress, we examined lung homogenates for changes in xanthine oxidase (XO), myeloperoxidase (MPO), and eNOS. The immunoblots revealed that the lungs from *apoA-I*$^{-/-}$ mice contained higher levels of XO, MPO, and eNOS than homogenates from control lungs. As XO generates hydrogen peroxide, MPO generates potent nitrogen- and chloro-oxidants, and eNOS is uncoupled in pro-oxidant environments; these data are consistent with the idea that the lungs of *apoA-I*$^{-/-}$ mice exist in chronic states of oxidative stress (Wang et al. 2010). Additional support comes from studies showing that even though the bronchial lavage fluid of *apoA-I*$^{-/-}$ mice contained higher levels of nitrite+nitrate than control mice, it oxidized dichlorodihydrofluorescein (DCF, an oxidant-sensitive fluorescent probe) to a greater extent than BALF from C57BL/6J mice (Wang et al. 2010). Thus, genetic deletion of apoA-I adversely impacts lung physiology and oxidant balance to create a new strain of mouse that is much more susceptible to airway inflammation. These observations provided the rationale for postulating that improving HDL functionality might be an effective strategy for reducing pulmonary inflammation.

In 2001, it was shown that the anti-inflammatory properties of 18A, an alpha-helical peptide derived from apoA-I, could be enhanced by strategic substitutions of phenylalanine (Datta et al. 2001). Subsequent studies showed that oral administration of D-4F could reduce atherosclerosis in mice in spite of chronically increased plasma cholesterol (Navab et al. 2002). Building on these findings, we observed that L-4F improved vasodilatation in hypercholesterolemic and sickle cell mice (Ou et al. 2003a) and restored endothelial cell nitric oxide and superoxide anion balance by recoupling eNOS activity (Ou et al. 2003b). One of the major mechanisms by which 4F was believed to reduce inflammation was by binding oxidized lipids with much greater affinity than apoA-I (Van Lenten et al. 2008) that would result in an efficient removal of the seeding molecules of the lipid hydroperoxides in HDL that impair functionality (Van Lenten et al. 1995; Navab et al. 1996). With this information as background, we reasoned that 4F might be useful for reducing airway inflammation in asthma.

4F Inhibits Airway Inflammation

To determine whether targeting HDL is an effective strategy for reducing airway inflammation, we developed an allergen-dependent murine model of asthma (Nandedkar et al. 2011). Ovalbumin (OVA) sensitization had no effect on total or HDL cholesterol levels but markedly increased p-HDL. Intranasal delivery of 4F, an apoA-I mimetic, reduced p-HDL in the OVA-sensitized mice to control levels. This is a major development since L-amino acid-containing peptides were thought not to work either orally or intranasal. Unfortunately, no studies were performed to determine plasma levels in mice that were treated with intranasal L-4F, which is an important piece of information in that, the effectiveness of L-4F could result from direct interactions with the inflamed airways or by a more efficient uptake into the circulation via the lungs than the gut. Either way, upon reaching the lung, its target organ, it was anticipated it would attenuate the proinflammatory effects of OVA which could also reduce the negative impact of asthma on HDL proinflammatory status. As p-HDL has been previously shown to be ineffective for function (Ansell et al. 2003), this marked increase in p-HDL in OVA-sensitized mice could be interpreted to mean that experimentally induced asthma impairs HDL function. More importantly, with 4F reducing p-HDL, any improvements in pulmonary function or decrease in inflammation of the lung could be legitimately credited, at least in part, to 4F's ability to improve HDL function. In contrast to the impact deleting apoA-I genetically on airway responses, OVA sensitization significantly increased airway resistance in response to methacholine challenge. In addition, OVA sensitization increased tissue dampening and elastance indicating that asthmatic mice had stiffer and less elastic lungs. The fact that 4F treatments reduced airway resistance as well as tissue dampening and elastance is consistent with the idea that apoA-I plays an important protective role in lung physiology by reducing inflammation which allows for greater movement of air in and out of the lung during breathing. Histological evidence revealed that OVA sensitization markedly increases in inflammatory cell influx and collagen deposition was observed in the mice. Intranasal 4F treatments markedly reduced inflammatory cell infiltration and collagen deposition. Further characterization revealed that OVA sensitization increases TGFβ and FSP-1 expression which are paralleled by marked increases in the levels of oxidized phospholipids (measured as anti-T15 antibodies Wool et al. 2010; Shaw et al. 2000) and 4-HNE formation in lung tissues. Again, 4F treatments reduced all of the biomarkers of inflammation, oxidative stress, and fibrosis in the lungs of OVA-sensitized mice.

One of the hallmarks of OVA sensitization is an increase in eosinophil peroxidase (EPO) activity in the bronchial lavage fluid (BALF) isolated from the mice which is paralleled by corresponding increases in eosinophil counts. Importantly, 4F treatments decreased EPO activity and the number of eosinophils in the BALF isolated from OVA-sensitized mice. ELISA studies showed that OVA sensitization increases total plasma levels of IgE in the mice which was partially attenuated by 4F treatments. These data are consistent with the idea that 4F decreases inflammation by binding and removing oxidized lipids. Recently, our laboratory showed that 4F can enter cells and bind to interferon response factor 5 (IRF5) in an irreversible fashion to decrease inflammation and cell death (Xu et al. 2012). Thus, apoA-I mimetics may have multiple mechanisms of action for reducing inflammation and immune responses that could also account for the observed improvements in airway inflammation in the OVA-sensitized mouse model.

Potential Mechanisms of Action

Studies from our laboratories suggest that 4F reduces inflammation by at least two distinct mechanisms. One mechanism familiar to experts in vascular biology and lipoprotein metabolism is mediated by 4F's unique ability to bind, inactivate, and remove proinflammatory oxidized lipids from the tissues. A second mechanism less well recognized but equally important is 4F's ability to bind IRF5. Recently, we reported that 4F bound IRF5 by an essentially irreversible biophysical mechanism (Xu et al. 2012). The importance of this observation lies in the fact that IRF5 has been called a molecular switch in immunology because it determines whether a macrophage promotes or inhibits inflammation (Xu et al. 2012; Chen et al. 2008; Krausgruber et al. 2011). The ability of 4F to bind and inhibit IRF5 begins to explain why 4F has such potent effects in murine models of autoimmune diseases (Weihrauch et al. 2007; McMahon and Brahn 2008; Woo et al. 2010; Charles-Schoeman et al. 2008). Whether 4F inhibits experimentally induced asthma by targeting IRF5 is unclear at this time. However, based on reports suggesting that macrophage responses to house-dust-mite allergens are also mediated by IRF5 (Draijer et al. 2013) and that polymorphisms in the IRF5 gene are associated with asthma (Wang et al. 2012), it is entirely possible that 4F could reduce inflammation in experimental asthma by targeting IRF5. Additional studies are required to determine if and the extent to which 4F targets IRF5 or other transcription factors to reduce airway inflammation.

Other Apolipoprotein Mimetics That Modulate Airway Inflammation

Although 4F is one of the most recognized mimetics for decreasing inflammation, other mimetics have been developed with varying anti-inflammatory properties. For example, as early as 2001, small peptides corresponding to the receptor-binding region of apoE were observed to decrease microglial inflammation (Laskowitz et al. 2001). Subsequently, Laskowitz and associates showed that these apoE mimetics reduce inflammation and injury in a number of neurological injury models such as traumatic brain injury, stroke, and spinal cord injury (Li et al. 2006; Wang et al. 2007; James et al. 2009; Laskowitz et al. 2010). Later they showed that the apoE mimetics were even effective for inhibiting inflammatory infiltrates in a murine model of multiple sclerosis (Li et al. 2006). In 2011, building on data showing that exposure to house-dust-mite (HDM) allergen increased apoE expression and armed with the knowledge that apoE protected against oxidative stress in brains, Yao et al. (2011) treated the HDM asthmatic mice with apoE (130–149) to inhibit airway inflammation. In addition, they looked at a structural analog of 37pA, called 5A, where five alanines are substituted for hydrophobic residues and then linked by a central proline. Asthmatic mice treated with 5A had reduced pulmonary inflammation compared to controls (Yao et al. 2011, 2012). As the COG113, an apoE mimetic, inhibits NFkB (Singh et al. 2011), it is possible that improvements after treatment resulted from the apoE mimetic's ability to inhibit NFkB more than its ability to bind, remove oxidized lipids, or interact with the apoE receptor. In contrast, 5A's mechanism of action appears to be by remodeling HDL. Taken together these data plus our work showing 4F interacts with IRF5 indicate that the apoA-I and apoE mimetics decrease inflammation by at least two mechanisms. If these data continue to hold up under further testing, then a great opportunity exists for developing new and novel therapeutics for decreasing inflammation in the lung that will be free of the side effects associated with corticosteroids.

Novel Apolipoprotein Mimetics

If apoA-I and apoE mimetics inhibit airway inflammation by improving HDL functionality and/or inhibiting proinflammatory transcription factors, then possibly other novel mimetics may also be of value for sorting out mechanisms. For example, earlier Getz and associates reported that b4F has greater binding affinity to HDL and anti-inflammatory properties than 4F (Wool et al. 2009). More recently, Zhao et al. (2014) showed that nanoparticles composed of small peptides covalently linked to form artificial dimer, trimer, and quad peptides appear to promote HDL remodeling and improve functionality. As we gain more experience with the mimetics and better understand their mechanisms of action, we should be able to design a whole series of alternative mimetics to test in murine models of inflammation. Outcomes from such studies could provide new insight into potential mechanisms of inflammation in asthma as well as the mechanisms by which the mimetics and nanostructure improve HDL functionality. It will be interesting to see if these new mimetics and nanostructures decrease airway inflammation as well as 4F and whether the mechanisms that decrease inflammation are mediated more by HDL-dependent mechanisms or whether they create novel intracellular mechanisms, such as those that target proinflammatory transcription factors.

The advancements made over the last 30 years provide great new opportunities for developing new therapeutic strategies and approaches for treating airway inflammation. Indeed, it may be very possible in the near future to develop a mimetic that could actually replace corticosteroids.

References

Ansell BJ, Navab M, Hama S, Kamranpour N, Fonarow G, Hough G, Rahmani S, Mottahedeh R, Dave R, Reddy ST, Fogelman AM (2003) Inflammatory/antiinflammatory properties of high-density lipoprotein distinguish patients from control subjects better than high-density lipoprotein cholesterol levels and are favorably affected by simvastatin treatment. Circulation 108(22):2751–2756

Chang FJ, Yuan HY, Hu XX, Ou ZJ, Fu L, Lin ZB, Wang ZP, Wang SM, Zhou L, Xu YQ, Wang CP, Xu Z, Zhang X, Zhang CX, Ou JS (2014) High density lipoprotein from patients with valvular heart disease uncouples endothelial nitric oxide synthase. J Mol Cell Cardiol 74:209–219. doi:10.1016/j.yjmcc.2014.05.015

Charles-Schoeman C, Banquerigo ML, Hama S, Navab M, Park GS, Van Lenten BJ, Wagner AC, Fogelman AM, Brahn E (2008) Treatment with an apolipoprotein A-1 mimetic peptide in combination with pravastatin inhibits collagen-induced arthritis. Clin Immunol 127(2):234–244. doi:10.1016/j.clim.2008.01.016

Chen W, Lam SS, Srinath H, Jiang Z, Correia JJ, Schiffer CA, Fitzgerald KA, Lin K, Royer WE Jr (2008) Insights into interferon regulatory factor activation from the crystal structure of dimeric IRF5. Nat Struct Mol Biol 15(11):1213–1220. doi:10.1038/nsmb.1496

Datta G, Chaddha M, Hama S, Navab M, Fogelman AM, Garber DW, Mishra VK, Epand RM, Epand RF, Lund-Katz S, Phillips MC, Segrest JP, Anantharamaiah GM (2001) Effects of increasing hydrophobicity on the physical-chemical and biological properties of a class A amphipathic helical peptide. J Lipid Res 42(7):1096–1104

Davidson WS, Silva RA, Chantepie S, Lagor WR, Chapman MJ, Kontush A (2009) Proteomic analysis of defined HDL subpopulations reveals particle-specific protein clusters: relevance to antioxidative function. Arterioscler Thromb Vasc Biol 29(6):870–876. doi:10.1161/ATVBAHA.109.186031, ATVBAHA.109.186031 [pii]

Draijer C, Robbe P, Boorsma CE, Hylkema MN, Melgert BN (2013) Characterization of macrophage phenotypes in three murine models of house-dust-mite-induced asthma. Mediators Inflamm 2013:632049. doi:10.1155/2013/632049

Gidding SS, Nehgme R, Heise C, Muscar C, Linton A, Hassink S (2004) Severe obesity associated with cardiovascular deconditioning, high prevalence of cardiovascular risk factors, diabetes mellitus/hyperinsulinemia, and respiratory compromise. J Pediatr 144(6):766–769. doi:10.1016/j.jpeds.2004.03.043

James ML, Sullivan PM, Lascola CD, Vitek MP, Laskowitz DT (2009) Pharmacogenomic effects of apolipoprotein e on intracerebral hemorrhage. Stroke 40(2):632–639. doi:10.1161/STROKEAHA.108.530402

Jefferys DB, Lessof MH, Mattock MB (1980) Corticosteroid treatment, serum lipids and coronary artery disease. Postgrad Med J 56(657):491–493

Kontush A, Chantepie S, Chapman MJ (2003) Small, dense HDL particles exert potent protection of atherogenic LDL against oxidative stress. Arterioscler Thromb Vasc Biol 23(10):1881–1888. doi:10.1161/01.ATV.0000091338.93223.E8, 01.ATV.0000091338.93223.E8 [pii]

Krausgruber T, Blazek K, Smallie T, Alzabin S, Lockstone H, Sahgal N, Hussell T, Feldmann M, Udalova IA (2011) IRF5 promotes inflammatory macrophage polarization and TH1-TH17 responses. Nat Immunol 12(3):231–238. doi:10.1038/ni.1990, ni.1990 [pii]

Laskowitz DT, Thekdi AD, Thekdi SD, Han SK, Myers JK, Pizzo SV, Bennett ER (2001) Downregulation of microglial activation by apolipoprotein E and apoE-mimetic peptides. Exp Neurol 167(1):74–85. doi:10.1006/exnr.2001.7541

Laskowitz DT, Song P, Wang H, Mace B, Sullivan PM, Vitek MP, Dawson HN (2010) Traumatic brain injury exacerbates neurodegenerative pathology: improvement with an apolipoprotein E-based therapeutic. J Neurotrauma 27(11):1983–1995. doi:10.1089/neu.2010.1396

Li FQ, Sempowski GD, McKenna SE, Laskowitz DT, Colton CA, Vitek MP (2006) Apolipoprotein E-derived peptides ameliorate clinical disability and inflammatory infiltrates into the spinal cord in a murine model of multiple sclerosis. J Pharmacol Exp Ther 318(3):956–965. doi:10.1124/jpet.106.103671

McMahon M, Brahn E (2008) Inflammatory lipids as a target for therapy in the rheumatic diseases. Expert Opin Investig Drugs 17(8):1213–1224. doi:10.1517/13543784.17.8.1213

Mineo C, Yuhanna IS, Quon MJ, Shaul PW (2003) High density lipoprotein-induced endothelial nitric-oxide synthase activation is mediated by Akt and MAP kinases. J Biol Chem 278(11):9142–9149

Nandedkar SD, Weihrauch D, Xu H, Shi Y, Feroah T, Hutchins W, Rickaby DA, Duzgunes N, Hillery CA, Konduri KS, Pritchard KA Jr (2011) D-4F, an apoA-1 mimetic, decreases airway hyperresponsiveness, inflammation, and oxidative stress in a murine model of asthma. J Lipid Res 52(3):499–508. doi:10.1194/jlr.M012724

Navab M, Berliner JA, Watson AD, Hama SY, Territo MC, Lusis AJ, Shih DM, Van Lenten BJ, Frank JS, Demer LL, Edwards PA, Fogelman AM (1996) The Yin and Yang of oxidation in the development of the fatty streak. A review based on the 1994 George Lyman Duff Memorial Lecture. Arterioscler Thromb Vasc Biol 16(7):831–842

Navab M, Anantharamaiah GM, Hama S, Garber DW, Chaddha M, Hough G, Lallone R, Fogelman AM (2002) Oral administration of an Apo A-I mimetic Peptide synthesized from D-amino acids dramatically reduces atherosclerosis in mice independent of plasma cholesterol. Circulation 105(3):290–292

Onufrak S, Abramson J, Vaccarino V (2007) Adult-onset asthma is associated with increased carotid atherosclerosis among women in the Atherosclerosis Risk in Communities (ARIC) study. Atherosclerosis 195(1):129–137. doi:10.1016/j.atherosclerosis.2006.09.004, S0021-9150(06)00547-8 [pii]

Ou J, Ou Z, Jones DW, Holzhauer S, Hatoum OA, Ackerman AW, Weihrauch DW, Gutterman DD, Guice K, Oldham KT, Hillery CA, Pritchard KA Jr (2003a) L-4F, an apolipoprotein A-1 mimetic, dramatically improves vasodilation in hypercholesterolemia and sickle cell disease. Circulation 107(18):2337–2341

Ou Z, Ou J, Ackerman AW, Oldham KT, Pritchard KA Jr (2003b) L-4F, an apolipoprotein A-1 mimetic, restores nitric oxide and superoxide anion balance in low-density lipoprotein-treated endothelial cells. Circulation 107(11):1520–1524

Ou J, Wang J, Xu H, Ou Z, Sorci-Thomas MG, Jones DW, Signorino P, Densmore JC, Kaul S, Oldham KT, Pritchard KA Jr (2005) Effects of D-4F on vasodilation and vessel wall thickness in hypercholesterolemic LDL receptor-null and LDL receptor/apolipoprotein A-I double-knockout mice on Western diet. Circ Res 97(11):1190–1197

Plump AS, Azrolan N, Odaka H, Wu L, Jiang X, Tall A, Eisenberg S, Breslow JL (1997) ApoA-I knockout mice: characterization of HDL metabolism in homozygotes and identification of a post-RNA mechanism of apoA-I up-regulation in heterozygotes. J Lipid Res 38(5):1033–1047

Pritchard KA Jr, Groszek L, Smalley DM, Sessa WC, Wu M, Villalon P, Wolin MS, Stemerman MB (1995) Native low-density lipoprotein increases endothelial cell nitric oxide synthase generation of superoxide anion. Circ Res 77(3):510–518

Pritchard KA, Ackerman AW, Ou J, Curtis M, Smalley DM, Fontana JT, Stemerman MB, Sessa WC (2002) Native low-density lipoprotein induces endothelial nitric oxide synthase dysfunction: role of heat shock protein 90 and caveolin-1. Free Radic Biol Med 33(1):52–62, doi:S0891584902008511 [pii]

Schafer T, Ruhdorfer S, Weigl L, Wessner D, Heinrich J, Doring A, Wichmann HE, Ring J (2003) Intake of unsaturated fatty acids and HDL cholesterol levels are associated with manifestations of atopy in adults. Clin Exp Allergy 33(10):1360–1367

Shaw PX, Horkko S, Chang MK, Curtiss LK, Palinski W, Silverman GJ, Witztum JL (2000) Natural antibodies with the T15 idiotype may act in atherosclerosis, apoptotic clearance, and protective immunity. J Clin Invest 105(12):1731–1740

Singh K, Chaturvedi R, Barry DP, Coburn LA, Asim M, Lewis ND, Piazuelo MB, Washington MK, Vitek MP, Wilson KT (2011) The apolipoprotein E-mimetic peptide COG112 inhibits NF-kappaB signaling, proinflammatory cytokine expression, and disease activity in murine models of colitis. J Biol Chem 286(5):3839–3850. doi:10.1074/jbc.M110.176719

Sorenson RC, Bisgaier CL, Aviram M, Hsu C, Billecke S, La Du BN (1999) Human serum Paraoxonase/Arylesterase's retained hydrophobic N-terminal leader sequence associates with HDLs by binding phospholipids : apolipoprotein A-I stabilizes activity. Arterioscler Thromb Vasc Biol 19(9):2214–2225

Van Lenten BJ, Hama SY, de Beer FC, Stafforini DM, McIntyre TM, Prescott SM, La Du BN, Fogelman AM, Navab M (1995) Anti-inflammatory HDL becomes pro-inflammatory during the acute phase response. Loss of protective effect of HDL against LDL oxidation in aortic wall cell cocultures. J Clin Invest 96(6):2758–2767

Van Lenten BJ, Wagner AC, Jung CL, Ruchala P, Waring AJ, Lehrer RI, Watson AD, Hama S, Navab M, Anantharamaiah GM, Fogelman AM (2008) Anti-inflammatory apoA-I-mimetic peptides bind oxidized lipids with much higher affinity than human apoA-I. J Lipid Res 49(11):2302–2311. doi:10.1194/jlr.M800075-JLR200, M800075-JLR200 [pii]

Wang H, Durham L, Dawson H, Song P, Warner DS, Sullivan PM, Vitek MP, Laskowitz DT (2007) An apolipoprotein E-based therapeutic improves outcome and reduces Alzheimer's disease pathology following closed head injury: evidence of pharmacogenomic interaction. Neuroscience 144(4):1324–1333. doi:10.1016/j.neuroscience.2006.11.017

Wang W, Xu H, Shi Y, Nandedkar S, Zhang H, Gao H, Feroah T, Weihrauch D, Schulte ML, Jones DW, Jarzembowski J, Sorci-Thomas M, Pritchard KA Jr (2010) Genetic deletion of apolipoprotein A-I increases airway hyperresponsiveness, inflammation, and collagen deposition in the lung. J Lipid Res 51(9):2560–2570. doi:10.1194/jlr.M004549, jlr.M004549 [pii]

Wang C, Rose-Zerilli MJ, Koppelman GH, Sandling JK, Holloway JW, Postma DS, Holgate ST, Bours V, Syvanen AC, Dideberg V (2012) Evidence of association between interferon regulatory factor 5 gene polymorphisms and asthma. Gene 504(2):220–225. doi:10.1016/j.gene.2012.05.021

Weihrauch D, Xu H, Shi Y, Wang J, Brien J, Jones DW, Kaul S, Komorowski RA, Csuka ME, Oldham KT, Pritchard KA (2007) Effects of D-4F on vasodilation, oxidative stress, angiostatin, myocardial inflammation and angiogenic potential in tight-skin mice. Am J Physiol Heart Circ Physiol 293(3):H1432–H1441

Woo JM, Lin Z, Navab M, Van Dyck C, Trejo-Lopez Y, Woo KM, Li H, Castellani LW, Wang X, Iikuni N, Rullo OJ, Wu H, La Cava A, Fogelman AM, Lusis AJ, Tsao BP (2010) Treatment with apolipoprotein A-1 mimetic peptide reduces lupus-like manifestations in a murine lupus model of accelerated atherosclerosis. Arthritis Res Ther 12(3):R93. doi:10.1186/ar3020

Wool GD, Vaisar T, Reardon CA, Getz GS (2009) An apoA-I mimetic peptide containing a proline residue has greater in vivo HDL binding and anti-inflammatory ability than the 4F peptide. J Lipid Res 50(9):1889–1900. doi:10.1194/jlr. M900151-JLR200

Wool GD, Cabana VG, Lukens J, Shaw PX, Binder CJ, Witztum JL, Reardon CA, Getz GS (2010) 4F peptide reduces nascent atherosclerosis and induces natural antibody production in apolipoprotein E-null mice. FASEB J 25:290–300. doi:10.1096/fj.10-165670, fj.10-165670 [pii]

Xu H, Krolikowski JG, Jones DW, Ge ZD, Pagel PS, Pritchard KA Jr, Weihrauch D (2012) 4F decreases IRF5 expression and activation in hearts of tight skin mice. PLoS One 7(12):e52046. doi:10.1371/journal.pone.0052046

Yao X, Remaley AT, Levine SJ (2011) New kids on the block: the emerging role of apolipoproteins in the pathogenesis and treatment of asthma. Chest 140(4):1048–1054. doi:10.1378/chest.11-0158

Yao X, Vitek MP, Remaley AT, Levine SJ (2012) Apolipoprotein mimetic peptides: a new approach for the treatment of asthma. Front Pharmacol 3:37. doi:10.3389/fphar.2012.00037

Zhao Y, Black AS, Bonnet DJ, Maryanoff BE, Curtiss LK, Leman LJ, Ghadiri MR (2014) In vivo efficacy of HDL-like nanolipid particles containing multivalent peptide mimetics of apolipoprotein A-I. J Lipid Res 55(10):2053–2063. doi:10.1194/jlr.M049262

Regulation of Macrophage Polarity by HDL, Apolipoproteins, and Apolipoprotein Mimetic Peptides

Samantha Giordano, Philip Kramer, Victor M. Darley-Usmar, and C. Roger White

Abstract Macrophages are a versatile and heterogeneous group of cells which vary in phenotype and function. M1-polarized macrophages play a key role in the host defense response via the production of inflammatory mediators and cytokines. The concept of macrophage plasticity proposes that these cells can be reprogrammed to an alternatively activated, M2-polarized state, thus allowing conversion of the initial inflammatory response to one of wound healing and repair. The focus of this chapter is to discuss mechanisms by which high-density lipoprotein (HDL) modulates macrophage phenotype and function. Specifically, recent studies are discussed suggesting that HDL reduces inflammatory tissue injury by inducing macrophages to undergo M2 polarization. This response may be mediated by both HDL-associated lipids and proteins. We additionally review recent studies suggesting that apolipoprotein A-I mimetic peptides replicate effects of HDL on macrophage polarization.

S. Giordano
Division of Cardiovascular Disease,
Department of Medicine, University of Alabama at Birmingham, Birmingham, Alabama

P. Kramer • V.M. Darley-Usmar
Mitochondrial Medicine Laboratory, Department of Pathology,
University of Alabama, Birmingham, AL, USA

C.R. White (✉)
Division of Cardiovascular Disease, Department of Medicine,
University of Alabama at Birmingham, Birmingham, AL 35294-0007, USA
e-mail: crwhite@uab.edu

G.M. Anantharamaiah, D. Goldberg (eds.), *Apolipoprotein Mimetics in the Management of Human Disease*, DOI 10.1007/978-3-319-17350-4_8

Introduction

Acute and chronic inflammations are associated with the infiltration of monocytes in tissues and their differentiation to form proinflammatory macrophages (Murray and Wynn 2011). High-density lipoprotein (HDL) plays an important role in reverse cholesterol transport (RCT) and also exerts prominent anti-inflammatory and antioxidant effects (Nofer et al. 2001; Li et al. 2005; Cao et al. 2004). HDL serves as a carrier for diverse proteins, including apolipoprotein (apo) A-I and apoE, that are thought to mediate anti-inflammatory effects of the lipoprotein particle (Barter et al. 2004). Recent studies show that these cytoprotective responses are related to modulation of immune cell function (Gaudreault et al. 2012a; Ali et al. 2005a). In the context of inflammation, however, HDL levels and function may become compromised, thus limiting the protective effects of the lipoprotein (Saemann et al. 2010).

Macrophage Polarization

Macrophages represent a heterogeneous group of cells that regulate the host defense response, wound healing, and immune cell regulation (Mosser and Edwards 2008; Martinez et al. 2008). Under normal physiological conditions, monocytes infiltrate the arterial wall to replenish tissue-resident macrophages (Randolph et al. 1998; Llodra et al. 2004). In the tissue microenvironment, local factors play an important role in regulating transcriptional responses of macrophages (Labonte et al. 2014). Macrophage polarization is a term used to describe the phenotypic and functional differentiation of these cells in response to local environmental stimuli (Mosser and Edwards 2008; Labonte et al. 2014; Lawrence and Natoli 2011). Two populations of activated macrophages have been identified that can be distinguished on the basis of their phenotypic differentiation, cell morphology, and function (Mosser 2003). These include the classically activated or M1 macrophage that is induced by Th1 cytokines (e.g., interferon-γ [IFN-γ], interleukin-2 [IL-2], tumor necrosis factor-α [TNF-α]) and bacterial products (e.g., lipopolysaccharide [LPS]) (Martinez et al. 2008; Lawrence and Natoli 2011; Romagnani 2000). These ligands activate the host defense response by stimulating expression of antigen-presenting molecules and inducible nitric oxide synthase (iNOS), formation of reactive oxygen and nitrogen species (ROS/RNS), and secretion of cytokines and chemokines (Porta et al. 2009). Interferon regulatory factor 5 (IRF5) and signal transducer and activation of transcription 1 (STAT1) are thought to be critical mediators of M1 macrophage polarization (Labonte et al. 2014; Lawrence and Natoli 2011; Krausgruber et al. 2011).

Alternatively activated or M2 macrophages represent the second phenotype. This state is induced by exposure to IL-4, IL-10, IL-13, and glucocorticoid hormones (Mosser and Edwards 2008; Martinez et al. 2008; Labonte et al. 2014; Lawrence and Natoli 2011). In contrast to M1 macrophages, M2 macrophages play an important role in the resolution of inflammation and injury by suppressing proinflammatory cytokine secretion and by promoting wound healing and tissue remodeling (Mosser and Edwards 2008; Martinez et al. 2008; Labonte et al. 2014; Lawrence and Natoli 2011). These functions are subserved by the transcription factors STAT3, STAT6, interferon regulatory factor 4 (IRF4), and peroxisome proliferator-activated receptor γ (PPARγ) (Labonte et al. 2014; Lawrence and Natoli 2011; Bouhlel et al. 2007a; Sanson et al. 2013). Additional data suggest that the DNA-binding protein Kruppel-like factor 4 (KLF4) induces M2 polarization by interacting with STAT6 to sequester coactivators required for NF-κB activation (Liao et al. 2011). IL-10 is an anti-inflammatory cytokine that is prominently expressed by M2 macrophages (Mosser and Edwards 2008; Martinez et al. 2008). It reduces expression of MHC Class II antigen-presenting molecules and the co-stimulatory molecule CD86 (Biswas and Lopez-Collazo 2009; Gordon 2003). Further, it downregulates proinflammatory gene expression via mechanisms involving activation of STAT3 (de Waal et al. 1991; Iyer and Cheng 2012; Lang et al. 2002). Subsets of M2 macrophages have been identified and are distinguished by patterns of gene expression and cytokine/chemokine secretion (Mosser and Edwards 2008; Porta et al. 2009). In addition to differences in their secreted products, M1 and M2 macrophages are commonly distinguished by their expression of cell surface markers. The reader is pointed to several excellent reviews that provide a detailed description of biomarkers for differentially polarized macrophages (Mosser and Edwards 2008; Martinez et al. 2008; Labonte et al. 2014).

Macrophage subtypes exhibit plasticity in that they can switch from one phenotypic state to another, thus ensuring that inflammatory responses and wound healing are tightly regulated (Martinez et al. 2008; Lawrence and Natoli 2011). The development of endotoxin tolerance is an example of this phenomenon (Lawrence and Natoli 2011; Biswas and Lopez-Collazo 2009). LPS activates macrophages through the binding of its lipid A subunit to Toll-like receptor 4 (TLR4). Macrophages initially respond to LPS stimulation by adopting an M1 phenotype characterized by an increase in cytokine/chemokine secretion and bactericidal activity. Endotoxin tolerance is characterized by a lack of response of macrophages to sequential LPS stimulation and is associated with the reprogramming of these cells to an M2-like phenotype (Lawrence and Natoli 2011; Biswas and Lopez-Collazo 2009). Endotoxin-tolerant cells are characterized by an increase in the expression of scavenger receptors (MARCO, CLEC4a), phagocytic molecules (CD68), and IL-10 (Biswas and Lopez-Collazo 2009). Further, the development of tolerance is associated with upregulation of acyloxyacyl hydrolase which hydrolyzes fatty acyl chains of lipid A resulting in diminished TLR4 activation (Biswas and Lopez-Collazo 2009). This reprogramming of M1 toward M2 macrophages reduces inflammatory injury and initiates wound healing and repair processes. The phenotypic switching of macrophages from an M2 to M1 phenotype has been described in the context of obesity (Mosser and Edwards 2008). In nonobese mice, adipose tissue macrophages normally display an anti-inflammatory M2 phenotype characterized by elevated production of IL-10 and arginase 1 (Arg1), which limits the activity of NOS isoforms (Lumeng et al. 2007). Diet-induced obesity in these animals results in the conversion of these cells to an M1 phenotype resulting in TNF-α secretion and upregulation of iNOS. This shift in macrophage polarity is associated with the development of insulin resistance (Lumeng et al. 2007). The phenotypic response of the macrophage is thus highly regulated by local environmental stimuli.

Macrophage Heterogeneity and Atherosclerosis

Atherosclerosis is a chronic inflammatory disorder that is characterized by macrophage accumulation in the arterial intima. Endothelial cell injury results in the upregulation of adhesion molecules (vascular cell adhesion molecule-1 [VCAM-1], intercellular adhesion molecule-1 [ICAM-1]) and the release of cytokines and chemokines (e.g., monocyte chemoattractant protein-1 [MCP-1]) that promote the homing of circulating monocytes to the blood vessel wall. In a hyperlipidemic environment, monocytes readily adopt an M1 phenotype and phagocytose modified lipoproteins to form foam cells (Moore and Tabas 2011a). These responses set the stage for the development of complex atherosclerotic lesions. The ongoing release of ROS/RNS, proteases, and tissue factor from M1 macrophages ultimately contributes to the destabilization and rupture of plaques and ensuing thrombosis (Wilson 2010).

Macrophage heterogeneity has been observed in atherosclerotic plaques of rodents and humans (Bouhlel et al. 2007a; Tacke et al. 2007; Waldo et al. 2008; Khallou-Laschet et al. 2010). Lymphocyte antigen 6C (Ly6C) is a glycoprotein that is commonly used to identify and differentiate monocyte subsets. Tacke and colleagues have identified Ly6C^{hi} and Ly6C^{lo} monocytes in the circulation of apoE$^{-/-}$ mice that express distinct chemokine receptors (Tacke et al. 2007). Ly6C^{hi} cells expressing CCR2, CCR5, and CX3CR1 accounted for approximately 75 % of circulating monocytes. Immunohistochemical studies showed a 20-fold increase in the accumulation of Ly6C^{hi} monocytes in atherosclerotic plaques of mice compared to Ly6C^{lo} cells (Tacke et al. 2007). Laser capture microdissection and quantitative RT-PCR have been used to specifically characterize lesional macrophage foam cells of apoE$^{-/-}$ mice (Trogan et al. 2002). These cells were shown to express high levels of CD68. Treatment of apoE$^{-/-}$ mice with LPS significantly induced mRNA expression for MCP-1, VCAM-1, and ICAM-1 in CD68^{+} cells compared to mRNA extracted from macrophages in non-lesioned tissue (Trogan et al. 2002). Distinct macrophage phenotypes with different inflammatory profiles are also present in arteries of patients with coronary artery disease (Waldo et al. 2008). Specifically, CD68^{+}/CD14^{+} macrophages were shown to be localized in fatty lesions, while CD68^{+}/CD14^{-} macrophages were observed in lesion-free sites (Waldo et al. 2008). Lesion-free (CD68^{+}/CD14^{-}) macrophages were further distinguished by an increase in the expression of genes (PPARγ, LXRα, ABCG1) that play a role in RCT (Waldo et al. 2008). These results suggest an important relationship between the cholesterol-handling capacity of the macrophage and its differentiated state.

Bouhlel and colleagues have identified specific markers for anti-inflammatory M2 macrophages in human atherosclerotic lesions (Bouhlel et al. 2007b). The macrophage marker CD36 was significantly upregulated in carotid plaques compared to lesion-free areas. RNA analyses revealed the presence of markers for both M1 (MCP-1, IL-6, TNF-α) and M2 (CD163, mannose receptor, IL-10) macrophages in plaques (Bouhlel et al. 2007b). Immunohistochemical studies confirmed that M1 markers were associated with foam cells, while M2 markers were spatially distinct. Further, PPARγ selectively co-localized with cells expressing M2 markers (Bouhlel et al. 2007b). Subsequent studies showed that treatment of humans with the PPARγ agonist pioglitazone induced circulating monocytes to adopt an M2 phenotype but did not increase the expression of M2 markers in macrophages that had already differentiated to an M1 phenotype (Bouhlel et al. 2007b). The authors concluded that PPARγ plays an important role in regulating inflammatory injury via its effects on monocyte differentiation per se (Bouhlel et al. 2007b). M1 and M2 macrophages coexist in atherosclerotic lesions. An increase in M1 macrophage content is associated with unstable plaques, while M2 macrophages are thought to play a role in stabilizing plaques (Shantsila and Lip 2009). The ratio of M1 to M2 macrophages may thus be an important determinant of plaque rupture and cardiovascular risk.

HDL Composition and Function

The ability of HDL to reduce inflammatory injury is thought to provide the basis for its protective effects in a wide array of disease states including sepsis, atherosclerosis, diabetes, Alzheimer's disease, arthritis, and infectious disease (Barter et al. 2004; White et al. 2012; Van Linthout et al. 2008; Lewis et al. 2010; Wu et al. 2014; Cruz et al. 2008). One of the principal functions of HDL is to mediate RCT, a process by which excess cholesterol is removed from non-hepatic tissues (especially cholesterol-laden, resident macrophages) and transferred to the liver for metabolism and excretion into the bile (Lewis and Rader 2005; Fazio and Linton 2006). HDL also possesses anti-inflammatory and antioxidant properties that are attributed, in large part, to its major protein constituent apoA-I (Ansell et al. 2005; Assmann and Nofer 2003; Dunbar and Rader 2005; Wu et al. 2004; Denis et al. 2004). Helical regions of apoA-I serve as a platform for the binding of antioxidant proteins, including paraoxonase 1 (PON1) and platelet-activating factor acetylhydrolase (PAF-AH) (Bashtovyy et al. 2011). Cytoprotective effects of apoE have also been observed in the context of coagulation, macrophage function, oxidative processes, central nervous system physiology, inflammation, and cell signaling (Davignon 2005; Gaudreault et al. 2012b). ApoE exerts anti-inflammatory effects that are independent of its cholesterol-lowering property (Gaudreault et al. 2012b; Ali et al. 2005b; Van Oosten et al. 2001; de Bont et al. 2000). These properties are discussed in detail in Chapter 8 of this edition.

The lipid composition of HDL is also an important determinant of its function (Ashby et al. 2001; Baker et al. 1999). Lipid species maintain the structural integrity of HDL and regulate the activities of HDL-associated proteins (Weisner et al. 2009). Among the phospholipids, phosphatidylcholine and sphingomyelin (SM) are well represented. SM is converted to ceramide (CER) by sphingomyelinase (Nixon 2009). Ceraminidase converts CER to sphingosine. Finally, the enzyme sphingosine kinase converts sphingosine to sphingosine 1-phosphate (S1P) (Nixon 2009). Anti-inflammatory and antioxidant properties are prominently expressed by small, dense HDL particles (preβ-HDL, HDL3) (Kontush et al. 2007). The S1P content in dense HDL particles is high but is reduced in more buoyant particles (HDL1, HDL2).

Dysfunctional HDL

HDL function is altered by dyslipidemia and is associated with changes in both the protein and lipid content of the particle (Schultz et al. 1993; Assmann and Gotto 2004). With respect to protein composition, reductions in both apolipoproteins and accessory proteins that regulate lipid metabolism have been reported. Specifically, the loss of apoA-I, PON1, and PAF-AH is associated with a decrease in the anti-inflammatory and antioxidant properties of HDL (Navab et al. 2005). Under these conditions, HDL may also adopt proinflammatory characteristics due to the incorporation of acute-phase reactants, including serum amyloid A, secretory phospholipase-A2, C-reactive protein, and ceruloplasmin (Cabana et al. 1989; Tietge et al. 2002). Additional studies show that overexpression of apoA-II relative to apoA-I in transgenic mice results in the formation of HDL particles that are pro-atherogenic (Boisfer et al. 1999).

Alterations in the S1P/SM ratio influence the putative anti-inflammatory effects of HDL-associated S1P (Kontush et al. 2007). Small, dense HDL3, characterized by an elevated S1P/SM ratio, is anti-inflammatory and antiapoptotic. In contrast, enrichment of HDL2 with SM and a reduced S1P/SM ratio negatively impact HDL surface fluidity and lecithin-cholesterol acyltransferase (LCAT) activity (Kontush et al. 2007). CER and S1P also act as opposing regulators of inflammation. In contrast to S1P, CER stimulates NF-κB, cyclooxygenase-2, and IL-6 secretion and is thought to serve as a biomarker for severe inflammation (Coroneos et al. 1996). Lipoprotein oxidation is also associated with a significant reduction in S1P levels and accumulation of the proinflammatory lipid species lysophosphatidylcholine (Kimura et al. 2001).

HDL-Associated S1P and Macrophage Phenotype

Several studies suggest that the S1P inhibits inflammation by activating the PI3-kinase/Akt signaling pathway in endothelial cells and macrophages (Theilmeier et al. 2006; Keul et al. 2007; Nofer et al. 2004; Argraves et al. 2008). Hughes and colleagues reported that pretreatment of bone marrow-derived macrophages (BMDMs) with S1P inhibits LPS-induced secretion of TNF-α, MCP-1, and IL-12, a response that was dependent on the activation of the S1P1 receptor isoform (Hughes et al. 2008). Further, S1P increased the activity of the M2 macrophage marker Arg1 and attenuated the NF-κB-mediated induction of iNOS (Hughes et al. 2008). These results suggested a role for S1P in the induction of an alternative, anti-inflammatory phenotype in macrophages. Other data show that S1P induces M2 macrophage polarization by stimulating the secretion of IL-4 (Park et al. 2014). This response was associated with upregulation of the IL-4 receptor α (IL-4Rα), STAT6 phosphorylation, and activation of the suppressor of cytokine signaling 1 (SOCS1) (s) (Park et al. 2014). FTY720 is a synthetic S1P analog that has been shown to modulate macrophage phenotype in low-density lipoprotein receptor-deficient (LDLR$^{-/-}$) mice in vivo (Nofer et al. 2007). While FTY720 administration did not alter plasma cholesterol levels in mice, it significantly reduced atheroma formation. This response was associated with a decrease in the ratio of M1/M2 macrophages in lesions (Nofer et al. 2007).

ABCA1 and Macrophage Polarization

Proinflammatory M1 macrophages contribute to atherogenesis by secreting cytokines/chemokines, by producing ROS/RNS, and by incorporating modified lipids to form foam cells. The observation that HDL/apoA-I administration inhibits foam cell formation in vitro and prevents aortic lesions in vivo may be related to their ability to modulate the differentiation of macrophages (Feig et al. 2011; Rader and Puré 2005; Moore and Tabas 2011b). Data suggest that a reduction in atheroma burden in experimental animals receiving HDL or lipid-lowering therapy is associated with a decrease in the ratio of M1/M2 macrophages in lesions (Wilson 2010; Feig et al. 2011). Further, the ATP-binding cassette transporter 1 (ABCA1) may play a critical role in shifting the balance toward M2 macrophage polarization.

ABCA1 is a critical mediator of RCT by mediating cholesterol efflux to lipid-poor HDL particles. Data suggest that proinflammatory Ly6C^{hi} monocytes express low levels of ABCA1 compared to Ly6C^{lo} cells and tissue-resident macrophages (Pradel et al. 2009). The localization of Ly6C^{hi} monocytes in atherosclerotic plaques has been linked to an impaired capacity of these cells to mediate RCT. Further, Ly6C^{hi} monocytes express traditional proinflammatory surface markers, while Ly6C^{lo} cells expressed higher levels of anti-inflammatory M2 markers (Arg1, CD163) (Pradel et al. 2009). A reduction in ABCA1 expression has been shown to stimulate STAT1 phosphorylation which is required for initiation of the M1 transcriptional program. Specifically, it was shown that treatment of peritoneal macrophages isolated from ABCA1$^{-/-}$ mice with IFNγ significantly increased pSTAT1 formation compared to ABCA1-expressing cells (Pradel et al. 2009).

Lipid rafts are cholesterol-enriched microdomains that play a critical role in mediating a variety of cellular responses (Yeung and Grinstein 2007; Fessler and Parks 2011). Cholesterol depletion and raft disruption are accompanied by the differentiation of macrophages to an anti-inflammatory phenotype (Cuschieri 2004). ABCA1 has been shown to facilitate lipid efflux to HDL/apoA-I by redistributing cholesterol from rafts to non-raft regions in the plasma membrane (Landry et al. 2006). It follows that ABCA1-deficient macrophages are characterized by cholesterol accumulation and an increase in lipid raft content (Zhu et al. 2008; Westerterp et al. 2013; Ma et al. 2012). The recruitment of proinflammatory TLRs to raft structures is increased in these cells and is associated with a significant increase in cytokine secretion (Westerterp et al. 2013; Ma et al. 2012).

Ma and colleagues reported that ABCA1 expression in BMDMs from C57Bl/6 mice is associated with an increase in IL-10 secretion and the adoption of an alternatively activated M2 phenotype (Ma et al. 2012). It follows that IL-10 secretion was negligible in BMDMs from ABCA1$^{-/-}$ mice, while TNF-α, IL-6, and IL12p40 release were significantly increased. The M2 phenotype in ABCA1-expressing cells was associated with not only IL-10 formation but also the activation of protein kinase A (PKA), a prominent inhibitor of NF-κB signaling (Ma et al. 2012). PKA activation also induces the phosphorylation of cAMP response element-binding protein (CREB) which is required for the transcription of IL-10 (Ma et al. 2012; Wen et al. 2010). PKA-dependent pCREB formation was mimicked by treating cells with the cholesterol-depleting agents methyl-β-cyclodextrin (MβCD) and filipin, suggesting an important role for cholesterol depletion in directing the phenotypic differentiation of macrophages (Ma et al. 2012). Conversely, cholesterol enrichment of BMDMs was associated with a reduction in PKA activity and the adoption of a proinflammatory M1 phenotype (Ma et al. 2012). It was concluded that ABCA1 expression was required for the disruption of lipid rafts, sites of cholesterol accumulation in the plasma membrane. Raft depletion thus facilitated the activation of PKA and the adoption of the M2 phenotype (Fig. 1) (Ma et al. 2012).

Tang and colleagues have suggested that ABCA1 acts as an anti-inflammatory receptor in macrophages (Tang et al. 2009). They showed that apoA-I interacts with ABCA1 to promote cholesterol efflux and the phosphorylation of Janus kinase 2 (JAK2) and STAT3 (Tang et al. 2009). ApoA-I inhibited LPS-induced cytokine secretion in J774 macrophages in a manner that was blocked by treatment of cells with STAT3 siRNA (Tang et al. 2009). It was shown that the binding of apoA-I to ABCA1 reveals docking sites for STAT3 (Fig. 1). At this site, STAT3 was phosphorylated by pJAK2. pSTAT3 then translocated to the nucleus where it suppressed the LPS-induced transcription of proinflammatory cytokines. It was concluded that ABCA1, independent of its lipid transport function, can inhibit inflammatory responses in macrophages via activation of the JAK2/STAT3 pathway (Tang et al. 2009). JAK2 is also reported to promote M2 polarization in murine BMDMs by a process requiring activation of STAT6 (Fig. 1) (Sanson et al. 2013).

HDL, Activating Transcription Factor, and Macrophage Polarization

Recent studies suggest that activating transcription factor 3 (ATF3), a member of the CREB family of transcription factors, plays a critical role in regulating macrophage phenotype and function (Gold et al. 2012; De Nardo et al. 2014; Chen et al. 1994).

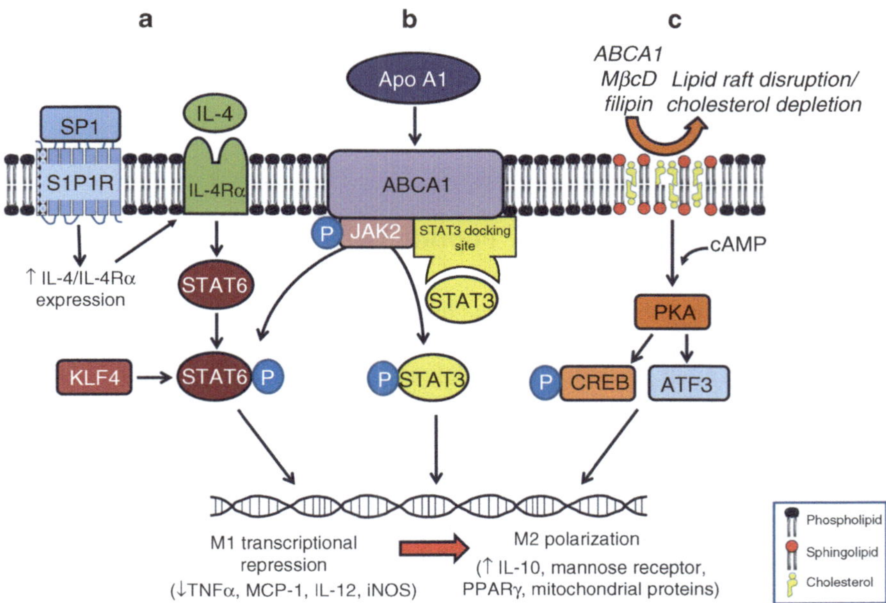

Fig. 1 HDL influences M2 macrophage polarization by multiple mechanisms. (**a**) Binding of HDL-associated S1P to the S1P1R isoform is associated with upregulation of the classical M2 activator IL-4 as well as IL-4Rα. Autocrine activation of macrophages by IL-4 induces STAT6 phosphorylation and the induction of an M2 polarization program. Kruppel-like factor 4 (KLF4) may interact cooperatively with STAT6 to induce an M2 genetic program. (**b**) ApoA-I binding to ABCA1 induces the phosphorylation and activation of JAK2. Binding of STAT3 to docking sites on ABCA1 allows the pJAK2-dependent phosphorylation of STAT3. pJAK2 is also implicated in the phosphorylation of STAT6. Translocation of pSTAT3 and pSTAT6 to the nucleus results in M1 transcriptional repression. (**c**) ABCA1 and cholesterol-depleting agents (MβCD/filipin) disrupt lipid raft structure. Destabilization of rafts is associated with the activation of PKA. The PKA-dependent activation of CREB and ATF3 induces the expression of M2 macrophage markers

Deletion of ATF3 promotes the formation of 25-hydroxycholesterol and foam cell formation in apoE$^{-/-}$ mice suggesting a role for the transcription factor in regulating macrophage lipid metabolism (Gold et al. 2012). More recently, it was shown that HDL induces an anti-inflammatory phenotype in macrophages by upregulating ATF3 (De Nardo et al. 2014). HDL attenuated cytokine formation in BMDMs in response to multiple TLR agonists. RNA profiling studies showed that HDL upregulated ATF3, a response that was associated with increased ATF3 binding to target gene promoters for IL-6, IL-12, and TNF-α (De Nardo et al. 2014). The authors concluded that HDL induces an anti-inflammatory program in macrophages by upregulating ATF3 which binds to promoters of proinflammatory genes and suppresses their transcription. The activation of ATF3 is likely dependent on the ABCA1-dependent activation of PKA, as described by Ma and colleagues (2012). As noted previously, the anti-inflammatory M2 macrophage phenotype associated with endotoxin tolerance requires the induction of ATF3 (Biswas and Lopez-Collazo 2009; Gilchrist et al. 2006). This response is similarly dependent on PKA activation, since it was shown that N6-benzoyladenosine-3,5-cAMP downregulated cytokine expression and upregulated IL-10 expression in endotoxin-treated rat microglia (Liu et al. 2011).

Apolipoprotein A-I Mimetic Peptide Design

Inflammation alters both HDL levels and function, thus limiting the atheroprotective effects of the lipoprotein (Asztalos and Schaefer 2003; Ansell et al. 2005). Attention has focused in recent years on the development of new therapies that increase the functional properties of HDL (Navab et al. 2004). One approach has been to develop synthetic, apolipoprotein A-I mimetic peptides. These peptides are functionally similar to native apolipoproteins but possess unique structural properties. A feature common to most apoA-I mimetic peptides is that they mediate cholesterol removal from cells and possess anti-inflammatory properties (Wool et al. 2009, 2011; Remaley et al. 2003; Ditiatkovski et al. 2013; Bielicki et al. 2010; Tabet et al. 2010; Yao et al. 2011). Segrest identified the class A amphipathic helix as a common structural motif present in exchangeable apolipoproteins (Segrest et al. 1974). The class A helix was defined as an α-helix with opposing polar and nonpolar faces that are hydrophilic and hydrophobic, respectively. This configuration resulted in the formation of a structure that was complementary to that of phospholipids and thus facilitated the formation of protein: lipid complexes (Segrest et al. 1974). Anantharamaiah went on to design the model peptide 18A that was composed of 18 amino acids (DWLKAFYDKVAEKLKEAF) and possessed a class A amphipathic structure (Anantharamaiah et al. 1985). 18A was shown to form small HDL-like particles in the presence of phospholipid and mimicked the properties of apoA-I (Anantharamaiah et al. 1985). A family of apoA-I mimetic peptides was developed that were structural variants of 18A. It was found that sequential substitution of aliphatic amino acids (Leu, Val) on the nonpolar face of 18A with phenylalanine (F) resulted in the formation of class A peptides with increased hydrophobicity and lipid-binding affinity (3F, 4F, 5F, 6F, 7F) (Datta et al. 2001; Garber et al. 2001; Chattopadhyay et al. 2013). Subsequent studies showed that apoA-I mimetic peptides reduced plasma lipid hydroperoxide content and atherogenic lesion formation when administered to atherosclerotic mice (Datta et al. 2001). These peptides also reduced the chemotactic activity of monocytes exposed to LDL (Garber et al. 2001; Chattopadhyay et al. 2013). A great deal of attention has focused on studying effects of the apoA-I mimetic peptide 4F in a variety of experimental models of acute and chronic inflammation. Most reports have ascribed the anti-inflammatory effects of 4F to its ability to bind and neutralize oxidized lipids (Van Lenten et al. 2008; Navab et al. 2010). This and other potential pharmacological effects of 4F are discussed in detail in other chapters in this edition.

Apolipoprotein A-I Mimetics and Macrophage Phenotype

The first study to suggest a direct modulatory effect of 4F on monocyte/macrophage function was reported by Van Lenten and colleagues (Van Lenten et al. 2002). They demonstrated that 4F, similar to apoA-I, inhibited the contact-mediated activation of monocytes by T lymphocytes under in vitro conditions (Van Lenten et al. 2002). The study showed that incubation of monocytes with T cells resulted in a prominent increase in IL-6 release that was inhibited in a concentration-dependent manner by 4F. Under the same conditions, 4F induced a significant increase in the secretion of the anti-inflammatory cytokine IL-10 (Van Lenten et al. 2002). We subsequently reported that 4F and apoA-I reduce proinflammatory responses of human monocytes (Smythies et al. 2010). Primary human monocytes were isolated and cultured in the presence of 4F, apoA-I, or saline vehicle. Treatment of monocytes with the peptide or apoA-I was subsequently shown to reduce the binding of these cells to LPS-primed human umbilical vein endothelial cells (Smythies et al. 2010). Transendothelial migration of 4F-treated monocytes was also reduced compared to vehicle treatment (Smythies et al. 2010). These responses were associated with a reduction in the expression of the integrin subunit CD49d which is required for binding to VCAM-1 on target cells. Furthermore, both treatments disrupted membrane-associated lipid rafts (Smythies et al. 2010).

The coordinated response of monocytes/macrophages to inflammatory stimuli is thought to be due to the localization of specific proteins in lipid rafts (Fessler and Parks 2011; Simons and Toomre 2000; Cuschieri 2004). Fcγ receptors, CD14, TLR4, HLA-DR, CD49d, CD11b, and CD11c are markers of proinflammatory macrophages that are localized to raft domains (Cuschieri 2004; Simons and Toomre 2000; Cuschieri 2004; Bournazos et al. 2009). We previously reported that treatment of human monocytes with 4F or apoA-I over a 7-day treatment period yielded an adherent population of cells that possessed a macrophage-like phenotype (Smythies et al. 2010). 4F or apoA-I treatment reduced cellular cholesterol content and expression of the raft-associated protein caveolin in these monocyte-derived macrophages (MDMs) (White et al. 2012; Smythies et al. 2010). CD14 and TLR4 are cell surface receptors for LPS and proinflammatory lipids that are known to localize in lipid rafts and are prominently expressed by M1 macrophages. Flow cytometry studies showed that 4F reduced the expression of both receptors in MDMs (Smythies et al. 2010). Functional analyses of MDMs revealed that 4F reduced LPS-dependent TLR4 recycling, phosphorylation of IκBα, and NF-κB activation/translocation (White et al. 2012). It followed that the secretion of TNF-α and IL-6 induced by LPS or lipoteichoic acid was significantly reduced by 4F treatment (White et al. 2012). Flow cytometry studies also showed that 4F reduced the surface expression of M1 macrophage markers including HLA-DR, CD86, CD11b, and CD11c, compared to control cells, suggesting an alteration in macrophage phenotype (Smythies et al. 2010). 4F also abolished the

LPS-induced upregulation of mRNA for MCP-1, macrophage inflammatory protein-1, RANTES , IL-6, and TNF-α. In contrast, expression levels for the M2 macrophage markers IL-10 and mannose receptor were significantly increased by 4F. Collectively, these changes reflect the adoption of an M2 phenotype (Smythies et al. 2010). Further, transcriptional profiling studies show that 4F regulates a number of macrophage genes that play a role in inflammation, including TLR5/6 and components of MyD88-dependent (MyD88, TRAF6, IRAK4, and IKBKB) and MyD88-independent (IRF3, TBK1, and TRIF) signaling pathways (White et al. 2012).

Cellular Bioenergetics and Macrophage Phenotype

Classically activated M1 and alternatively activated M2 macrophages possess different metabolic profiles (Vats et al. 2006). Glycolytic activity is enhanced in M1 macrophages due to the increased requirement for the rapid generation of ATP for cellular processes such as respiratory burst activity (Rodriguez-Prados et al. 2010). In contrast, an increase in oxidative phosphorylation in M2 macrophages is thought to facilitate secretion of proteins that facilitate wound repair and healing, processes that require the sustained but not necessarily rapid generation of ATP (Odegaard et al. 2007, 2008). As a result, mitochondrial oxygen consumption is significantly increased in M2 compared to M1 macrophages (Tavakoli et al. 2013). Further, treatment of tissue-resident macrophages with inhibitors of oxidative phosphorylation prevents M2 macrophage differentiation, as revealed by a reduction in Arg1 expression and upregulation of proinflammatory cytokines (Vats et al. 2006). PPARγ is thought to play a critical role in M2 macrophage differentiation via stimulatory effects on mitochondrial respiration (Vats et al. 2006; Bensinger and Tontonoz 2008). This response is dependent on the expression of the PPARγ coactivator PGC-1β and its transcriptional regulator STAT6 (Vats et al. 2006). PPARγ also facilitates cholesterol removal by inducing ABCA1 expression and suppresses M1 macrophage activation by downregulating iNOS, IL-6, cyclooxygenase-2, and components of the NF-κB pathway (Vats et al. 2006; Alleva et al. 2002; Rigamonti et al. 2008).

The adoption of an M2-like phenotype in 4F-treated, human macrophages is associated with an increase in mitochondrial respiration. Specifically, 4F increased basal and ATP-linked oxygen consumption rates (OCR) as well as maximal uncoupled mitochondrial respiration compared to cells treated with saline (Fig. 2). The 4F-mediated increase in oligomycin-sensitive OCR (ATP-linked OCR) reflects a stimulatory effect of 4F on mitochondrial ATP formation, while the increased maximal OCR induced by the uncoupling agent FCCP reveals an increase in the overall activity of the electron transport chain (Brand and Nicholls 2011). The observation that cellular cholesterol depletion upregulates PPARγ suggests a possible signaling mechanism to explain the effect of 4F on M2 macrophage differentiation (Fajas et al. 1999).

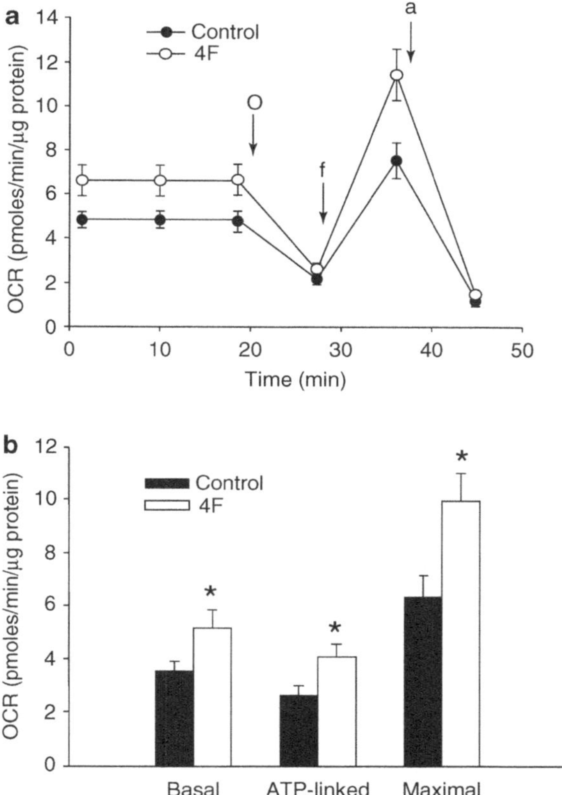

Fig. 2 The apolipoprotein A-I mimetic peptide 4F increases mitochondrial oxygen consumption in human macrophages. (**a**) Oxygen consumption rates (OCR) were measured using extracellular flux technology in macrophages treated with 4F or saline control for 7 days. After measuring basal OCR, the bioenergetic profile for 4F or saline-treated macrophages was determined by sequential addition of oligomycin (o), FCCP (f), and antimycin A (**a**). These treatments inhibit ATP synthase, uncouple the mitochondrial proton gradient, and inhibit complex III of the electron transport chain, respectively. (**b**) Changes in OCR induced by these reagents were used to measure bioenergetic endpoints. 4F treatment significantly increased basal, ATP-linked, and the maximal theoretical OCR compared to saline controls. OCR was normalized to protein per well and is presented as the mean ± SEM (N=3–5 wells per experiment). * (P<0.05) denotes a significant difference compared to control

Summary

Macrophages are a heterogeneous group of cells which mediate a variety of responses. The concept of macrophage plasticity proposes that M1 macrophages can be reprogrammed to an M2 polarized state, thus allowing conversion of the initial inflammatory response to one of wound healing and repair. Evidence cited in this chapter suggests that HDL plays an important role in directing M2 macrophage polarization and, in doing so, reduces inflammatory tissue injury. Several mechanisms have been proposed to explain this HDL-mediated response. First, HDL-associated S1P may activate the S1P1 receptor isoform resulting in the induction of an IL-4-dependent transcriptional program that suppresses proinflammatory pathways while activating M2 phenotypic/functional markers. Second, the binding of apoA-I to ABCA1 may lead to the JAK2-dependent activation of STAT3 and STAT6 which both induce an M2 transcriptional program. ABCA1 may also promote M2 macrophage polarization by mediating cellular cholesterol efflux, lipid raft disruption, and the activation of PKA-dependent signaling pathways (CREB, ATF3). The ability of HDL to modulate macrophage phenotype and resolve inflammatory injury, however, may be limited by reduced plasma levels of the lipoprotein that accompany numerous pathologic conditions. The observation that HDL may also become dysfunctional in some disease states has generated interest in the development of new therapies that improve the functional properties of HDL. The availability of pharmacological agents that modulate macrophage phenotype, however, is limited. While PPARγ agonists have been shown to induce M2 macrophage differentiation, administration of thiazolidinediones can produce untoward effects. ApoA-I mimetic peptides mimic effects of apoA-I/ABCA1 in mediating cholesterol efflux, lipid raft disruption, and the adoption of an M2-like phenotype. These observations may provide the rationale for the use of apoA-I mimetic peptides as an anti-inflammatory therapy.

References

Ali K, Middleton M, Pure E, Rader DJ (2005) Apolipoprotein E suppresses the type I inflammatory response *in vivo*. Circ Res 97:922–927

Alleva DG, Johnson EB, Lio FM, Boehme SA, Conlon PJ, Crowe PD (2002) Regulation of murine macrophage proinflammatory and anti-inflammatory cytokines by ligands for peroxisome proliferator-activated receptor-γ: counter-regulatory activity by IFN-γ. J Leukoc Biol 71: 677–685

Anantharamaiah GM, Jones JL, Brouillette CG, Schmidt CF, Chung BH, Hughes TA, Bhown AS, Segrest JP (1985) Studies of synthetic peptide analogs of the amphipathic helix. Structure of complexes with dimyristoyl phosphatidylcholine. J Biol Chem 260:10248–10255

Ansell BJ, Watson KE, Fogelman AM, Navab M, Fonarow GC (2005) High-density lipoprotein function: recent advances. J Am Coll Cardiol 46:1792–1798

Argraves KM, Gazzolo PJ, Groh EM, Wilkerson BA, Matsuura BS, Twal WO, Hammad SM, Argraves WS (2008) High density lipoprotein-associated sphingosine 1-phosphate promotes endothelial barrier function. J Biol Chem 283:25,074–25,081

Ashby D, Gamble J, Vadas M, Fidge N, Siggins S, Rye KA, Barter PJ (2001) Lack of an effect of serum amyloid A (SAA) on the ability of high-density lipoproteins to inhibit endothelial cell adhesion molecular expression. Atherosclerosis 154:113–121

Assmann G, Gotto AM (2004) HDL cholesterol and protective factors in atherosclerosis. Circulation III-8

Assmann G, Nofer JR (2003) Atheroprotective effects of high-density lipoproteins. Annu Rev Med 54:321–341

Asztalos BF, Schaefer EJ (2003) HDL in atherosclerosis: actor or bystander? Atherosclerosis 4:21–29

Baker PW, Rye KA, Gamble JR, Vadas MA, Barter PJ (1999) Ability of reconstituted high density lipoproteins to inhibit cytokine-induced expression of vascular cell adhesion molecule-1 in human umbilical vein endothelial cells. J Lipid Res 40:345–353

Barter PJ, Nicholls S, Rye KA, Anantharamaiah GM, Navab M, Fogelman AM (2004) Antiinflammatory properties of HDL. Circ Res 95:764–772

Bashtovyy D, Jones MK, Anantharamaiah GM, Segrest JP (2011) Sequence conservation of apolipoprotein A-I affords novel insights into HDL structure-function. J Lipid Res 52:435–450

Bensinger SJ, Tontonoz P (2008) Integration of metabolism and inflammation by lipid-activated nuclear receptors. Nature 454:470–477

Bielicki JK, Zhang H, Cortez Y, Zheng Y, Narayanaswami V, Patel A, Johansson J, Azhar S (2010) A new HDL mimetic peptide that stimulates cellular cholesterol efflux with high efficiency greatly reduces atherosclerosis in mice. J Lipid Res 51:1496–1503

Biswas SK, Lopez-Collazo E (2009) Endotoxin tolerance: new mechanisms, molecules and clinical significance. Trends Immunol 30:475–487

Boisfer E, Lambert G, Atger V, Tran NQ, Pastier D, Benetollo C, Trottier JF, Beaucamps I, Antonuccii M, Laplaudi M, Griglioi S, Chambaz J, Kalopissis AD (1999) Overexpression of human apolipoprotein A-II in mice induces hypertriglyceridemia due to defective very low density lipoprotein hydrolysis. J Biol Chem 274:11564–11572

Bouhlel MA, Derudas B, Rigamonti E, Dièvart R, Brozek J, Haulon S, Zawadzki C, Jude B, Torpier G, Marx N, Staels B, Chinetti-Gbaguidi G (2007) PPARγ activation primes human monocytes into alternative M2 macrophages with anti-inflammatory properties. Cell Metab 6:137–143

Bournazos S, Hart SP, Chamberlain LH, Glennie MJ, Dransfield I (2009) Association of FcgammaRIIa (CD32a) with lipid rafts regulates ligand binding activity. J Immunol 182:8026–8036

Brand MD, Nicholls DG (2011) Assessing mitochondrial dysfunction in cells. Biochem J 435:297–312

Cabana VG, Siegel JN, Sabesin SM (1989) Effects of the acute phase response on the concentration and density distribution of plasma lipids and apolipoproteins. J Lipid Res 30:39–49

Cao WM, Murao K, Imachi H, Yu X, Abe H, Yamauchi A, Niimi M, Miyauchi A, Wong NC, Ishida T (2004) A mutant high-density lipoprotein receptor inhibits proliferation of human breast cancer cells. Cancer Res 64:1515–1521

Chattopadhyay A, Navab M, Hough G, Gao F, Meriwether D, Grijalva V, Springstead JR, Palgnachari MN, Namiri-Kalantari R, Su F, Van Lenten BJ, Wagner AC, Anantharamaiah GM, Farias-Eisner R, Reddy ST, Fogelman AM (2013) A novel approach to oral apoA-I mimetic therapy. J Lipid Res 54:995–1010

Chen BPC, Liang G, Whelan J, Hai T (1994) ATF3 and ATF3AZip – transcriptional repression versus activation by alternatively spliced isoforms. J Biol Chem 269:15819–15826

Coroneos E, Wang Y, Panuska JR, Templeton DJ, Kester M (1996) Sphingolipid metabolites differentially regulate extracellular signal-regulated kinase and stress-activated protein kinase cascades. Biochem J 316:13–17

Cruz D, Watson AD, Miller CS, Montoya D, Ochoa MT, Sieling PA, Gutierrez MA, Navab M, Reddy ST, Witztum JL, Fogelman AM, Rea TH, Eisenberg D, Berliner J, Modlin RL (2008) Host-derived oxidized phospholipids and HDL regulate innate immunity in human leprosy. J Clin Invest 118:2917–2928

Cuschieri J (2004) Implications of lipid raft disintegration: enhanced anti-inflammatory macrophage phenotype. Surgery 136:169–175

Datta G, Chaddha M, Hama S, Navab M, Fogelman AM, Garber DW, Mishra VK, Epand RM, Epand RF, Lund-Katz S, Phillips MC, Segrest JP, Anantharamaiah GM (2001) Effects of increasing hydrophobicity on the physical-chemical and biological properties of a class A amphipathic helical peptide. J Lipid Res 42:1096–1104

Davignon J (2005) Apolipoprotein E and atherosclerosis-beyond lipid effect. Arterioscler Thromb Vasc Biol 25:267–269 de Bont N, Netea MG, Demacker PNM, Kullberg BJ, van der Meer JW, Stalenhoef AF (2000) Apolipoprotein E-deficient mice have an impaired immune response to *Klebsiella pneumoniae*. Eur J Clin Invest 30:818–822

De Nardo D, Labzin LI, Kono H, Seki R, Schmidt SV, Beyer M, Xu D, Zimmer S, Lahrmann C, Schildberg FA, Vogelhuber J, Kraut M, Ulas T, Kerksiek A, Krebs W, Bode N, Grebe A, Fitzgerald ML, Hernandez NJ, Williams BRG, Knolle P, Kneilling M, Röcken M, Lütjohann D, Wright SD, Schultze JL, Latz E (2014) High-density lipoprotein mediates anti-inflammatory reprogramming of macrophages via the transcriptional regulator ATF3. Nat Immunol 15:152–160

de Waal MR, Abrams J, Bennett B, Figdor CG, de Vries JE (1991) Interleukin 10(IL-10) inhibits cytokine synthesis by human monocytes: an autoregulatory role of IL-10 produced by monocytes. JEM 174:1209–1220

Denis M, Haidar B, Marcil M, Bouvier M, Krimbou L, Genest J Jr (2004) Molecular and cellular physiology of apolipoprotein A-I lipidation by the ATP-binding cassette transporter A1 (ABCA1). J Biol Chem 279:7384–7394

Ditiatkovski M, D'Souza W, Kesani R, Chin-Dusting J, de Haan JB, Remaley A, Sviridov D (2013) An apolipoprotein A-I mimetic peptide designed with a reductionist approach stimulates reverse cholesterol transport and reduces atherosclerosis in mice. PLoS One 8:e68802. doi:10.1371/journal.pone.0068802

Dunbar RL, Rader DJ (2005) Current drug options for raising HDL cholesterol. Curr Treat Options Cardiovasc Med 7:15–23

Fajas L, Schoonjans K, Gelman L, Kim JB, Najib J, Martin G, Fruchart JC, Briggs M, Spiegelman BM, Auwerx J (1999) Regulation of peroxisome proliferator-activated receptor gamma expression by adipocyte differentiation and determination factor 1/sterol regulatory element binding protein 1: implications for adipocyte differentiation and metabolism. Mol Cell Biol 19:5495–5503

Fazio S, Linton MF (2006) Sorting out the complexities of reverse cholesterol transport: CETP polymorphisms, HDL, and coronary disease. J Clin Endocrinol Metab 91:3273–3275

Feig JE, Rong JX, Shamir R, Sanson M, Vengrenyuk Y, Liu J, Rayner K, Moore K, Garabedian M, Fisher EA (2011) HDL promotes rapid atherosclerosis regression in mice and alters inflammatory properties of plaque monocyte-derived cells. Proc Natl Acad Sci U S A 108:7166–7171

Fessler MB, Parks JS (2011) Intracellular lipid flux and membrane microdomains as organizing principles in inflammatory cell signaling. J Immunol 187:1529–1535

Garber DW, Datta G, Chaddha M, Palgunachari MN, Hama SY, Navab M, Fogelman AM, Segrest JP, Anantharamaiah GM (2001) A new synthetic class A amphipathic peptide analogue protects mice from diet-induced atherosclerosis. J Lipid Res 42:545–552

Gaudreault N, Kumar N, Posada JM, Stephens KB, de Mochel SN R, Eberle D, Olivas VR, Kim RY, Harms MJ, Johnson S, Messina LM, Rapp JH, Raffai RI (2012) ApoE suppresses atherosclerosis by reducing lipid accumulation in circulating monocytes and the expression of inflammatory monocytes on monocytes and vascular endothelium. Arterioscler Thromb Vasc Biol 32:264–272

Gilchrist M, Thorsson V, Li B, Rust AG, Korb M, Roach JC, Kennedy K, Hai T, Bolouri H, Aderem A (2006) Systems biology approaches identify ATF3 as a negative regulator of toll-like receptor 4. Nature 441:173–178

Gold ES, Ramsey SA, Sartain MJ, Selinummi J, Podolsky I, Rodriguez DJ, Moritz RL, Aderem A (2012) ATF3 protects against atherosclerosis by suppressing 25-hydroxycholesterol-induced lipid body formation. JEM 209:807–817

Gordon S (2003) Alternative activation of macrophages. Nat Rev Immunol 3:23–35

Hughes JE, Srinivasan S, Lynch KR, Proia RL, Ferdek P, Hedrick CC (2008) Sphingosine-1-phosphate induces an antiinflammatory phenotype in macrophages. Circ Res 102:950–958

Iyer SS, Cheng G (2012) Role of interleukin 10 transcriptional regulation in inflammation and autoimmune disease. Crit Rev Immunol 32:23–63

Keul P, Sattler K, Levkau B (2007) HDL and its sphingosine-1-phosphate content in cardioprotection. Heart Fail Rev 12:301–306

Khallou-Laschet J, Varthaman A, Fornasa G, Compain C, Gaston AT, Clement M, Dussiot M, Levillain O, Graff-Dubois S, Nicoletti A, Caligiuri G (2010) Macrophage plasticity in experimental atherosclerosis. PLoS One 5(1):e8852. doi:10.1371/ journal.pone.0008852

Kimura T, Sato K, Kuwabara A, Tomura H, Ishiwara M, Kobayashi I, Ui M, Okajima F (2001) Sphingosine 1-phosphate may be a major component of plasma lipoproteins responsible for the cytoprotective actions in human umbilical vein endothelial cells. J Biol Chem 276: 31,780–31,785

Kontush A, Therond P, Zerrad A, Couturier M, Négre-Salvayre A, de Souza JA, Chantepie S, Chapman MJ (2007) Preferential sphingosine-1-phosphate enrichment and sphingomyelin depletion are key features of small dense HDL3 particles: relevance to antiapoptotic and antioxidative activities. Arterioscler Thromb Vasc Biol 27:1843–1849

Krausgruber T, Blazek K, Smallie T, Alzabin S, Lockstone H, Sahgal N, Hussell T, Feldmann M, Udalova IA (2011) IRF5 promotes inflammatory macrophage polarization and TH1-TH17 responses. Nat Immunol 12:231–239

Labonte AC, Tosello-Trampont AC, Hahn YS (2014) The role of macrophage polarization in infectious and inflammatory diseases. Mol Cells 37:275–285

Landry YD, Denis M, Nandi S, Bell S, Vaughan AM, Zha X (2006) ATP-binding cassette transporter A1 expression disrupts raft membrane microdomains through its ATPase-related functions. J Biol Chem 281:36091–36101

Lang R, Patel D, Morris JJ, Rutschman RL, Murray PJ (2002) Shaping gene expression in activated and resting primary macrophages by IL-10. J Immunol 169:2253–2263

Lawrence T, Natoli G (2011) Transcriptional regulation of macrophage polarization: enabling diversity with identity. Nat Rev Immunol 11:750–761

Lewis GF, Rader DJ (2005) New insights into the regulation of HDL metabolism and reverse cholesterol transport. Circ Res 96:1221–1232

Lewis TL, Cao D, Lu H, Mans RA, Su YR, Jungbauer L, Linton MF, Fazio S, LaDu MJ, Li L (2010) Overexpression of human apolipoprotein A-I preserves cognitive function and attenuates neuroinflammation and cerebral amyloid angiopathy in a mouse model of Alzheimer disease. J Biol Chem 285:36958–36968

Li XA, Guo L, Dressman JL, Asmis R, Smart EJ (2005) A novel ligand-independent apoptotic pathway induced by scavenger receptor class B, type I and suppressed by endothelial nitric-oxide synthase and high density lipoprotein. J Biol Chem 280:19087–19096

Liao X, Sharma N, Kapadia F, Zhou G, Lu Y, Hong H, Paruchuri K, Mahabeleshwar GH, Dalmas E, Venteclef N, Flask CA, Kim J, Doreian BW, Lu KQ, Kaestner KH, Hamik A, Clément K, Jain MK (2011) Krüppel-like factor 4 regulates macrophage polarization. J Clin Invest 121:2736–2749

Liu J, Zhao X, Cao J, Xue Q, Feng X, Liu X, Zhang F, Yu B (2011) Differential roles of PKA and Epac on the production of cytokines in the endotoxin-stimulated primary cultured microglia. J Mol Neurosci 45:186–193

Llodra J, Angeli V, Liu J, Trogan E, Fisher EA, Randolph GJ (2004) Emigration of monocyte-derived cells from atherosclerotic lesions characterizes regressive, but not progressive, plaques. Proc Natl Acad Sci U S A 101:11779–11784

Lumeng CN, Bodzin JL, Saltiel AR (2007) Obesity induces a phenotypic switch in adipose tissue macrophage polarization. J Clin Invest 117:175–184

Ma L, Dong F, Zaid M, Kumar A, Zha X (2012) ABCA1 protein enhances toll-like receptor 4 (TLR4)-stimulated Interleukin-10 (IL-10) secretion through Protein Kinase A (PKA) activation. J Biol Chem 287:40502–40512

Martinez FO, Sica A, Mantovani A, Locati M (2008) Macrophage activation and polarization. Front Biosci 13:453–461

Moore KJ, Tabas I (2011) The cellular biology of macrophages in atherosclerosis. Cell 145:341–355

Mosser DM (2003) The many faces of macrophage activation. J Leukoc Biol 73:209–212

Mosser DM, Edwards JP (2008) Exploring the full spectrum of macrophage activation. Nat Rev Immunol 8:958–969

Murray PJ, Wynn TA (2011) Protective and pathogenic functions of macrophage subsets. Nat Rev Immunol 11:723–737

Navab M, Anantharamaiah GM, Reddy ST, Hama S, Hough G, Grijalva VR, Wagner AC, Frank JS, Datta G, Garber D, Fogelman AM (2004) Oral D-4F causes formation of pre-beta high-density lipoprotein and improves high-density lipoprotein-mediated cholesterol efflux and reverse cholesterol transport from macrophages in apolipoprotein E-null mice. Circulation 109:3215–3220

Navab M, Anantharamaiah GM, Fogelman AM (2005) The role of high-density lipoprotein in inflammation. Trends Cardiovasc Med 15:158–161

Navab M, Shechter I, Anantharamaiah GM, Reddy ST, Van Lenten BJ, Fogelman AM (2010) Structure and function of HDL mimetics. Arterioscler Thromb Vasc Biol 30:164–168

Nixon GF (2009) Sphingolipids in inflammation: pathological implications and potential therapeutic targets. Br J Pharmacol 158:982–993

Nofer JR, Levkau B, Wolinska I, Junker R, Fobker M, von Eckardstein A, Seedorf U, Assmann G (2001) Suppression of endothelial cell apoptosis by high density lipoproteins (HDL) and HDL-associated lysosphingolipids. J Biol Chem 276:34480–34485

Nofer JR, van der Giet M, Tölle M, Wolinska I, von Wnuck LK, Baba HA, Tietge UJ, Gödecke A, Ishii I, Kleuser B, Schäfers M, Fobker M, Zidek W, Assmann G, Chun J, Levkau B (2004) HDL induces NO-dependent vasorelaxation via the lysophospholipid receptor S1P3. J Clin Invest 113:569–581

Nofer JR, Bot M, Brodde M, Taylor PJ, Salm P, Brinkmann V, van Berkel T, Assmann G, Biessen EA (2007) FTY720, a synthetic sphingosine 1 phosphate analogue, inhibits development of atherosclerosis in low-density lipoprotein receptor-deficient mice. Circulation 115:501–508

Odegaard JI, Ricardo-Gonzalez RR, Goforth MH, Morel CR, Subramanian V, Mukundan L, Red Eagle A, Vats D, Brombacher F, Ferrante AW, Chawla A (2007) Macrophage-specific PPARγ controls alternative activation and improves insulin resistance. Nature 447:1116–1120

Odegaard JI, Ricardo-Gonzalez RR, Red Eagle A, Vats D, Morel CR, Goforth MH, Subramanian V, Mukundan L, Ferrante AW, Chawla A (2008) Alternative M2 activation of Kupffer cells by PPARdelta ameliorates obesity-induced insulin resistance. Cell Metab 7:496–507

Park SJ, Lee KP, Kang S, Lee J, Dato K, Chung HY, Okajima F, Im DS (2014) Sphingosine 1-phosphate induced anti-atherogenic and atheroprotective M2 macrophage polarization through IL-4. Cell Signal 26:2249–2258

Porta C, Rimoldi M, Raes G, Brys L, Ghezzi P, Di Liberto D, Dieli F, Ghisletti S, Natoli G, De Baetselier P, Mantovani A, Sica A (2009) Tolerance and M2 (alternative) macrophage polarization are related processes orchestrated by p50 nuclear factor κB. Proc Natl Acad Sci U S A 106:14978–14983

Pradel LC, Mitchell AJ, Zarubica A, Dufort L, Chasson L, Naquet P, Broccardo C, Chimini G (2009) ATP-binding cassette transporter hallmarks tissue macrophages and modulates cytokine-triggered polarization programs. Eur J Immunol 39:2270–2280

Rader DJ, Puré E (2005) Lipoproteins, macrophage function, and atherosclerosis: beyond the foam cell? Cell Metab 1:223–230

Randolph GJ, Beaulieu S, Lebecque S, Steinman RM, Muller WA (1998) Differentiation of monocytes into dendritic cells in a model of transendothelial trafficking. Science 282:480–483

Remaley AT, Thomas F, Stonik JA, Demosky SJ, Bark SE, Neufeld EB, Bocharov AV, Vishnyakova TG, Patterson AP, Eggerman TL, Santamarina-Fojo S, Brewer HB (2003) Synthetic amphipathic helical peptides promote lipid efflux from cells by an ABCA1-dependent and an ABCA1-independent pathway. J Lipid Res 44:828–836

Rigamonti E, Chinetti-Gbaguidi G, Staels B (2008) Regulation of macrophage functions by PPAR-α, PPAR-γ, and LXRs in mice and men. Arterioscler Thromb Vasc Biol 28:1050–1059

Rodriguez-Prados JC, Traves PG, Cuenca J, Rico D, Aragones J, Martin-Sanz P, Cascante M, Bosca L (2010) Substrate fate in activated macrophages: a comparison between innate, classic, and alternative activation. J Immunol 185:605–614

Romagnani S (2000) T-cell subsets (Th1 versus Th2). Ann Allergy Asthma Immunol 85:9–18

Saemann MD, Poglitsch M, Kopecky C, Haidinger M, Horl WH, Weichhart T (2010) The versatility of HDL: a crucial anti-inflammatory regulator. Eur J Clin Invest 40:1131–1143

Sanson M, Distel E, Fisher EA (2013) HDL induces the expression of the M2 macrophage markers arginase 1 and Fizz-1 in a STAT6-dependent process. PLoS One 8(8):e74676. doi:10.1371/journal.pone.0074676

Schultz JR, Verstuyft JG, Gong EL, Nichols AV, Rubin EM (1993) Protein composition determines the anti-atherogenic properties of HDL in transgenic mice. Nature 365:762–764

Segrest JP, Jackson RL, Morrisett JD, Gotto AM (1974) A molecular theory of lipid-protein interactions in the plasma lipoproteins. FEBS Lett 38:247–253

Shantsila E, Lip GYH (2009) Monocytes in acute coronary syndromes. Arterioscler Thromb Vasc Biol 29:1433–1438

Simons K, Toomre D (2000) Lipid rafts and signal transduction. Nat Rev 1:31–40

Smythies L, White CR, Maheshwari A, Palgunachari M, Anantharamaiah GM, Chaddha M, Kurundkar AR, Datta G (2010) The apolipoprotein A-I mimetic, 4F, alters the function of human monocyte-derived macrophages. Am J Physiol 298:C1538–C1548

Tabet F, Remaley AT, Segaliny AI, Millet J, Yan L, Nakhla S, Barter PJ, Rye KA, Lambert G (2010) The 5A apolipoprotein A-I mimetic peptide displays antiinflammatory and antioxidant properties *in vivo* and *in vitro*. Arterioscler Thromb Vasc Biol 30:246–252

Tacke F, Alvarez D, Kaplan TJ et al (2007) Monocyte subsets differentially employ CCR2, CCR5 and CX3CR1 to accumulate within atherosclerotic plaques. J Clin Invest 117:185–194

Tang C, Liu Y, Kessler PS, Vaughan AM, Oram JF (2009) The macrophage cholesterol exporter ABCA1 functions as an anti-inflammatory receptor. J Biol Chem 284:32336–32343

Tavakoli S, Zamora D, Ullevig S, Asmis R (2013) Bioenergetic profiles diverge during macrophage polarization: implications for the interpretation of 18F-FDG PET imaging of atherosclerosis. J Nucl Med 54:1661–1667

Theilmeier G, Schmidt C, Herrmann J, Keul P, Schäfers M, Herrgott I, Mersmann J, Larmann J, Hermann S, Stypmann J, Schober O, Hildebrand R, Schulz R, Heusch G, Haude M, von Wnuck LK, Herzog C, Schmitz M, Erbel R, Chun J, Levkau B (2006) High-density lipoproteins and their constituent, sphingosine-1-phosphate, directly protect the heart again ischemia/reperfusion injury *in vivo* via the S1P3 lysophospholipid receptor. Circulation 114:1403–1409

Tietge UJF, Maugeais C, Lund-Katz S, Grass D, deBeer FC, Rader DJ (2002) Human secretory phospholipase A2 mediates decreased plasma levels of HDL cholesterol and apoA-I in response to inflammation in human apoA-I transgenic mice. Arterioscler Thromb Vasc Biol 22:1213–1218

Trogan E, Choudhury RP, Dansky HM, Rong JX, Breslow JL, Fisher EA (2002) Laser capture microdissection analysis of gene expression in macrophages from atherosclerotic lesions of apolipoprotein E-deficient mice. Proc Acad Natl Sci USA 99:2234–2239

Van Lenten BJ, Wagner AC, Anantharamaiah GM, Garber DW, Fishbein MC, Adhikary L, Nayak DP, Hama S, Navab M, Fogelman AM (2002) Influenza infection promotes macrophage traffic into arteries of mice that is prevented by D-4F, an apolipoprotein a-i mimetic peptide. Circulation 106:1127–1132

Van Lenten BJ, Wagner AC, Jung CL, Ruchala P, Waring AJ, Lehrer RI, Watson AD, Hama S, Navab M, Anantharamaiah GM, Fogelman AM (2008) Anti-inflammatory apoA-I-mimetic peptides bind oxidized lipids with much higher affinity than human apoA-I. J Lipid Res 49:2302–2311

Van Linthout S, Spillmann F, Riad A, Trimpert C, Lievens J, Meloni M, Escher F, Filenberg E, Demir O, Li J, Shakibaei M, Schimke I, Staudt A, Felix SB, Schultheiss HP, De Geest B, Tschöpe C (2008) Human apolipoprotein A-I gene transfer reduces the development of experimental diabetic cardiomyopathy. Circulation 117:1563–1573

Van Oosten M, Rensen PCN, Van Amersfoort ES, Van Eck M, Van Dami AM, Breve JJP, Vogel T, Panet A, Van Berkel TJC, Kuiper J (2001) Apolipoprotein E protects against bacterial lipopolysaccharide-induced lethality. J Biol Chem 276:8820–8824

Vats D, Mukundan L, Odegaard JI, Zhang L, Smith KL, Morel CR, Wagner RA, Greaves DR, Murray PJ, Chawla A (2006) Oxidative metabolism and PGC-1β attenuate macrophage-mediated inflammation. Cell Metab 4:13–24

Waldo SW, Buono C, Zhao B et al (2008) Heterogeneity of human macrophages in culture and in atherosclerotic plaques. Am J Pathol 172:1112–1126

Weisner P, Leidl K, Boettcher A, Schmitz G, Liebisch G (2009) Lipid profiling of FPLC-separated lipoprotein fractions by electrospray ionization tandem mass spectrometry. J Lipid Res 50:574–585

Wen AY, Sakamoto KM, Miller LS (2010) The role of the transcription factor CREB in immune function. J Immunol 185:6413–6419

Westerterp M, Murphy AJ, Wang M, Pagler TA, Vengrenyuk Y, Kappus MS, Gorman DJ, Nagareddy PR, Zhu X, Abramowicz S, Parks JS, Welch CL, Fisher EA, Wang N, Yvan-Charvet L, Tall AR (2013) Deficiency of ABCA1 and ABCG1 in macrophages increases inflammation and accelerates atherosclerosis in mice. Circ Res 112:1456–1465

White CR, Smythies LE, Crossman DK, Palgunachari M, Anantharamaiah GM, Datta G (2012) Regulation of pattern recognition receptors by the apolipoprotein A-I mimetic peptide 4F. Arterioscler Thromb Vasc Biol 32:2631–2639

Wilson HM (2010) Macrophage heterogeneity in atherosclerosis-implications for therapy. J Cell Mol Med 14:2055–2065

Wool GD, Vaisar T, Reardon CA, Getz GS (2009) An apoA-I mimetic peptide containing a proline residue has greater *in vivo* HDL binding and anti-inflammatory ability than the 4F peptide. J Lipid Res 50:1889–1900

Wool GD, Cabana VG, Lukens J, Shaw PX, Binder CJ, Witztum JL, Reardon CA, Getz GS (2011) 4F Peptide reduces nascent atherosclerosis and induces natural antibody production in apolipoprotein E-null mice. FASEB J 25:290–300

Wu A, Hinds CJ, Thiemermann C (2004) High-density lipoproteins in sepsis and septic shock: metabolism, actions, and therapeutic applications. Shock 21:210–221

Wu BJ, Ong KL, Shrestha S, Chen K, Tabet F, Barter PJ, Rye KA (2014) Inhibition of arthritis in the Lewis rat by apolipoprotein A-I and reconstituted high-density lipoproteins. Arterioscler Thromb Vasc Biol 34:543–551

Yao X, Dai C, Fredriksson K, Dagur PK, McCoy JP, Qu X, Yu ZX, Keeran KJ, Zywicke GJ, Amar MJ, Remaley AT, Levine SJ (2011) 5A, an apolipoprotein A-I mimetic peptide, attenuates the induction of house dust mite-induced asthma. J Immunol 186:576–583

Yeung T, Grinstein S (2007) Lipid signaling and the modulation of surface charge during phagocytosis. Immunol Rev 219:17–36

Zhu X, Lee JY, Timmins JM, Brown JM, Boudyguina E, Mulya A, Gebre AK, Willingham MC, Hiltbold EM, Mishra N, Maeda N, Parks JS (2008) Increased cellular free cholesterol in macrophage-specific ABCA1 knock-out mice enhances pro-inflammatory response of macrophages. J Biol Chem 283:22930–22941

Apolipoprotein E and Atherosclerosis: Beyond Lipid Effects

Robert L. Raffai

Abstract Apolipoprotein (apo) E is recognized for its unparalleled ability to suppress atherosclerosis (Davignon 2005). Beyond its participation in the removal of atherogenic remnant lipoproteins from plasma, apoE is known to exert a direct influence on numerous cells including those of the vessel wall, the immune system, and the bone marrow. The expression of apoE in the macrophage has long been recognized to suppress atherosclerosis by enhancing the efflux of cellular cholesterol, thereby preventing foam cell formation in the vessel wall (Fazio et al. 1997; Curtiss and Boisvert 2000). More recent findings have added to the list of apoE's antiatherogenic properties that include an ability to suppress myelopoiesis (Murphy et al. 2011) and the activation of circulating monocytes in hyperlipidemic mice (Gaudreault et al. 2012a). The underlying mechanisms of these new protective properties have largely been ascribed to the lipid efflux capacity of apoE both through its cellular expression (Murphy et al. 2011) and by its ability to enhance the cholesterol efflux capacity of plasma HDL (Gaudreault et al. 2012a). ApoE is also known to control cellular signaling via its interaction with apoE receptors and heparan sulfate proteoglycans, which has been shown to control biological effects ranging from macrophage plasticity and smooth muscle cell proliferation to endothelial cell activation (Curtiss and Boisvert 2000). An exciting new cell signaling property of apoE has recently emerged, introducing a novel paradigm for apoE-mediated cellular control in the cardiovascular system. Lipoprotein-associated apoE has been shown to suppress smooth muscle cell proliferation and aortic stiffening by regulating the expression of key microRNA (Kothapalli et al. 2012, 2013). More recent observations from the author's laboratory show that apoE can influence microRNA levels in monocytes and macrophages to suppress NF-κB-driven inflammation and atherosclerosis in hyper-

R.L. Raffai, PhD
Department of Surgery, University of California San Francisco & Veterans Affairs Medical Center, 4150 Clement Street, San Francisco, CA 94121, USA
e-mail: robert.raffai@ucsfmedctr.org

G.M. Anantharamaiah, D. Goldberg (eds.), *Apolipoprotein Mimetics in the Management of Human Disease*, DOI 10.1007/978-3-319-17350-4_9

lipidemic mice. Collectively, such recent findings introduce a new dimension to our understanding of how apoE can suppress atherosclerosis beyond modulating plasma and cellular lipid levels and introduce potential new apoE-based therapeutic targets for this rampant cardiovascular disease.

ApoE and Atherosclerosis

ApoE and Plasma Lipid Homeostasis

Apolipoprotein (apo) E is a multifunctional protein, privileged among plasma apolipoproteins in its capacity to suppress atherosclerosis (Curtiss 2000; Raffai 2012). Decades of research conducted by R.W. Mahley and K.H. Weisgraber along with their coworkers at the J. David Gladstone Foundation laboratories in San Francisco, California, led to seminal findings that revealed structural and functional components of apoE that contribute to its ability to promote the clearance of cholesterol-rich plasma lipoproteins by the liver (Mahley 1988; Hussain et al. 1989; Mahley et al. 1990). The "secretion-capture" process of apoE was identified as a fundamental property of hepatocyte-derived apoE that enables the protein to efficiently clear atherogenic plasma lipoproteins within the space of Disse in the liver (Mahley and Ji 1999). Although extrahepatic sources of apoE have been shown to contribute to lipoprotein clearance by the liver (Hasty et al. 1999a), studies conducted by Gladstone investigators demonstrated that even a very small amount of hepatocyte-derived apoE is highly effective in clearing atherogenic lipoproteins from plasma (Raffai et al. 2003). The central role of apoE in the clearance of remnant lipoproteins from plasma was more recently highlighted in studies exploring the role of PCSK-9 blockade to control hyperlipidemia in mice (Ason et al. 2014). Results of that study underscore the importance of apoE for the success of this new therapeutic lipid management strategy among hyperlipidemic individuals who are refractory to existing therapies.

ApoE and Lipid Homeostasis in Cells of the Hematopoietic System

Another well-understood antiatherogenic property of apoE lies in its ability to promote cellular cholesterol efflux in macrophages, including via interactions with ATP-binding cassettes A1 and G1. Both cell-derived and lipoprotein-associated apoE reduce macrophage lipid accumulation that contributes to suppression of foam cell formation in the arterial wall (Curtiss and Boisvert 2000). More recently, cell-derived apoE expression was shown to reduce cholesterol accumulation in hematopoietic stem and progenitor cells of mice-fed lipid-rich diets that reduced proliferative signaling, monocytosis, and atherosclerosis (Murphy et al. 2011). Moreover, apoE accumulation in hyperlipidemic mouse plasma was shown to suppress atherosclerosis by enhancing the cholesterol efflux capacity of high-density lipoprotein (HDL) and by reducing lipid accumulation and the expansion of activated monocytes in circulation (Gaudreault et al. 2012a).

Pleiotropic Properties of ApoE in Atherosclerosis

Beyond its pivotal role in lipoprotein cholesterol transport and in regulating cellular lipid levels in myeloid cells, apoE is recognized for its capacity to suppress atherosclerosis by exerting multiple anti-inflammatory properties on almost every cell type found in the arterial wall (Davigonon 2005; Curtiss and Boisvert 2000; Kottapalli et al. 2012). Macrophages are the main source of apoE in the arterial wall, where it contributes to suppress atherosclerosis (Fazio et al. 1997, 2002; Hasty et al. 1999b). Cellular cholesterol accumulation in macrophages leads to oxysterol-mediated upregulation of liver X receptor (LXR) target genes that include apoE, ABCA1, and ABCG1 that participate in eliminating pools of cellular cholesterol and increasing a local pool of extracellular apoE in the artery (Venkateshwaran et al. 2000; Chawla et al. 2001; Yvan-Charvet et al. 2010a). ApoE is known to reduce lipid oxidation (Miyata and Smith 1996), the activation of endothelial cells (Stannard et al. 2001) and platelets (Riddle et al. 1997), and the phagocytotic clearance of apoptotic bodies (Grainger et al. 2004) and suppresses the migration and proliferation of vascular smooth muscle cells (Swertfeger and Hui 2001, 2002). Remarkably, these protective effects persist even when apoE is present at sub-physiological levels that lead to hyperlipidemia (Hasty et al. 1999b; Bellosta et al. 1995; Thorngate et al. 2000; Wientgen et al. 2004). Studies have also shown that apoE can suppress mitogen-activated proliferation of CD4 and CD8 T cells (Hui et al. 1980; Pepe and Curtiss 1986; Kelly et al. 1994) and antigen-dependent T-cell activation by reducing the density of major histocompatibility (MHC) class II molecules and co-stimulatory molecules on macrophages (Tenger and Zow 2003). ApoE is also known to regulate innate immunity (Ali et al. 2005) and the susceptibility to bacterial infections (Roselaar et al. 1998; de Bont et al. 2000) and sepsis (Van Oosten et al. 2001; Kattan et al. 2008). Interestingly, apoE expression by macrophages is itself subject to regulation by inflammatory cytokines. While TNFα increases apoE expression (Duan et al. 1995), IFNγ reduces apoE expression (Brand et al. 1993). Thus, the diversity of cytokines generated within the arterial wall may impact on the protective potential of apoE on atherosclerosis development.

ApoE Regulation of Macrophage Polarity and Inflammatory Phenotypes

Macrophages are plastic cells that exist as heterogeneous populations in atherosclerotic lesions (Martinez et al. 2008; Mantovani et al. 2009). Their polarity is driven through environmental cues including plasma lipid levels, cytokines, and oxidized

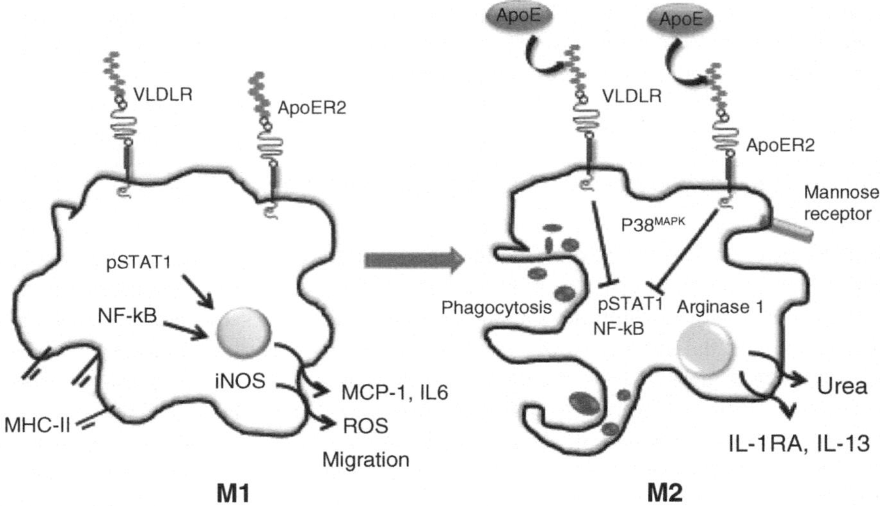

Fig. 1 ApoE promotes macrophage switching from an M1 to an M2 phenotype. Binding of apoE to the VLDLR or ApoER2 results in intracellular signaling through $P38^{MAPK}$ reducing the activation of STAT1 and NF-κB and the production of pro-inflammatory cytokines. ApoE-induced polarization also reduces cell migration and iNOS-derived reactive oxygen species. M2-polarized cells display enhanced phagocytosis, secretion of anti-inflammatory cytokines, and production of urea through the activity of arginase

lipids (Adamson and Leitinger 2011). Pro-inflammatory M1 and the more recently described Mox macrophages contribute to plaque growth and instability (Kadl et al. 2010; Khallou-Laschet et al. 2010), while alternatively activated M2 and Mres macrophages have been shown to participate in the regression of atherosclerosis (Feig et al. 2011a, b) and resolution of inflammation (Serhan et al. 2009).

A recent study introduces apoE as a regulator of macrophage polarity and effector function (Baitsch et al. 2011). Using transformed murine RAW264 cells expressing human VLDLR or ApoER2 transgenes but not apoE, the investigators demonstrated that apoE can downregulate the expression of M1 macrophage markers including iNOS while increasing the expression of M2 markers including arginase-1. Genetic reprogramming of macrophages by apoE was concentration dependent and reduced the output of reactive oxygen and nitrogen species while increasing the output of urea (Fig. 1). ApoE reduced their sensitivity to Poly (I:C) and IFNγ, leading to reduced secretion of pro-inflammatory cytokines and a propensity for migration. In contrast, apoE enhanced the secretion of anti-inflammatory cytokines and promoted phagocytosis, all features of M2 macrophages (Martinez et al. 2008).

ApoE-mediated signaling through the VLDLR and ApoER2 has previously been shown to result in the activation of protein kinase AKT via the activity of intracellular adapter protein disabled-1 (DAB1) (Schneider and Nimpf 2003). Primary murine macrophages express VLDLR but not DAB1 (Baitsch et al. 2011). Thus, apoE-mediated signal transduction in primary macrophages was found to derive from tyrosine kinase-dependent activation of $p38^{MAPK}$, which led to reduced activation of the transcription factors STAT1 and NF-κB and downstream cytokine production (Fig. 1).

ApoE Drives M2 Macrophage Polarization In Vivo

In vivo evidence of apoE signaling on macrophage polarity was demonstrated by increased anti-inflammatory cytokine levels in *Apoe*$^{-/-}$ mice that received bone marrow (BM) from WT mice but not *Apoe*$^{-/-}$ mice (Baitsch et al. 2011). Peritoneal macrophages prepared from recipient animals revealed that apoE reduced M1 cytokine production and cell surface MHC-II expression, while increasing the expression of M2 cytokines and cell surface expression of the mannose receptor (Fig. 1). The impact of apoE on macrophage polarity was not cell autonomous as primary macrophages derived from *Apoe*$^{-/-}$ mice were receptive to the M2-polarizing effects of circulating apoE in WT mice. Together, these findings highlight apoE as a potent inducer of macrophage polarity that could impact favorably in regulating the progression and stability of atherosclerotic lesions.

ApoE Controls Lipid-Induced Monocytosis

Studies by Murphy et al. (2011) uncovered yet another property through which apoE suppresses atherosclerosis beyond reducing plasma cholesterol levels. The authors previously reported that impaired cellular cholesterol efflux caused by the combined genetic deletion of ABCA1 and ABCG1 in mice resulted in the hyperproliferation of hematopoietic stem and multipotential progenitor cells (HSPCs) in the bone marrow, causing myeloproliferation and monocytosis (Yvan-Charvet et al. 2010a, b). HSPC hyperproliferation was linked to increased cholesterol-rich lipid rafts and the common beta-subunit (CBS) of the IL-3/GM-CSF receptor in the plasma membrane that led to enhanced proliferative signaling (Yvan-Charvet et al. 2010a, b). Because both apoA-I and apoE participate in mediating cellular cholesterol efflux (Yvan-Charvet et al. 2010a), their participation in controlling lipid-driven HSPC proliferation and monocytosis was investigated. *Apoe*$^{-/-}$ mice fed a high-fat diet displayed robust HSPC proliferation in the bone marrow and developed neutrophilia and monocytosis. In contrast, hyperlipidemic *Ldlr*$^{-/-}$ mice and *Apoa-I*$^{-/-}$ mice displayed only moderately increased HSPC proliferation and monocytosis (Murphy et al. 2011). These findings demonstrated that apoE but not apoA-I participates to actively suppress HSPC proliferation in mice fed a lipid-rich diet.

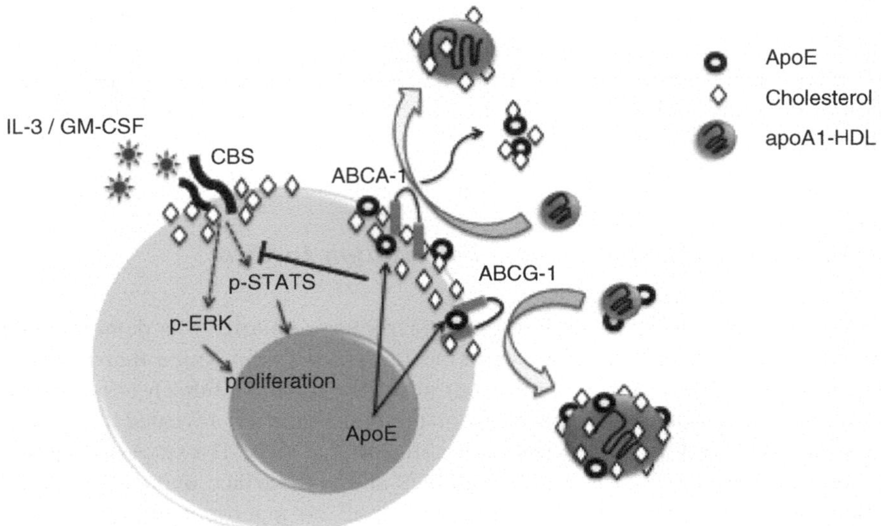

Fig. 2 ApoE suppression of lipid-induced HSPC hyperproliferation. Hyperlipidemia promotes HSPC proliferation by enriching the plasma membrane with cholesterol-rich lipid rafts and the common beta-subunit (*CBS*) of the IL-3 and GM-CSF receptor and thereby growth signaling via p-ERK and p-STAT. ApoE produced by HSPC can become anchored to the cell membrane where it promotes cholesterol efflux via ABCA-1 and ABCG-1 reducing cell surface lipid rafts, the CBS, and growth signaling. HDL containing apoA1 in plasma can also suppress HSPC proliferation by promoting cholesterol efflux via ABCA-1. HDL containing apoE could also suppress HSPC proliferation by promoting cholesterol efflux via ABCG-1

Cell-Derived ApoE Controls Lipid-Induced HSPC Proliferation via ABCA-1/ABCG-1

ApoE was found to be expressed by HSPCs, which could be induced by LXR activators that had previously been shown to suppress their proliferation (Yvan-Charvet et al. 2010b). ApoE expression by HSPCs led to its becoming anchored on the cell surface through interactions with HSPG, similar to how it is known to occur on hepatocytes (Mahley and Ji 1999) and macrophages (Lin et al. 2001) where it participates in cellular lipid transport. The importance of cell surface pools of apoE in controlling HSPC proliferation was demonstrated by reduced cellular proliferation following heparinase treatment even after stimulation with LXR activators and IL3. Importantly, apoE-mediated HSPC proliferative control was shown to be mediated through ABCA1 and ABCG1, as in their absence pools of cell surface apoE no longer suppressed proliferation (Murphy et al. 2011) (Fig. 2).

A series of competitive cell transfer experiments demonstrated that cell-derived but not circulating apoE plays a key role in suppressing diet-induced HSPC proliferation and myeloproliferation. ApoE-deficient HSPCs displayed enhanced proliferation when infused into hyperlipidemic *Ldlr*$^{-/-}$ mice that contributed to more monocytes and neutrophils in the circulation and the spleen. Moreover, greater proportions of monocytes derived from apoE-deficient BM displayed markers of cellular activation including the Ly6C antigen and VLA-4 adhesion molecule, which led to their preferential recruitment into established atheroma (Murphy et al. 2011).

Finally, the authors demonstrated that endogenous apoE controlled lipid-induced HSPC proliferation by reducing cellular cholesterol levels and thereby lipid rafts and the CBS on the cell surface and thereby signaling via p-ERK1/2 and p-STAT5 (Fig. 2). Interestingly, although physiological levels of circulating apoE and apoA-I were not capable of suppressing HSPC proliferation in hyperlipidemic *Ldlr*$^{-/-}$ mice, infusions of larger amounts of recombinant apoA-I containing HDL particles did reduce HSPC proliferation and concomitant monocytosis. The "therapeutic" effect of HDL infusion on suppressing HSPC proliferation was associated with reduced plasma membrane lipid rafts and the CBS (Murphy et al. 2011).

Plasma ApoE Reduces Neutral Lipids and Activation of Monocytes in Spontaneously Hyperlipidemic Mice

Human hyperlipidemia often results in apoE accumulation in plasma and atheroma (Mahley 1988; Rosenfeld et al. 1993). Because of its potent ability to reduce plasma lipid levels in rodents, investigating how elevated apoE levels contribute to regulate atherosclerosis in the setting of hyperlipidemia has been challenging. Work from the author's laboratory introduced new strains of mice that spontaneously display similarly elevated plasma lipid levels in the presence and absence of apoE accumulation in the plasma (Gaudreault et al. 2012a). Hypomorphic apoE (*Apoe*$^{h/h}$) mice, also termed HypoE mice, have previously been reported to express reduced levels of apoE in all tissues due to a genetic alteration in the *Apoe* locus (Raffai and Weisgraber 2002). Deleting LDL receptor expression in HypoE mice to generate *Apoe*$^{h/h}$*Ldlr*$^{-/-}$ mice led to spontaneous hyperlipidemia that was similar to levels seen in *Apoe*$^{-/-}$*Ldlr*$^{-/-}$ mice that completely lack apoE. Remarkably, chow-fed *Apoe*$^{h/h}$*Ldlr*$^{-/-}$ mice displayed plasma apoE levels that exceeded those of *Ldlr*$^{-/-}$ mice, suggesting a defect in remnant lipoprotein clearance (Gaudreault et al. 2012a).

Elevated levels of circulating apoE in the hyperlipidemic plasma of *Apoe*$^{h/h}$*Ldlr*$^{-/-}$ mice led to a significant reduction in atherosclerosis in both the aortic root and the abdominal aorta of 5-month-old mice (Gaudreault et al. 2012a). At that time point, apoE reduced blood leukocyte counts by 25 % and led to a twofold reduction in pro-inflammatory Ly6C^{high} monocytes. ApoE accumulation in hyperlipidemic plasma led to reduced neutral lipid levels in monocytes, especially among Ly6C^{high} monocytes that also displayed reduced levels of the adhesion molecules CD62L, CD54, and CD49d involved in vascular recruitment.

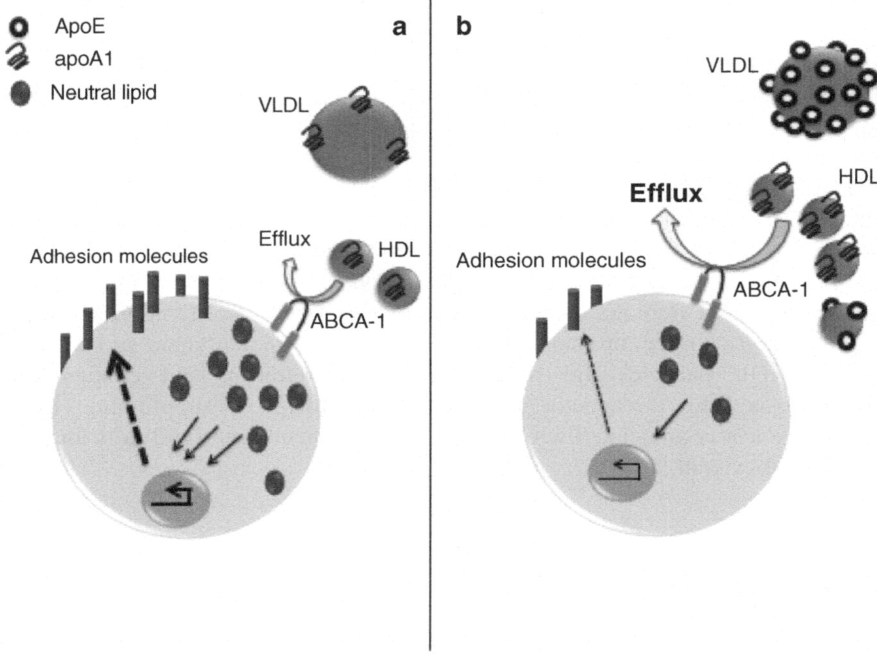

Fig. 3 ApoE reduces lipid accumulation and the activation of monocytes in hyperlipidemic plasma. (**a**) In the absence of apoE, apoA1 distributes to VLDL and HDL. (**b**) Accumulation of apoE in hyperlipidemic plasma leads to its preferential binding to VLDL causing the displacement of apoA1 that distributes mainly to HDL. This increases apoA1-rich HDL in plasma that more effectively removes cellular lipids from circulating monocytes, reducing cellular activation and the expression of cell surface adhesion molecules that contribute to vascular recruitment

ApoE Increases ApoA-I HDL and Improves Their Function in Hyperlipidemia

The protective effects of apoE on reducing blood leukocyte counts and monocyte lipid accumulation and activation were initially linked to its impact on plasma lipoprotein remodeling. In contrast to $Apoe^{-/-}Ldlr^{-/-}$ mouse plasma where apoA-I distributed among all classes of plasma lipoproteins, apoE distributed almost exclusively to VLDL, and apoA-I was present only among HDL in $Apoe^{h/h}Ldlr^{-/-}$ mouse plasma (Gaudreault et al. 2012a). This resulted in a twofold increase in HDL-associated cholesterol and apoA-I in $Apoe^{h/h}Ldlr^{-/-}$ mice. ApoE's affinity for larger triglyceride-rich lipoproteins likely displaced apoA-I from VLDL, concentrating it onto HDL (Fig. 3). $Apoe^{h/h}Ldlr^{-/-}$ mouse HDL were more potent at promoting cholesterol efflux form cultured macrophages, and this effect was proposed to protect monocytes from lipid excess. The beneficial impact of apoE on lipoprotein remodeling and plasma HDL elevation also led to reduced endothelial cell activation that could have contributed to further reduce atherosclerosis in $Apoe^{h/h}Ldlr^{-/-}$ mice (Gaudreault et al. 2012a).

Results of studies by Murphy et al. and Gaudreault et al. clearly illustrate apoE's ability to control lipid-driven monocytosis and thereby atherosclerosis. However, unlike the former study that did not find an effect of endogenous circulating apoE or apoA-I on monocytosis (Murhpy et al. 2011), the latter study did provide evidence that these two apolipoproteins can cooperate in the circulation to suppress lipid-induced monocytosis and monocyte activation (Gaudreault et al. 2012a). Moreover, by increasing apoA-I-rich HDL in the plasma, circulating apoE could have also impacted to suppress HSPC hyperproliferation in *Apoe*$^{h/h}$*Ldlr*$^{-/-}$ mice (Fig. 2). Indeed, minor apoE-only HDL such as γLpE could have exerted profound protective effects on reducing cell membrane cholesterol and lipid rafts and thereby growth signaling in HSPCs from these mice.

Conversely, the reduced expression of apoE in *Apoe*$^{h/h}$*Ldlr*$^{-/-}$ mice likely extended to HSPCs and could explain the more modest reduction in monocytosis observed in that study (Gaudreault et al. 2012a). Interestingly, conditional repair of the hypomorphic *Apoe*$^{h/h}$ allele has recently provided new insights into the role of apoE derived from Kupffer cells and macrophages in diet-induced hyperlipidemia and atherosclerosis (Gaudreault et al. 2012b). Thus, future studies of conditional apoE expression in this model may prove useful to dissect the importance of the source of apoE in controlling myeloid-derived cell hyperproliferation and activation in hyperlipidemia.

Spontaneous and Diet-Induced Hyperlipidemia: Impact on Lipoprotein Biology and Atherosclerosis

Discordances between the conclusions of both studies may also lie with a more pronounced hyperlipidemia and use of a lipid-rich diet by Murphy et al. (2011). Diet-induced hyperlipidemia in *Apoe*$^{-/-}$ and *Ldlr*$^{-/-}$ mice has been shown to be accompanied by a loss of plasma HDL and accumulation of VLDL (Getz and Reardon 2006). Such effects could in part explain why elevated circulating apoE and apoA-I levels did not impact on restraining monocytosis in those studies. In contrast, the hyperlipidemic plasma of chow-fed *Apoe*$^{-/-}$ *Ldlr*$^{-/-}$ mice and *Apoe*$^{h/h}$*Ldlr*$^{-/-}$ mice provided an opportunity to assess biological properties of HDL with differing levels of functionality (Gaudreault et al. 2012a). In that vein, it is interesting to question whether the beneficial effects of apoE on suppressing monocytosis and their activation derived solely from cellular lipid loss or whether protective effects could have also derived from cellular signaling via receptors including VLDLR as described by Baitsch et al. (2011).

ApoE4 Domain Interaction and Atherosclerosis

Another caveat that could explain the differences in conclusions formulated from the two studies may lie with the isoform of mouse apoE that was studied by Gaudreault et al. (2012a). *Apoe*$^{h/h}$*Ldlr*$^{-/-}$ mice used in that study expressed an apoE4-like form of mouse apoE called Arg-61 apoE, engineered to reproduce a unique biophysical property of apoE4 called domain interaction (Raffai et al. 2001). Prior studies have shown that Arg-61 apoE reproduces the VLDL preference of apoE4 while retaining high affinity to the LDLR (Raffai et al. 2001).

Recent studies by Eberlé et al. (2012) demonstrated that apoE4 domain interaction in Arg-61 apoE contributes to accelerate diet-induced atherosclerosis. Domain interaction raised plasma apoB-lipoprotein levels and reduced apoE secretion in peritoneal macrophages while enhancing their cellular activation, including by raising cell surface MHC-II expression (Eberle et al. 2012). Thus, the beneficial effects of circulating apoE on reducing atherosclerosis could have been even more pronounced had the *Apoe*$^{h/h}$*Ldlr*$^{-/-}$ mice expressed WT mouse apoE. Like human apoE3, WT mouse apoE displays a preference for HDL (Raffai et al. 2001), which could have further improved the cholesterol efflux properties of plasma HDL and suppressed monocytosis more profoundly. Moreover, additional detrimental effects of domain interaction including reduced cellular secretion of Arg-61 apoE by HSPC could have impacted negatively in suppressing their hyperproliferation.

ApoE Regulation of Myeloid Cells via MicroRNA: Impact on Atherosclerosis

MicroRNAs have emerged as key regulators of inflammation and inflammatory diseases including atherosclerosis (Sun et al. 2014; Nazari-Jahantigh et al. 2012). Studies from the author's laboratory have recently uncovered evidence linking cellular apoE expression to enhanced miR-146a levels in macrophages and monocytes that suppress inflammation and atherosclerosis in hyperlipidemic mice (Fig. 4). Indeed, among the numerous microRNA that are known to regulate inflammation, miR-146a is established as a critical regulator of myeloid cell activation and expansion (Zhao et al. 2011; Boldin et al. 2011; Taganov et al. 2006). It also controls the balance between pro- and anti-inflammatory monocytes by downregulating the expression of the transcription factor RelB that controls the proliferation of Ly-6C^{high} monocytes, which are recognized for their inflammatory (Etzrodt et al. 2012) and atherogenic properties (Swirski et al. 2007). MiR-146a is also recognized for its ability to potently suppress acute inflammatory challenges by reducing TLR-driven NF-κB signaling in macrophages and in hematopoietic stem cells (Zhao et al. 2011, 2013; Taganov et al. 2006). This function is crucial to prevent an immunological overload and fatal inflammation following a bout of sepsis or LPS injection (Boldin et al. 2011). However, prior to our studies, the relevance of miR-146a in controlling immunity during prolonged periods of chronic inflammation such as hyperlipidemia and its impact on atherosclerosis had not been reported. Our findings therefore provide new insight to explain the susceptibility to atherosclerosis (Plump et al. 1992; Zhang et al. 1992) and sepsis (Ali et al. 2005; de Bont et al. 1999) reported in *Apoe*$^{-/-}$ mice.

Interestingly, the ability of apoE to regulate cellular microRNA levels is not limited to myeloid cells. A study has recently reported that apoE can control miR-145

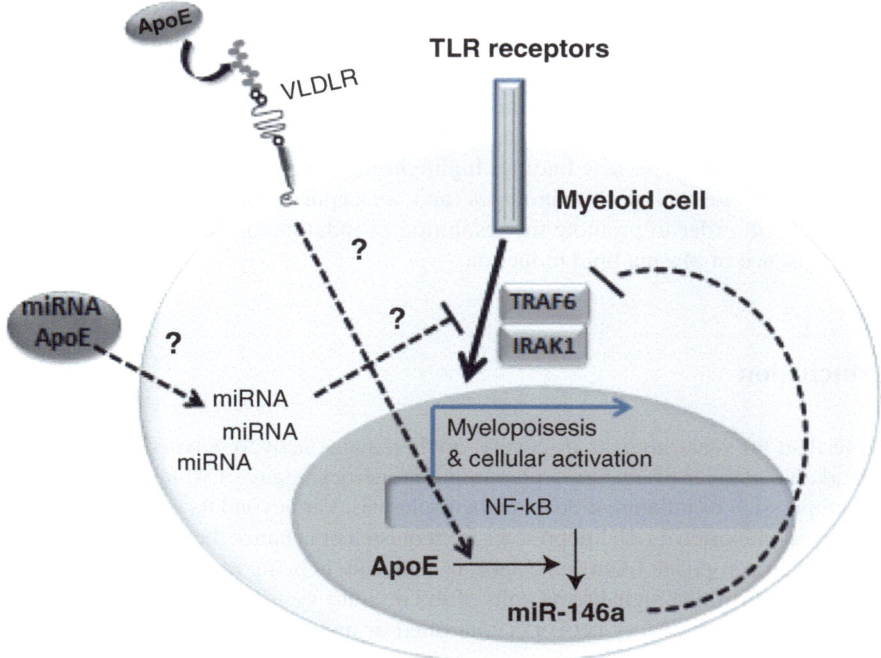

Fig. 4 Activation of NF-κB signaling in myeloid cells, including via ligations of Toll-like receptors (*TLR*), causes cellular activation and proliferation. MicroRNA-146a normally emerges from NF-κB activation to attenuate this signaling pathway by destabilizing target mRNA including TRAF6 and IRAK1. Findings from our laboratory show that apoE suppresses myeloid cell activation and myelopoiesis by increasing cellular miR-146a levels to suppress NF-κB-mediated activation of myeloid cells. This effect contributes to suppress atherosclerosis progression in hyperlipidemic mice. Whether lipoprotein-associated apoE can contribute to microRNA regulation through receptor-mediated cellular signaling via the VLDLR or other cell surface receptors is currently under investigation. Also whether apoE can alter the microRNA content of plasma lipoproteins and enable their cellular uptake via cell surface receptors is also being explored

to suppress smooth muscle cell activation and aortic stiffness (Kothapalli et al. 2013). Because apoE is known to suppress endothelial cell activation, it is possible that it could be doing so in part by raising cellular miR-146a levels that are known to significantly suppress endothelial dysfunction (Cheng et al. 2013). Collectively, these findings provide a new mechanistic link to explain how apoE suppresses atherosclerosis beyond reducing plasma lipid levels or enhancing cellular lipid efflux. In fact, this new mode of cellular regulation by apoE could explain results of earlier reports that documented its capacity to suppress type I inflammation (Ali et al. 2005) and promote atherosclerosis regression beyond reducing plasma lipid levels (Eberle et al. 2013). Also, because apoE participates in remodeling the lipid and protein components of plasma lipoproteins (Gaudreault et al. 2012a), it could also have a major impact in shaping their microRNA repertoire and ultimately their delivery to target cells (Fig. 4), a process that has recently been shown to suppress vascular inflammation in mice (Tabet et al. 2014). Indeed, preliminary data from the author's laboratory support this possibility that could in part explain the observed reduced endothelial activation (Gaudreault et al. 2012a) and atherosclerosis in hyperlipidemic mice that accumulate apoE in the plasma.

Taken together, these new findings highlight the potential utility of apoE to profoundly regulate cellular phenotypes and susceptibility to inflammation via microRNA in order to promote the resolution of inflammation and atherosclerosis in the absence of plasma lipid reduction.

Conclusion

More than 40 years after its discovery, apoE remains actively studied owing to its remarkable number of emerging pleiotropic properties, many of which contribute to the suppression of inflammation and atherosclerosis. Far beyond its well-known ability to clear cholesterol-rich lipoproteins from plasma or enhance the release of cellular lipid from macrophage foam cells, apoE is increasingly being recognized for its ability to control cellular signaling in cells of the immune system. Our understanding of the vast cellular regulatory networks controlled by apoE is just beginning to emerge. Past and more recent evidence demonstrates that apoE can impact numerous forms of cellular signaling that now include microRNA-controlled cellular gene expression, including in monocytes and macrophages. The profound impact that apoE can exert on suppressing systemic and vascular inflammation in hyperlipidemic mice is a testament to the value of targeting apoE and its cell signaling properties as a means to control human atherosclerosis. The lessons learned of failed therapeutic trials centered on apoA-I should invigorate a desire to focus attention on apoE and its mimetic peptides to harness the regal powers vested in this apolipoprotein.

References

Adamson S, Leitinger N (2011) Phenotypic modulation of macrophages in response to plaque lipids. Curr Opin Lipidol 22(5):335–342

Ali K, Middleton M, Pure E, Rader DJ (2005) Apolipoprotein E suppresses the type I inflammatory response in vivo. Circ Res 97(9):922–927

Ason B, van der Hoorn JW, Chan J, Lee E, Pieterman EJ, Nguyen KK et al (2014) PCSK9 inhibition fails to alter hepatic LDLR, circulating cholesterol, and atherosclerosis in the absence of ApoE. J Lipid Res 55(11):2370–2379, Epub 2014/09/27

Baitsch D, Bock HH, Engel T, Telgmann R, Muller-Tidow C, Varga G et al (2011) Apolipoprotein E induces antiinflammatory phenotype in macrophages. Arterioscler Thromb Vasc Biol 31(5): 1160–1168

Bellosta S, Mahley RW, Sanan DA, Murata J, Newland DL, Taylor JM et al (1995) Macrophage-specific expression of human apolipoprotein E reduces atherosclerosis in hypercholesterolemic apolipoprotein E–null mice. J Clin Invest 96:2170–2179

Boldin MP, Taganov KD, Rao DS, Yang L, Zhao JL, Kalwani M et al (2011) miR-146a is a significant brake on autoimmunity, myeloproliferation, and cancer in mice. J Exp Med 208(6): 1189–1201

Brand K, Mackman N, Curtiss LK (1993) Interferon-g inhibits macrophage apolipoprotein E production by posttranslational mechanisms. J Clin Invest 91:2031–2039

Chawla A, Boisvert WA, Lee CH, Laffitte BA, Barak Y, Joseph SB et al (2001) A PPAR gamma-LXR-ABCA1 pathway in macrophages is involved in cholesterol efflux and atherogenesis. Mol Cell 7(1):161–171

Cheng HS, Sivachandran N, Lau A, Boudreau E, Zhao JL, Baltimore D et al (2013) MicroRNA-146 represses endothelial activation by inhibiting pro-inflammatory pathways. EMBO Mol Med 5(7):949–966, Epub 2013/06/05

Curtiss LK (2000) ApoE in atherosclerosis. A protein with multiple hats. Arterioscler Thromb Vasc Biol 20:1852–1853

Curtiss LK, Boisvert WA (2000) Apolipoprotein E and atherosclerosis. Curr Opin Lipidol 11(3):243–251, Epub 2000/07/06

Davignon J (2005) Apolipoprotein E, and atherosclerosis: beyond lipid effect. Arterioscler Thromb Vasc Biol 25(2):267–269

de Bont N, Netea MG, Demacker PN, Verschueren I, Kullberg BJ, van Dijk KW et al (1999) Apolipoprotein E knock-out mice are highly susceptible to endotoxemia and Klebsiella pneumoniae infection. J Lipid Res 40(4):680–685

de Bont N, Netea MG, Demacker PNM, Kullberg BJ, van der Meer JWM, Stalenhoef AFH (2000) Apolipoprotein E-deficient mice have an impaired immune response to *Klebsiella pneumoniae*. Eur J Clin Invest 30:818–822

Duan H, Li Z, Mazzone T (1995) Tumor necrosis factor-a modulates monocyte/macrophage apoprotein E gene expression. J Clin Invest 96:915–922

Eberle D, Kim RY, Luk FS, de Mochel NS, Gaudreault N, Olivas VR et al (2012) Apolipoprotein e4 domain interaction accelerates diet-induced atherosclerosis in hypomorphic arg-61 apoe mice. Arterioscler Thromb Vasc Biol 32(5):1116–1123

Eberle D, Luk FS, Kim RY, Olivas VR, Kumar N, Posada JM et al (2013) Inducible apoe gene repair in hypomorphic apoE mice deficient in the low-density lipoprotein receptor promotes atheroma stabilization with a human-like lipoprotein profile. Arterioscler Thromb Vasc Biol 33(8):1759–1767, Epub 2013/06/22

Etzrodt M, Cortez-Retamozo V, Newton A, Zhao J, Ng A, Wildgruber M et al (2012) Regulation of monocyte functional heterogeneity by miR-146a and Relb. Cell Rep 1(4):317–324, Epub 2012/05/01

Fazio S, Babaev VR, Murray AB, Hasty AH, Carter KJ, Gleaves LA et al (1997) Increased atherosclerosis in mice reconstituted with apolipoprotein E null macrophages. Proc Natl Acad Sci U S A 94(9):4647–4652, Epub 1997/04/29

Fazio S, Babaev VR, Burleigh ME, Major AS, Hasty AH, Linton MF (2002) Physiological expression of macrophage apoE in the artery wall reduces atherosclerosis in severely hyperlipidemic mice. J Lipid Res 43(10):1602–1609

Feig JE, Parathath S, Rong JX, Mick SL, Vengrenyuk Y, Grauer L et al (2011a) Reversal of hyperlipidemia with a genetic switch favorably affects the content and inflammatory state of macrophages in atherosclerotic plaques. Circulation 123(9):989–998

Feig JE, Rong JX, Shamir R, Sanson M, Vengrenyuk Y, Liu J et al (2011b) HDL promotes rapid atherosclerosis regression in mice and alters inflammatory properties of plaque monocyte-derived cells. Proc Natl Acad Sci U S A 108(17):7166–7171

Gaudreault N, Kumar N, Posada JM, Stephens KB, Reyes de Mochel NS, Eberle D et al (2012a) ApoE suppresses atherosclerosis by reducing lipid accumulation in circulating monocytes and the expression of inflammatory molecules on monocytes and vascular endothelium. Arterioscler Thromb Vasc Biol 32(2):264–272

Gaudreault N, Kumar N, Olivas VR, Eberle D, Rapp JH, Raffai RL (2012b) Macrophage-specific apoE gene repair reduces diet-induced hyperlipidemia and atherosclerosis in hypomorphic apoe mice. PLoS One 7(5):e35816

Getz GS, Reardon CA (2006) Diet and murine atherosclerosis. Arterioscler Thromb Vasc Biol 26(2):242–249
Getz GS, Reardon CA (2009) Apoprotein E as a lipid transport and signaling protein in the blood, liver, and artery wall. J Lipid Res 50(Suppl):S156–S161
Grainger DJ, Reckless J, McKilligin E (2004) Apolipoprotein E modulates clearance of apoptotic bodies in vitro and in vivo, resulting in a systemic proinflammatory state in apolipoprotein E-deficient mice. J Immunol 173(10):6366–6375
Hasty AH, Linton MF, Swift LL, Fazio S (1999a) Determination of the lower threshold of apolipoprotein E resulting in remnant lipoprotein clearance. J Lipid Res 40:1529–1538
Hasty AH, Linton MF, Brandt SJ, Babaev VR, Gleaves LA, Fazio S (1999b) Retroviral gene therapy in apoE-deficient mice. ApoE expression in the artery wall reduces early foam cell lesion formation. Circulation 99:2571–2576
Hui DY, Harmony JAK, Innerarity TL, Mahley RW (1980) Immunoregulatory plasma lipoproteins. Role of apoprotein E and apoprotein B. J Biol Chem 255:11775–11781
Hussain MM, Mahley RW, Boyles JK, Fainaru M, Brecht WJ, Lindquist PA (1989) Chylomicron-chylomicron remnant clearance by liver and bone marrow in rabbits. Factors that modify tissue-specific uptake. J Biol Chem 264:9571–9582
Kadl A, Meher AK, Sharma PR, Lee MY, Doran AC, Johnstone SR et al (2010) Identification of a novel macrophage phenotype that develops in response to atherogenic phospholipids via Nrf2. Circ Res 107(6):737–746
Kattan OM, Kasravi FB, Elford EL, Schell MT, Harris HW (2008) Apolipoprotein E-mediated immune regulation in sepsis. J Immunol 181(2):1399–1408
Kelly ME, Clay MA, Mistry MJ, Hsieh-Li H-M, Harmony JAK (1994) Apolipoprotein E inhibition of proliferation of mitogen-activated T lymphocytes: production of interleukin 2 with reduced biological activity. Cell Immunol 159:124–139
Khallou-Laschet J, Varthaman A, Fornasa G, Compain C, Gaston AT, Clement M et al (2010) Macrophage plasticity in experimental atherosclerosis. PLoS One 5(1):e8852
Kothapalli D, Liu SL, Bae YH, Monslow J, Xu T, Hawthorne EA et al (2012) Cardiovascular protection by ApoE and ApoE-HDL linked to suppression of ECM gene expression and arterial stiffening. Cell Rep 2(5):1259–1271, Epub 2012/10/30
Kothapalli D, Castagnino P, Rader DJ, Phillips MC, Lund-Katz S, Assoian RK (2013) Apolipoprotein E-mediated cell cycle arrest linked to p27 and the Cox2-dependent repression of miR221/222. Atherosclerosis 227(1):65–71
Lin C-Y, Huang ZH, Mazzone T (2001) Interaction with proteoglycans enhances the sterol efflux produced by endogenous expression of macrophage apoE. J Lipid Res 42:1125–1133
Mahley RW (1988) Apolipoprotein E: cholesterol transport protein with expanding role in cell biology. Science 240:622–630
Mahley RW, Ji ZS (1999) Remnant lipoprotein metabolism: key pathways involving cell-surface heparan sulfate proteoglycans and apolipoprotein E. J Lipid Res 40(1):1–16
Mahley RW, Innerarity TL, Rall SC Jr, Weisgraber KH, Taylor JM (1990) Apolipoprotein E: genetic variants provide insights into its structure and function. Curr Opin Lipidol 1:87–95
Mantovani A, Garlanda C, Locati M (2009) Macrophage diversity and polarization in atherosclerosis: a question of balance. Arterioscler Thromb Vasc Biol 29(10):1419–1423
Martinez FO, Sica A, Mantovani A, Locati M (2008) Macrophage activation and polarization. Front Biosci 13:453–461
Miyata M, Smith JD (1996) Apolipoprotein E allele-specific antioxidant activity and effects on cytotoxicity by oxidative insults and b-amyloid peptides. Nat Genet 14:55–61
Murphy AJ, Akhtari M, Tolani S, Pagler T, Bijl N, Kuo CL et al (2011) ApoE regulates hematopoietic stem cell proliferation, monocytosis, and monocyte accumulation in atherosclerotic lesions in mice. J Clin Invest 121(10):4138–4149
Nazari-Jahantigh M, Wei Y, Noels H, Akhtar S, Zhou Z, Koenen RR et al (2012) MicroRNA-155 promotes atherosclerosis by repressing Bcl6 in macrophages. J Clin Invest 122(11):4190–4202
Pepe MG, Curtiss LK (1986) Apolipoprotein E is a biologically active constituent of the normal immunoregulatory lipoprotein, LDL-In. J Immunol 136:3716–3723

Plump AS, Smith JD, Hayek T, Aalto-Setala K, Walsh A, Verstuyft JG et al (1992) Severe hypercholesterolemia and atherosclerosis in apolipoprotein E-deficient mice created by homologous recombination in ES cells. Cell 71(2):343–353, Epub 1992/10/16

Raffai RL (2012) Apolipoprotein E, regulation of myeloid cell plasticity in atherosclerosis. Curr Opin Lipidol 23(5):471–478

Raffaï RL, Weisgraber KH (2002) Hypomorphic apolipoprotein E mice. A new model of conditional gene repair to examine apolipoprotein E-mediated metabolism. J Biol Chem 277:11064–11068

Raffaï RL, Dong L-M, Farese RV Jr, Weisgraber KH (2001) Introduction of human apolipoprotein E4 "domain interaction" into mouse apolipoprotein E. Proc Natl Acad Sci U S A 98:11587–11591

Raffaï RL, Hasty AH, Wang Y, Mettler SE, Sanan DA, Linton MF et al (2003) Hepatocyte-derived apoE is more effective than non-hepatocyte-derived apoE in remnant lipoprotein clearance. J Biol Chem 278:11670–11675

Riddell DR, Graham A, Owen JS (1997) Apolipoprotein E inhibits platelet aggregation through the L-arginine: nitric oxide pathway. Implications for vascular disease. J Biol Chem 272:89–95

Roselaar SE, Daugherty A (1998) Apolipoprotein E-deficient mice have impaired innate immune responses to *Listeria monocytogenes* in vivo. J Lipid Res 39:1740–1743

Rosenfeld ME, Butler S, Ord VA, Lipton BA, Dyer CA, Curtiss LK et al (1993) Abundant expression of apoprotein E by macrophages in human and rabbit atherosclerotic lesions. Arterioscler Thromb 13:1382–1389

Schneider WJ, Nimpf J (2003) LDL receptor relatives at the crossroad of endocytosis and signaling. Cell Mol Life Sci 60(5):892–903

Serhan CN, Yang R, Martinod K, Kasuga K, Pillai PS, Porter TF et al (2009) Maresins: novel macrophage mediators with potent antiinflammatory and proresolving actions. J Exp Med 206(1):15–23

Stannard AK, Riddell DR, Sacre SM, Tagalakis AD, Langer C, von Eckardstein A et al (2001) Cell-derived apolipoprotein E (apoE) particles inhibit vascular cell adhesion molecule-1 (VCAM-1) expression in human endothelial cells. J Biol Chem 276:46011–46016

Sun X, He S, Wara AK, Icli B, Shvartz E, Tesmenitsky Y et al (2014) Systemic delivery of microRNA-181b inhibits nuclear factor-kappaB activation, vascular inflammation, and atherosclerosis in apolipoprotein E-deficient mice. Circ Res 114(1):32–40, Epub 2013/10/03

Swertfeger DK, Hui DY (2001) Apolipoprotein E receptor binding *versus* heparan sulfate proteoglycan binding in its regulation of smooth muscle cell migration and proliferation. J Biol Chem 276:25043–25048

Swertfeger DK, Bu G, Hui DY (2002) Low density lipoprotein receptor-related protein mediates apolipoprotein E inhibition of smooth muscle cell migration. J Biol Chem 277:4141–4146

Swirski FK, Libby P, Aikawa E, Alcaide P, Luscinskas FW, Weissleder R et al (2007) Ly-6Chi monocytes dominate hypercholesterolemia-associated monocytosis and give rise to macrophages in atheromata. J Clin Invest 117(1):195–205, Epub 2007/01/04

Tabet F, Vickers KC, Cuesta Torres LF, Wiese CB, Shoucri BM, Lambert G et al (2014) HDL-transferred microRNA-223 regulates ICAM-1 expression in endothelial cells. Nat Commun 5:3292, Epub 2014/03/01

Taganov KD, Boldin MP, Chang KJ, Baltimore D (2006) NF-kappaB-dependent induction of microRNA miR-146, an inhibitor targeted to signaling proteins of innate immune responses. Proc Natl Acad Sci U S A 103(33):12481–12486, Epub 2006/08/04

Tenger C, Zhou X (2003) Apolipoprotein E modulates immune activation by acting on the antigen-presenting cell. Immunology 109(3):392–397

Thorngate FE, Rudel LL, Walzem RL, Williams DL (2000) Low levels of extrahepatic nonmacrophage apoE inhibit atherosclerosis without correcting hypercholesterolemia in apoE-deficient mice. Arterioscler Thromb Vasc Biol 20:1939–1945

Van Oosten M, Rensen PC, Van Amersfoort ES, Van Eck M, Van Dam AM, Breve JJ et al (2001) Apolipoprotein E protects against bacterial lipopolysaccharide-induced lethality. A new therapeutic approach to treat gram-negative sepsis. J Biol Chem 276(12):8820–8824

Venkateswaran A, Laffitte BA, Joseph SB, Mak PA, Wilpitz DC, Edwards PA et al (2000) Control of cellular cholesterol efflux by the nuclear oxysterol receptor LXR alpha. Proc Natl Acad Sci U S A 97(22):12097–12102

Wientgen H, Thorngate FE, Omerhodzic S, Rolnitzky L, Fallon JT, Williams DL et al (2004) Subphysiologic apolipoprotein E (apoE) plasma levels inhibit neointimal formation after arterial injury in apoE-deficient mice. Arterioscler Thromb Vasc Biol 24(8):1460–1465

Yvan-Charvet L, Wang N, Tall AR (2010a) Role of HDL, ABCA1, and ABCG1 transporters in cholesterol efflux and immune responses. Arterioscler Thromb Vasc Biol 30:139–143

Yvan-Charvet L, Pagler T, Gautier EL, Avagyan S, Siry RL, Han S et al (2010b) ATP-binding cassette transporters and HDL suppress hematopoietic stem cell proliferation. Science 328(5986): 1689–1693

Zhang SH, Reddick RL, Piedrahita JA, Maeda N (1992) Spontaneous hypercholesterolemia and arterial lesions in mice lacking apolipoprotein E. Science 258(5081):468–471, Epub 1992/10/16

Zhao JL, Rao DS, Boldin MP, Taganov KD, O'Connell RM, Baltimore D (2011) NF-kappaB dysregulation in microRNA-146a-deficient mice drives the development of myeloid malignancies. Proc Natl Acad Sci U S A 108(22):9184–9189, Epub 2011/05/18

Zhao JL, Rao DS, O'Connell RM, Garcia-Flores Y, Baltimore D (2013) MicroRNA-146a acts as a guardian of the quality and longevity of hematopoietic stem cells in mice. ELife 2:e00537, Epub 2013/05/25

Apolipoprotein E Mimetic Peptides: Cholesterol-Dependent and Cholesterol-Independent Properties

David W. Garber, Dennis Goldberg, and G.M. Anantharamaiah

Abstract Apolipoprotein E (apoE) has a dual-domain structure, with a four-helix bundle containing the receptor-binding region in the amino terminal domain and a carboxyl terminal lipid-binding domain. Peptides derived from the LDL receptor (LDL-R)-binding region of apoE have been studied by a number of groups, with the primary focus being on the binding of the peptides to LDL-R. Based on the dual-domain structure, a peptide was designed with the highly cationic residues 141–150 from human apoE (hE) covalently bound to the lipid-associating class A α-helical peptide 18A and the amino and carboxyl termini blocked with acetyl and amide groups, respectively. This peptide, called Ac-hE18A-NH_2 (in clinical development as AEM-28), was found to have striking cholesterol- and triglyceride-reducing and anti-inflammatory properties. Unlike statin drugs and proprotein convertase subtilisin/kexin type-9 (PCSK-9) inhibitors, these properties exist even in the absence of a functional LDL-R, with cholesterol reduction being mediated by binding to heparan sulfate proteoglycans (HSPG). Ac-hE18A-NH_2 is currently undergoing phase 1a/1b clinical trials and has shown acceptable tolerability and promising efficacy. Thus, this

---

Conflicts of Interest LipimetiX Development LLC has licensed the peptide described in this study, and Dennis Goldberg is president of this company. All authors have intellectual property in these peptides.

D.W. Garber (✉)
Department of Medicine, University of Alabama at Birmingham,
BDB Room D-654, 1720 2nd Ave S, Birmingham, AL 35294-0012, USA
e-mail: dgarber@uab.edu

D. Goldberg
LipimetiX Development LLC, 5 Commonwealth Rd, Suite 2A, Natick, MA, USA

G.M. Anantharamaiah
Department of Medicine, Department of Biochemistry and Molecular Biology,
University of Alabama at Birmingham, Birmingham, AL, USA
e-mail: ganantha@uabmc.edu

G.M. Anantharamaiah, D. Goldberg (eds.), *Apolipoprotein Mimetics in the Management of Human Disease*, DOI 10.1007/978-3-319-17350-4_10

and similar peptides have great potential for treatment of statin-resistant conditions such as familial hypercholesterolemia and acute hypertriglyceridemic pancreatitis.

Current Approaches to Cholesterol Reduction

It has long been recognized that elevated levels of plasma cholesterol, especially those of low-density lipoprotein (LDL), are associated with an increased risk of cardiovascular disease (CVD) (Gordon et al. 1981). A major mechanism by which LDL levels are regulated was first described by Brown and Goldstein (1986), for which they were awarded the Nobel Prize in 1985. While studying patients with familial hypercholesterolemia (FH), where LDL levels are dramatically increased leading to very premature CVD, they identified the LDL receptor (LDL-R). This is a cell surface protein that binds LDL through its ligand, apolipoprotein (apo) B100, leading to the clearance of LDL from the plasma primarily by the liver. When defective (as in FH), either binding or internalization is reduced or eliminated and LDL plasma levels are increased.

Perhaps the most effective pharmacological intervention to lower plasma LDL levels has been the development of statin drugs. These inhibit HMG-CoA reductase, reducing cholesterol synthesis (Endo 1992). However, this alone is not sufficient to markedly decrease plasma LDL levels. Instead, reduced cellular cholesterol leads to upregulation of LDL-R synthesis which then leads to increased clearance of LDL from the plasma (Ma et al. 1986). Unfortunately, these drugs are either totally (in the case of homozygous LDL-R deficiency) or partially (in the case of heterozygosity) ineffective in FH patients.

Recently, a new modulator of LDL-R levels has been described. Proprotein convertase subtilisin/kexin type-9 (PCSK-9) has been identified in the last decade as a chaperone that directs LDL-R to the lysosome for degradation (Zhang et al. 2007; for review see Lagace 2014). Increased activity of PCSK-9 reduces LDL-R on the cell surface with a resulting increase in plasma cholesterol levels (Abifadel et al. 2003). Both internal and external pathways of LDL-R degradation exist (Zhang et al. 2007; Poirier et al. 2009). In the intracellular route, nascent PCSK-9 binds to LDL-R and directs it to the lysosome for degradation (Poirier et al. 2009). In the extracellular route, PCSK-9 is secreted from the cell and binds to LDL-R at the cell surface, inhibiting its function and again directing it for degradation (Zhang et al. 2007). A number of approaches to the inhibition of PCSK-9 activity are being investigated (Hooper and Burnett 2013). One approach is the use of monoclonal antibodies to secreted PCSK-9, such as alirocumab (Roth et al. 2014) or evolocumab (Blom et al. 2014). Clinical trials with antisense oligonucleotides to inhibit PCSK-9 have been terminated (Hooper and Burnett 2013), although this approach is continuing to be experimentally pursued. Finally, small interfering RNA (siRNA) directed at PCSK-9 synthesis has successfully reduced LDL cholesterol in a mouse model (Ason et al. 2011), and clinical trials have begun in humans (Fitzgerald et al. 2012). Importantly, PCSK-9 inhibition does not alter plasma cholesterol in the absence of a functional LDL receptor or apoE, at least in LDL-R null or apolipoprotein E (apoE) null mice (Ason et al. 2014). Thus, anti-PCSK-9 therapy is dependent on both a functional LDL receptor as well as an appropriate ligand. This is in contrast to the mechanism of cholesterol reduction by the peptide Ac-hE18A-NH_2, which does not require either a functional LDL receptor or apoE (as will be discussed later).

Studies of Cationic Domain Peptides

ApoE is a second ligand for LDL-R (Bradley et al. 1984) but also mediates the clearance of triglyceride-rich lipoproteins such as chylomicrons, very-low-density lipoprotein (VLDL), and intermediate-density lipoprotein (IDL). It binds to a number of alternate receptors such as the LDL-R-related protein (LRP) and heparan sulfate proteoglycans (HSPG) (Mahley and Ji 1999; Gonzsales et al. 2013). Thus, even when the LDL-R pathway is defective, apoE can mediate removal of atherogenic lipoproteins to some degree. It can also modulate LDL levels by clearing the intermediates involved in LDL production, including VLDL and IDL. ApoE can be generally considered to have two domains, a receptor-binding domain toward the amino terminus and a lipid-binding domain toward the carboxyl terminus. The receptor-binding domain in the region of residues 136–150 (Weisgraber 1994) is highly cationic, leading to an early name for apoE, arginine-rich protein or ARP (Shore and Shore 1973; Danielsson et al. 1978). Mice which have been genetically modified to lack apoE (apoE null) are hypercholesterolemic and spontaneously develop atherosclerosis, which is accelerated by a Western diet (Zhang et al. 1992; Plump et al. 1992). Surprisingly, transplant of hematopoietic bone marrow from wild-type mice can prevent or reverse the atherogenesis without markedly reducing plasma cholesterol levels (Zhu et al. 1998; Linton et al. 1995). As noted in a previous chapter, apoE has many atheroprotective properties independent of its cholesterol-lowering ability (Mahley 1988; Davignon 2005).

Initial studies of the functional domains of apoE were done using proteolytic fragments produced by thrombin cleavage. Innerarity et al. reported that two large thrombolytic peptides were created, an amino terminal and a carboxyl terminal peptide (Innerarity et al. 1983). When mixed with the phospholipid dimyristoylphosphatidyl choline (DMPC), the amino terminal peptide was as effective as intact apoE in competing with LDL binding to the LDL receptor, while the carboxyl terminal region mediated association with the lipid surface of lipoproteins (Innerarity et al. 1983; Gianturco et al. 1983). Cyanogen bromide cleavage peptides defined the binding region to residues 126–218. If the positively charged residues Arg and Lys were chemically modified, receptor-binding activity was lost (Innerarity et al. 1983; Zaiou et al. 2000). The use of monoclonal antibodies further narrowed the binding region to residues 139–169, with a probable refinement of the binding region to residues 140–150 (Weisgraber et al. 1983).

Studies using synthetic peptides derived from the apoE sequence were first reported in 1985 by Sparrow et al. who demonstrated that peptide 129–160 had an α-helical structure when mixed with DMPC, while peptides which were more narrowly restricted to the previously identified receptor-binding region did not show an increase in α-helicity when mixed with DMPC (Sparrow et al. 1985). However, this peptide had low affinity for lipid surfaces and had no effect on LDL uptake by fibroblasts unless lipid affinity was increased by adding acyl groups to the amino terminus (Mims et al. 1994). Dyer and Curtiss studied the binding activity of peptides consisting of residues 141–155 and found that the monomeric peptide had no inhibitory activity against LDL degradation by human fibroblasts or THP-1 monocytes. A dimeric tandem repeat of these residues was effective in inhibiting LDL degradation, while a trimer had 20-fold greater inhibitory activity than the dimer (Dyer and Curtiss 1991). The same group also found that peptides 141–155 or 141–150 dimers had similar receptor-binding activity, while deletion of the three cationic residues at the N-terminus of either peptide of abolished this (Dyer et al. 1995). Although the monomer of peptide 141–155 did not have receptor-binding activity, acetylation of the amino terminal of this peptide enhanced LDL clearance in vivo (Nikoulin and Curtiss 1998).

ApoE is anti-inflammatory and is a strong inhibitor of T lymphocyte proliferation in vitro (Avila et al. 1982; Pepe and Curtiss 1986; Kelly et al. 1994) and of proliferation of interleukin 2-dependent T lymphocytes (Mistry et al. 1995). Monomeric peptides 130–149 or 130–155 inhibited T lymphocyte proliferation without cytotoxicity, while monomeric peptide 130–169 and dimeric peptides 141–155 or 141–149 inhibited proliferation and also had considerable cytotoxicity (Clay et al. 1995). ApoE also exhibited antioxidant properties. These were localized to the receptor-binding region using either monomeric or dimeric peptide 141–155, which inhibited Cu^{2+}-induced LDL oxidation (Pham et al. 2005).

Ac-hE18A-NH_2

Design

As previously noted, apoE can be considered to have two functional domains, an amino terminal receptor-binding region and a carboxyl terminal lipid-associating region. Our laboratory designed a dual-domain peptide to mimic this, with the amino terminal consisting of residues 141–150 of human apoE (LRKLRKRLLR) covalently attached on the carboxyl end to the well-studied lipid-associating peptide 18A (Anantharamaiah et al. 1985) which mimics some structural and functional properties of apoA-I (Fig. 1). This peptide was referred to as hE18A, with the h

Fig. 1 Design of the dual-domain cationic peptide Ac-hE18A-NH_2. (**a**) The upper portion is the amino residue sequence of human apoE. Residues in *bold* represent amphipathic helices. Underlined residues in *red* (residues 141–150) represent the LDL receptor and heparan sulfate proteoglycan (*HSPG*)-binding site; this portion, designated hE, is covalently bound to the amino terminus of the class A amphipathic peptide 18A (illustrated by the helical wheel). Blocking of the amino and carboxyl termini increases helicity and atheroprotective efficacy. The control peptide, Ac-nhE18A-NH_2, which is not cationic and does not bind to HSPG, is formed by attaching residues 151–160 (shown in *red* but not underlined) to 18A. (**b**) Space-filling model for AEM-28 showing that the N-terminal is rich in positively charged Lys and Arg residues, shown in *blue*. The 18A portion is the lipid-binding domain. When several copies of this peptide associate with atherogenic lipoproteins, the lipoproteins are decorated with highly positively charged residues and thus associate with HSPG on the liver surface, resulting in a dramatic clearance of plasma cholesterol

a

10	20	30	40	50
KVEQAVETEP	EPELRQQTEW	QSGQRWELAL	GRFWDYLRWV	QTLSEQVQEE
60	70	80	90	100
LLSSQVTQEL	RALMDETMKE	LKAYKSELEE	QLTPVAEETR	ARLSKELQAA
110	120	130	140	hE 150
QARLGADMED	VCGRLVQYRG	EVQAMLGQST	EELRVRLASH	LRKLRKRLLR
nhE 160	170	180	190	200
DADDLQKRLA	VYQAGAREGA	ERGLSAIRER	LGPLVEQGRV	RAATVGSLAG
210	220	230	240	250
QP**LQERAQAW**	**GERLRARMEE**	**MGSRTRDRLD**	**EVKEQVAEVR**	**AKLEEQAQQI**
260	270	280	290	299
RLQAEAFQAR	**LKSWF**EPLVE	DMQRQWAGLV	**EVKQAAVGTS**	AAPVPSDNH

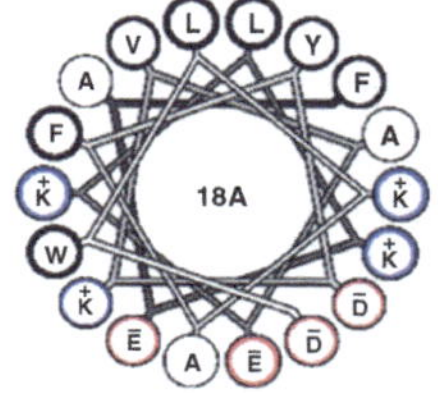

hE

Ac-L-R-K-L-R-K-R-L-L-R-D-W-L-K-A-F-Y-D-K-V-A-E-K-L-K-E-A-F-NH_2

Ac-hE18A-NH_2

b

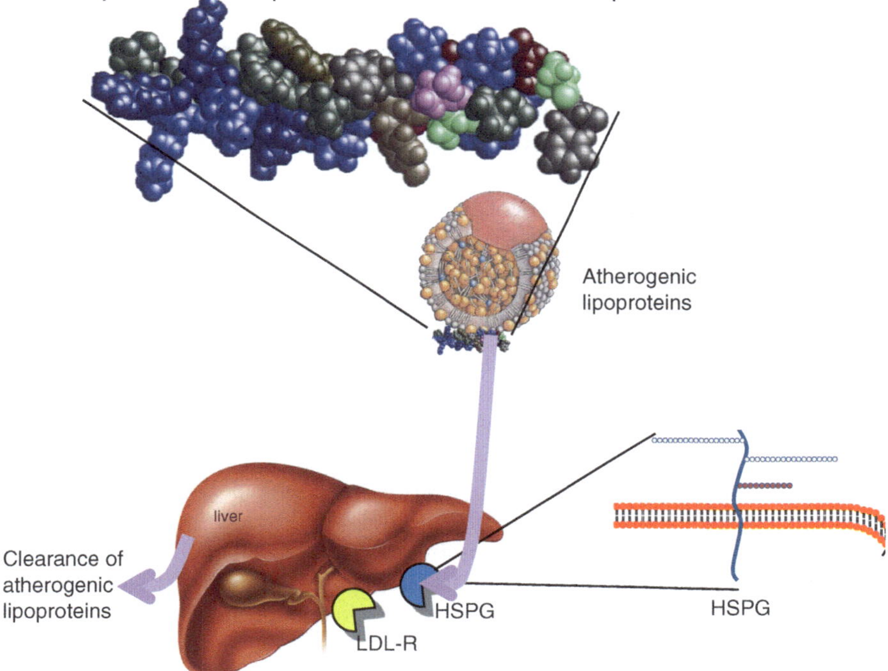

signifying human apoE. It was subsequently found that efficacy of the peptide was increased when the amino and carboxyl termini were blocked with acetyl and amide groups, respectively, resulting in Ac-hE18A-NH_2. This is also referred to as AEM-28 (where AEM stands for apoE mimetic) by the group pursuing human clinical trials, as will be discussed.

Initial Studies and Mechanism of Plasma Cholesterol Clearance

Initial studies of the effects of Ac-hE18A-NH_2 were performed in mouse embryonic fibroblasts using human lipoproteins (Datta et al. 2000). In these studies, human LDL was radioiodinated and uptake and degradation were determined in the absence and presence of peptide. Peptide Ac-hE18A-NH_2 was shown to associate with human LDL using agarose gel electrophoresis. In the presence of the peptide, the electronegativity of LDL was reduced in a peptide dose-dependent manner. Additional peptides studied were Ac-hE(R)18A-NH_2 (where the apoE peptide lysine residues were all replaced with arginine; LRRLRRRLLR) and Ac-mE18A-NH_2 (where the apoE-derived peptide was replaced with the mouse sequence, LRKMRKRLMR). It was found that all three peptides significantly increased uptake and degradation of [^{125}I]LDL by fibroblasts, with degradation being similar for all peptides in the conditions used, while uptake was greater in the presence of Ac-hE(R)18A-NH_2 and less with Ac-mR18A-NH_2. Incubation of [^{125}I]LDL in the absence of peptide with fibroblasts from dual LDL-R/LRP null or LRP null fibroblasts reduced internalization by half, while the increase in internalization induced by Ac-hE81A-NH_2 was not markedly decreased in the knockout cells. This suggested that the increased internalization induced by the peptide was not dependent on either LDL-R or LRP. However, pretreatment of fibroblasts with heparinase/heparitinase essentially abolished the peptide-mediated increased LDL uptake, suggesting that this effect was dependent on heparan sulfate proteoglycan (HSPG).

Similar results were obtained in studies using radiolabeled human LDL and VLDL in HepG2 (human liver carcinoma) cells, a cell model of hepatocytes (Datta et al. 2001a). Incubation of Ac-hE18A-NH_2 with [^{125}I]LDL or [^{125}I]VLDL dramatically increased cellular uptake of the lipoproteins. In the case of VLDL, treatment with heparinase/heparitinase again abolished the effect. Also with VLDL, the labeled lipoprotein mixed with Ac-18A-NH_2 (which lacked the apoE residues) had no effect on uptake; this was not reported for LDL. It was also observed that Ac-hE18A-NH_2 incubated in increasing proportion with VLDL displaced apoE from the lipoprotein. Finally, the peptide was injected into apoE null mice intravenously at a dose of 5 mg/kg. At 6 h, plasma cholesterol was reduced by 88 % and remained significantly lower than the baseline level at 24 h, although it had increased compared with the 6 h level. The reduction was primarily in the VLDL and IDL/LDL regions of the profile, with essentially no reduction in HDL. Injection of Ac-18A-NH_2 had an effect on plasma cholesterol nearly identical to injection of saline alone.

In vivo studies of the cholesterol-reducing effect of Ac-hE18A-NH_2 were continued and extended into other mouse models (Garber et al. 2003). In order to determine the time course of cholesterol reduction, [^{125}I]Ac-hE18A-NH_2 was injected into apoE null mice and sequential blood samples were taken. Both peptide and plasma cholesterol were cleared in a biphasic manner. The halftimes for the rapid phase of clearance were 12.24 min for cholesterol and 1.57 min for peptide, while the slow-phase halftimes were 6.05 h for cholesterol and 1.61 h for peptide. When the lipoprotein-associated radioactivity profile was measured at 2 min following injection, 61 % was associated with the combined VLDL + IDL/LDL peak and 39 % was in the HDL peak. After 6 h, radioactivity in the VLDL + IDL/LDL peak was reduced by 59 %, while the reduction in the HDL peak was 30 %. When plasma cholesterol profiles were compared at baseline and 30 min, all of the reduction was in the VLDL + IDL/LDL peak, with essentially no apparent reduction in the HDL peak. Similar results were found in C57BL/6J mice fed the Paigen atherogenic diet. However, no reduction in plasma cholesterol was seen in C57BL/6J mice fed chow, or LDL-R null mice fed either chow or Western diet. As this was in conflict with results using human lipoproteins in cell culture (Datta et al. 2000, 2001a), it was initially assumed that the cholesterol clearance was dependent on the LDL receptor. However, plasma distributions of [^{125}I]Ac-hE18A-NH_2 in LDL-R null mice fed either diet showed no association of the peptide with LDL in these animals, perhaps due to a higher surface pressure of mouse LDL. When the peptide was injected into apoE null/LDL-R null dual-knockout mice, plasma cholesterol was cleared in a similar manner to the apoE null single-knockout mice. Thus, the LDL receptor was not required for the cholesterol-reducing effect of the peptide. Human [^{125}I]lipoproteins with and without peptide were injected into LDL-R null mice fed normal chow. VLDL radioactivity and LDL radioactivity were reduced at 2 min in the presence of peptide, but clearance of HDL was not different with peptide vs. saline. Organ distribution of radioactivity was determined, and 80–90 % of the radiolabel was in the liver. VLDL and LDL with peptide had significantly greater hepatic uptake of radiolabel compared with those lipoproteins without peptide, while there was no difference in HDL uptake with or without peptide.

Effects on Plasma Cholesterol in WHHL and Cholesterol-Fed Rabbits

Most of the earlier studies to determine the ability of the peptide to reduce plasma cholesterol were done in mice, especially apoE null mice. As mentioned earlier, a rapid reduction of plasma cholesterol to more than 70 % was observed within 15 min after injection with Ac-hE18A-NH_2. However, the plasma cholesterol levels returned back almost to the original levels by 24 h. New Zealand white rabbits are sensitive to cholesterol-rich diets and develop hypercholesterolemia within 15 days and eventually develop atherosclerosis. When a resident at the UAB Medical Center, Dr. Himanshu Gupta, approached one of the authors to study the effect of the peptide on

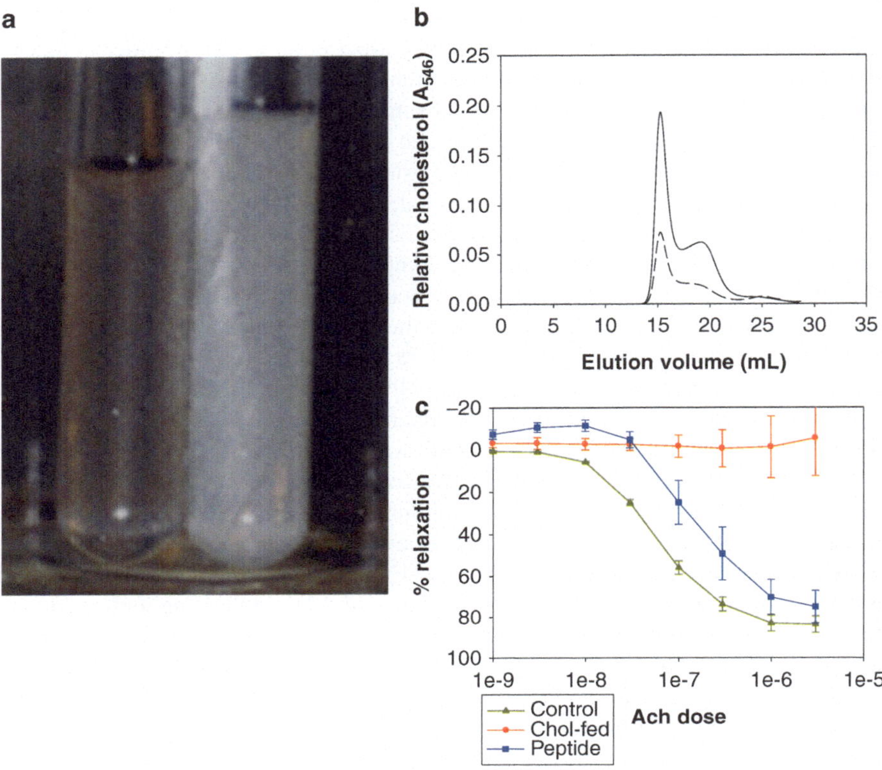

Fig. 2 (**a**) New Zealand white rabbits ($n=3$) fed a high (1 %)-cholesterol diet. After 1 month on the 1 % cholesterol diet, 3 mg of Ac-hE18A-NH_2 was administered via the ear vein. 14 days later, plasma from peptide-administered rabbits showed clear plasma, whereas the plasma from the control group on high-cholesterol diet was turbid. (**b**) Representative cholesterol profiles of the cholesterol-fed rabbits administered Ac-hE18A-NH_2 showed significantly less atherogenic lipoproteins compared to control. (**c**) Endothelial function experiments (measured as described previously; Gupta et al. 2005) showed almost complete restoration of the endothelial function in the peptide-administered rabbits (*squares*) compared to cholesterol-fed control rabbits (*circles*), which exhibited essentially no relaxation with acetylcholine. Control chow-fed rabbits are represented by triangles (From Dr. C. Roger White; used with permission)

plasma cholesterol in New Zealand white rabbits fed a cholesterol-supplemented diet (0.5 % cholesterol modified diet, 58HP, Test Diet Inc.) for 20 days, 3 mg/kg peptide was i.v. administered and plasma cholesterol measured at time points similar to the experiments with apoE null mice. At these earlier time points, all of the plasma looked turbid and there was no change in plasma cholesterol levels. However, 15 days later, a second peptide injection was done with a blood sample taken before and after peptide injection. Surprisingly, the sample taken before injection lacked turbidity (Fig. 2a). Thus, although no acute effect was observed, cholesterol was reduced 2 weeks following injection. Column lipoprotein profiles (Garber et al. 2000) indicated a clear reduction in plasma VLDL and LDL cholesterol for more than a week after each injection (Fig. 2b; Sharifov et al. 2011). The mechanism of this sustained effect remains unknown, although other sustained effects have been demonstrated in mice, as will be discussed later. These rabbits also had profound vascular dysfunction, as demonstrated by acetylcholine-mediated endothelium-dependent relaxation of perfused aortae. However, the aortae from peptide-treated rabbits had this vascular function restored to nearly normal levels (Fig. 2c).

Studies of Ac-hE18A-NH_2 were done in Watanabe heritable hyperlipidemic (WHHL) rabbits (Gupta et al. 2005), which lack a functional LDL receptor (Kita et al. 1981). Again using radioiodinated peptide, plasma clearance of cholesterol and peptide was determined to be biphasic. The rapid phase had halftimes of 37.1 min for cholesterol and 38.6 min for peptide, while the slow-phase halftimes were 48.9 h for cholesterol and 17.0 h for peptide. Cholesterol was reduced approximately 40 % by 5 h and remained at that level for 24 h; triglyceride was also reduced by about 40 %, but the reduction was much more rapid, reaching a minimum by 30 min and remaining at that level for 12 h. Unlike cholesterol, triglyceride returned to baseline levels by 24 h. The antioxidative enzyme paraoxonase-1 (PON) activity and lipid hydroperoxide (LOOH) levels were measured following peptide administration. PON activity increased approximately fivefold by 2 h, while LOOH levels decreased by half at the same time point. As with human LDL (Datta et al. 2000), the electronegativity of LDL from these rabbits was reduced in peptide-injected animals. Finally, endothelium- dependent and endothelium-independent relaxation was determined in aortic ring segments taken 18 h after injection with either saline or Ac-hE18A-NH_2. Aortic response to acetylcholine of segments from saline-injected WHHL rabbits was significantly impaired compared with those from normal rabbits, while segments from peptide-injected rabbits had a normal response. There was no difference in response to sodium nitroprusside, indicating that the endothelium was the site of vascular dysfunction. Superoxide anion formation was also measured in the aortic ring segments, with those from peptide-injected rabbits having significantly less.

Atheroprotective Properties

It was hypothesized that the cationic nature of the amino terminal apoE-derived portion of Ac-hE18A-NH_2 drove the rapid plasma cholesterol clearance due to its ability to interact with HSPG. A control peptide was synthesized with the apoE-derived portion consisting of the next ten residues of human apoE (residues 151–160; DADDLQKRLA) bound to peptide 18A to form Ac-nhE18A-NH_2 (Nayyar et al. 2010), where the n refers to its lack of HSPG binding. In contrast to Ac-hE18A-NH_2, the apoE-derived portion of Ac-nhE18A-NH_2 consisted of negatively charged residues and the hydrophobic residue Leu. Both peptides rapidly cleared phospholipid suspensions, and both readily bound to human LDL. However, Ac-hE18A-NH_2 mediated increased uptake of LDL by HepG2 cells, while Ac-nhE18A-NH_2 did not. In addition, Ac-hE18A-NH_2 mediated a reduction in the LDL content of LOOH in vitro, while Ac-nhE18A-NH_2 actually increased the LDL LOOH content. Injection of the peptides into apoE null mice again showed rapid reduction of plasma cholesterol in Ac-hE18A-NH_2-injected mice, while injection of Ac-nhE18A-NH_2 had no effect. Finally, female apoE null mice were administered either peptide three times a week for 6 weeks, starting at 16 weeks of age. Only Ac-hE18A-NH_2 reduced plasma cholesterol and triglyceride levels and increased PON-1 activity at the end of the treatment period. When aortic sinus lesions were measured, mice injected with Ac-hE18A-NH_2 had significantly lower lesion areas compared with controls, while Ac-nhE18A-NH_2 actually had significantly greater lesion area, in line with the changes in the levels of lipid hydroperoxide. Thus, the supposed control peptide Ac-nhE18A-NH_2 was actually proinflammatory and atherogenic.

In these studies (Nayyar et al. 2010), the involvement of HSPG was further shown by injecting heparinase either before or after injection of the peptide Ac-hE18A-NH_2. When heparinase was injected 5 min before the peptide, the cholesterol-reducing effect was entirely abolished. When injected 15 min after the peptide, heparinase had no effect on the peptide-mediated cholesterol reduction. Thus, the mechanism of apoE mimetic-mediated clearance of atherogenic lipoproteins via the HSPG pathway appears to be rapid and not reversible by removal of HSPG after peptide injection.

Reduction of Oxidative Processes

The abilities of the peptide to recycle, modify HDL profiles, and inhibit lipopolysaccharide (LPS) effects were investigated in vitro (Datta et al. 2010a). Recycling was studied in THP-1 monocyte-derived macrophages and in HepG2 cells. Cells were incubated with [^{125}I]Ac-hE18A-NH_2 for 2 h, after which cell-surface-bound peptide was removed by heparin treatment. Radioactivity in cells and media was determined at time points up to 24 h. Cell peptide content initially declined over 1 h, then increased over the next 4 h, with a concomitant increase in the media for 1–2 h, followed by a decrease the next 4 h, and finally increasing again at 24 h with a decrease in cellular radioactivity at the same time point. The radioactivity in the media at the 24 h time point was found to be intact peptide as determined by HPLC. This indicated that the peptide, like apoE, could be recycled after uptake. Secretion of preβ-HDL from HepG2 cells was stimulated by peptide incubation, while cells which were not exposed to peptide secreted primarily α-HDL. However, the total mass of apoA-I secreted was similar in both conditions. The enhanced preβ-HDL secretion persisted for at least 2 days even after removal of the peptide. Additionally, incubation of α-HDL (secreted from HepG2 cells) with peptide displaced apoA-I to form preβ-HDL. Incubation with the peptide also released surface-bound apoE from THP-1 cells, although synthesis of apoE (as determined by apoE mRNA levels) was not changed. At the same time, incubation with peptide stimulated cholesterol efflux from THP-1 cells in a dose-dependent manner. LPS-induced inflammatory responses were then studied. LPS induces vascular cell adhesion molecule-1 (VCAM-1) synthesis in human umbilical vascular endothelial cells (HUVEC); incubation with the peptide inhibited synthesis of VCAM-1 in a dose-dependent manner. Peptide incubation also inhibited LPS-induced interleukin-6 (IL-6) and monocyte chemotactic protein-1 (MCP-1) secretion from THP-1 macrophages with co-incubation, preincubation, and post-incubation of the peptide with LPS.

Further investigations into the anti-inflammatory properties of Ac-hE18A-NH_2 were carried out both in vivo and in vitro (Datta et al. 2010b; Sharifov et al. 2014). In these studies, Ac-hE18A-NH_2 properties were compared with L-4F, a well-studied apoA-I peptide mimetic (Datta et al. 2001b). These peptides were incubated with isolated human blood in the presence and absence of LPS. As expected, endotoxin activity as measured by the limulus amoebocyte lysate (LAL) assay was increased when LPS alone was added, but both peptides dramatically decreased this activity. LPS induced TNF-α and IL-6 in plasma from these samples and this was also reduced by both peptides, although not to the same degree as endotoxin activity. In the case of IL-6, Ac-hE18A-NH_2 induced a significantly greater reduction than L-4F. LPS-induced superoxide production from isolated human leukocytes was also reduced by both peptides, but again, the reduction in the presence of Ac-hE18A-NH_2 was significantly greater than that induced by L-4F. Similar results were obtained when studying the LPS-mediated inflammatory response in THP-1 monocyte-derived macrophages using LPS of various types. Again, Ac-hE18A-NH_2 reduced TNF-α and IL-6 secretion to a significantly greater degree than did L-4F. The active state of LPS has been postulated to be aggregated. Both peptides caused disaggregation of LPS, but L-4F did so to a lesser extent. Experiments in THP-1 cells, in which the cells were pretreated with peptide and then treated with LPS after the peptide was removed, demonstrated that Ac-hE18A-NH_2, but not L-4F, had strong cell-dependent anti-inflammatory properties as determined by reduced TNF-α secretion. Similar results were obtained from in vivo experiments using C57BL/6J mice. Peptides or saline were administered 5 min after LPS, and both peptides reduced plasma IL-6, interferon-γ (INF-γ), and serum amyloid A (SAA). Again, Ac-hE18A-NH_2 was superior to L-4F in suppressing IL-6 and IFN-γ, but was equivalent in the reduction of SAA.

Sustained Effects

Longer-term studies of the atheroprotective effects of Ac-hE18A-NH_2 have identified a striking sustained effect, lasting weeks to months after peptide administration was stopped (Goldberg et al. 2013). The protocol for the experiment is described schematically in Fig. 3. Female apoE null mice were fed a Western diet for 6 weeks beginning at 14 weeks of age, after which the diet was changed to normal chow for 2 weeks and mice were randomized into two groups. One group was administered Ac-hE18A-NH_2 in saline (100 μg/100 μL) retro-orbitally three times a week, while the control group was administered an equal volume of saline three times a week for 1 month. One month after the final peptide treatment, blood was collected and organs were harvested. In a second experiment, blood was collected and organs were harvested from a subgroup at the end of the peptide treatment and from a second group 1 month after the final peptide treatment. Blood was also collected from

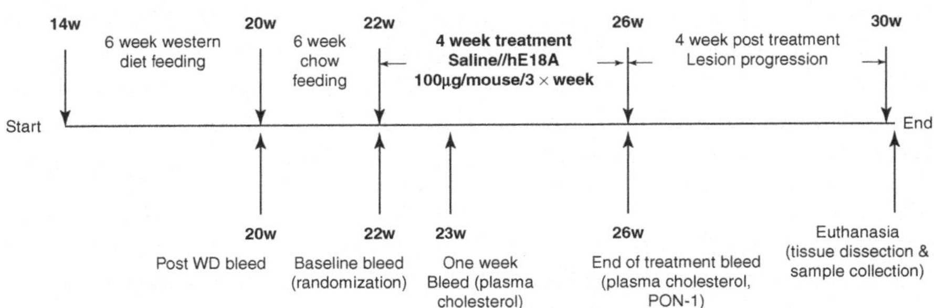

Fig. 3 Experimental protocol for determining sustained effect of apoE mimetic peptide Ac-hE18A-NH_2

the retro-orbital sinus under anesthesia at time points mentioned in Fig. 3. As expected, during the feeding of the Western diet, plasma cholesterol increased to approximately 1,400 mg/dL, but by the end on the subsequent 2-week period on normal chow, levels had fallen to approximately 475 mg/dL. At 4 weeks post-peptide treatment, both groups had similar cholesterol levels. In the second experiment, en face aortic lesions were assessed in a subgroup of animals at the end of the peptide treatment period and were not found to be different. However, when lesions were assessed 4 weeks after peptide treatment was ended, lesions had progressed compared to the end of the peptide period, but in both experiments lesions in the peptide group were significantly less than in the control group. There was no correlation between cholesterol reduction during the peptide treatment and final lesion areas. PON-1 activity was significantly higher in the peptide group compared with the control group both at the end of the peptide treatment period and at the termination of the experiment.

The mechanism of this sustained peptide effect is unknown. In other experiments in which a sustained effect was observed, it was hypothesized that the peptide treatment was related to a sustained increase in apoE secretion or levels, but as this experiment was performed in apoE null mice, the mechanism clearly is apoE independent. It seems likely that a fuller understanding of the mechanisms involved in this sustained effect will require gene array analyses to determine which, if any, genetic or signaling pathways are responsible for these properties.

Comparisons with Other Peptides

Peptide L-4F, an apoA-I peptide mimetic, has been shown to have significant atheroprotective properties without reducing plasma cholesterol (White et al. 2014). A comparison of these properties was made between L-4F and Ac-hE18A-NH_2 in older female apoE null mice, starting at 22–24 weeks of age (Nayyar et al. 2012). Three experiments were done with different dosing regimens, although doses per administration were all 100 μg/dose. In the first, L-4F was administered daily intraperitoneally, while Ac-hE18A-NH_2 was administered twice weekly retro-orbitally, both for 8 weeks. In the second, L-4F was again administered daily, while Ac-hE18A-NH_2 was given three times weekly, both for 6 weeks. In the third, both peptides were given three times weekly retro-orbitally for 6 weeks. Similar results were obtained in all three regimens. Plasma cholesterol and triglyceride was reduced only in mice receiving Ac-hE18A-NH_2. Both peptides reduced aortic lesion area, but in the third experiment, the reduction in mice receiving Ac-hE18A-NH_2 was significantly greater than in those receiving L-4F. Both peptide groups had reduced plasma lipid hydroperoxides to a similar extent, but only mice receiving Ac-hE18A-NH_2 had a significant reduction in SAA.

In order to produce a smaller peptide with similar anti-inflammatory and cholesterol-reducing properties, modifications to the lytic cationic peptide 18L (Tytler et al. 1993) were made to eliminate its lytic properties (Handattu et al. 2010). Phe and Trp residues were added to the center of the hydrophobic face to increase anti-inflammatory properties, similar to 4F (Datta et al. 2004; Van Lenten et al. 2008), and Arg replaced Lys residues to maintain cationic properties but reduce the lytic wedge shape. This new cationic 18-residue peptide, mR18L, was compared with peptide m18L, in which the Lys residues were not replaced by Arg residues (Handattu et al. 2010). Both peptides cleared POPC suspensions, although mR18L cleared to a slightly greater extent. Both peptides enhanced the uptake of [^{125}I]LDL by HepG2 cells, although mR18L was twice as effective as m18L in enhancing uptake. When injected intravenously into apoE null mice, again both peptides mediated reduction of plasma cholesterol, but mR18L produced a small but significantly greater reduction at 6 h. Pretreatment with heparinase reduced this with both peptides. When [^{14}C]-labeled peptides were administered by gavage, both peptides were found intact in the blood. Thus, atheroprotective properties of the peptides were determined by mixing peptide with powdered rodent chow which was re-pelleted and fed to apoE null mice for 6 weeks. At 3 and 6 weeks, only mR18L had significantly reduced plasma cholesterol compared with baseline, and at the conclusion of the experiment, only mR18L had significantly reduced aortic sinus lesions. Finally, monocyte adhesion to bovine aortic endothelial cells (BAEC) was tested, and compared with control plasma, only plasma from mR18L-treated mice had reduced monocyte adhesion.

Peptide mR18L was then compared with the dual-domain peptide Ac-hE18A-NH_2 (Handattu et al. 2013a). As noted before (Garber et al. 2003), a single intravenous administration of Ac-hE18A-NH_2 did not reduce plasma cholesterol in LDL-R mice, although administration of mR18L did induce a significant reduction. However, when administered retro-orbitally two times a week for 8 weeks, both peptides induced nearly identical reductions at each time point measured, beginning at 2 weeks. These reductions were primarily in the VLDL and LDL regions of the cholesterol profile, with smaller but significant reductions in HDL. When reactive oxygen species in the plasma were measured at euthanasia, Ac-hE81A-NH_2 induced a large and significant reduction, while mR18L did not. Both peptides reduced aortic sinus and whole aorta lesions compared with control animals, but the reduction induced by Ac-hE18A-NH_2 was significantly greater than that induced by mR18L. As the similar reduction in cholesterol alone was not sufficient to account for the difference in atheroprotection, in vitro studies of apoE from HepG2 and THP-1 cells were performed. It was found that exposure to the cells of oxidized POPC (ox-POPC) inhibited apoE secretion, while co-incubation of ox-POPC with Ac-hE18A-NH_2 rescued this. Peptide mR18L was much less effective in rescuing apoE secretion from the ox-POPC-mediated inhibition.

Alzheimer's Disease

It has been convincingly demonstrated that Ac-hE18A-NH_2 has anti-inflammatory properties beyond its ability to lower cholesterol. As Alzheimer's disease (AD) has a major inflammatory component, studies were done in an animal model of AD (APP/PS1ΔE9 transgenic mice, referred to here as AD mice) to determine if the peptide could attenuate the effects of the disease (Handattu et al. 2013b). Since these animals are normolipidemic, it was anticipated that the peptide would have no effect on plasma cholesterol, similar to chow-fed C57BL/6J mice (Garber et al. 2003), and this in fact was the case. In a chronic experiment, AD mice were administered Ac-hE18A-NH_2 retro-orbitally three times a week for 6 weeks, beginning at 4 months of age. At the end of the experimental period, cognitive function was assessed by the Morris water maze (Brandeis et al. 1989). AD mice which received the peptide were significantly faster in finding the hidden platform, and demonstrated improved memory retention, although this did not reach statistical significance. Immunohistochemical analysis of amyloid-β deposition in the brain demonstrated a significant reduction in peptide-treated mice. This was also true for reactive astrocytes and activated microglia. Analysis of inflammatory factors in brain homogenates showed significantly decreased IL-6 and TNF-α levels. Brain apoE levels were also substantially increased in peptide-treated mice. In vitro studies showed that the peptide increased amyloid-β uptake by THP-1 monocyte-derived macrophages in a dose-dependent manner. As was observed in HepG2 and THP-1 cells (Handattu et al. 2013a), oxidized phospholipid substantially inhibited apoE secretion in astrocytes; this was again rescued by treatment with Ac-hE18A-NH_2.

Modes of Administration

Several modes of administration of Ac-hE18A-NH_2 were investigated using cholesterol reduction as the endpoint. Initial experiments were done using tail vein intravascular injections in mice. As this is a tedious procedure, intraperitoneal and subcutaneous injections were performed. With a single injection, no change in plasma cholesterol was observed. It is speculated that the avid binding of the peptide to HSPG occurred before entry of the peptide into the blood stream. Chronic administrations using these routes have not been tested. On the suggestion of a university veterinarian, retro-orbital injections were studied as an alternative to tail vein injections. Direct comparisons of tail vein vs. retro-orbital injections in apoE null mice were then performed and demonstrated nearly identical reductions in cholesterol at 5 min and 5 h (Handattu et al. 2013b). Thus, in all subsequent mouse studies, the retro-orbital route was employed.

In one set of experiments, Ac-hE18A-NH_2 was incorporated into a proprietary phospholipid multivesicular liposome and injected subcutaneously into apoE null mice (Ramprasad et al. 2002). Following a single injection of the liposome/peptide mixture, cholesterol was decreased over 8 days, with the maximum decrease of approximately 18 % occurring at day 6. When the free peptide was injected subcutaneously, the maximum reduction in plasma cholesterol of 43 % occurred at 4 h postinjection, and levels returned to baseline by 24 h. This is in contrast with previous subcutaneous injections, in which no change in plasma cholesterol was observed. However, in this case, a very large dose of peptide was injected (30 mg/kg) compared with the usual dose of 5 mg/kg in the majority of experiments.

Ac-hE18A-NH_2 Clinical Studies: LPX-112

LPX-112 was the initial clinical study with Ac-hE18A-NH_2 (referred to here as AEM-28). These studies were designed as a blended phase 1a/1b, single/multiple ascending dose (SAD/MAD) protocol. The SAD arm of the study examined the safety and tolerability of six ascending doses of AEM-28, ranging from 0.032 to 3.54 mg/kg. There were two placebo and four active drug recipients in each cohort. All subjects were pre-dosed with methylprednisolone and an H1 and H2 antagonist. The design of the study is displayed in Fig. 4.

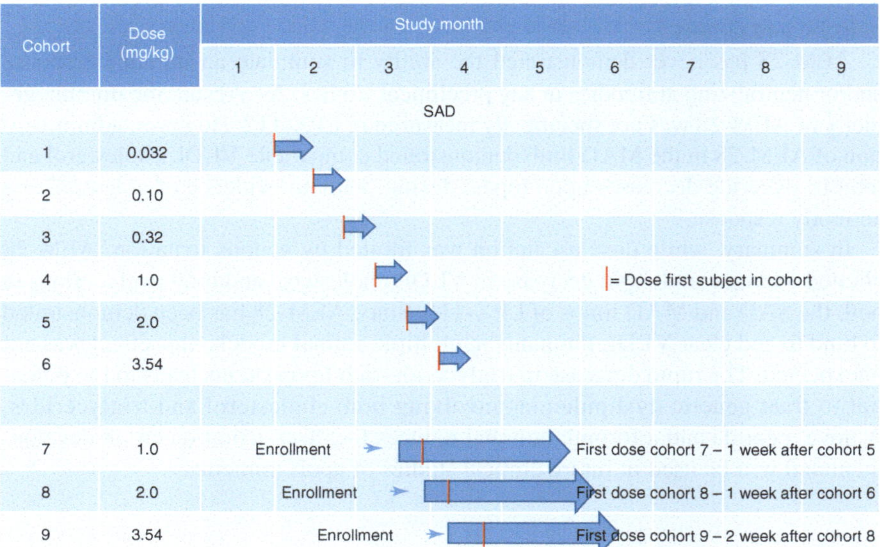

Fig. 4 Blended phase 1a/1b single/multiple ascending dose (SAD/MAD) protocol design for AEM-28

Normolipidemic volunteer subjects participated in the SAD limb of the study. Inclusion criteria for the MAD limb included subjects with elevated cholesterol while on statin therapy and were expanded to include nondiabetic subjects with elevated fasting triglycerides in response to the pharmacodynamic effects observed in the SAD limb. There was one placebo and four active drug recipients in each MAD limb cohort.

AEM-28 was generally well tolerated. Local venous irritation was observed at the highest doses, precluding further dose escalation. There were no significant systemic adverse reactions to the peptide. The MAD subjects received three doses, spaced 2 weeks apart. Each dose escalation began after the subjects in a previous cohort had received their second dose. Due to venous irritation at the 3.54 mg/kg dose, the study was terminated after all subjects in cohort 9 had received at least one dose.

Since the subjects in the SAD limb were fasted overnight and for 2 h following the start of drug administration, plasma VLDL cholesterol and total triglycerides were low at the start of infusion and continued to decline during the remainder of the fasting period. Nonetheless, rapid and substantial dose-dependent decreases in VLDL cholesterol and total triglycerides were observed. The effects of AEM-28 on VLDL cholesterol and total triglycerides at the 3.54 mg dose are displayed in Fig. 5a, b.

While the subjects in the MAD limb were also fasted overnight, initial VLDL cholesterol and total triglycerides were higher, and the decline during drug administration was not as steep due to the inclusion of subjects with elevated fasting triglycerides (Fig. 6a, b). AEM-28 elicited a similar, rapid decline in both VLDL cholesterol and total triglycerides, resulting in a 75 % decrease from baseline in the active drug recipients in cohort 9. The decrease in VLDL cholesterol and total triglycerides in cohorts 8 and 9 was significantly greater than in placebo and cohort 7.

AEM-28 has never demonstrated the ability to stimulate an immune response and/or neutralizing antibodies in any preclinical studies. As a result, the immunogenicity of AEM-28 was not specifically measured in LPX-112. However, administration of AEM-28 in the MAD limb demonstrated comparable VLDL cholesterol and total triglyceride decreases upon repeat dosing, with no evidence of a neutralizing antibody response.

In summary, while dose escalation was limited by venous irritation, AEM-28 elicited a unique and rapid decrease in VLDL cholesterol and total triglycerides in both the SAD and MAD limbs of LPX-112. Since AEM-28 has been demonstrated to bind to and clear VLDL remnants in multiple animal models, this effect was not unexpected. The rapid decrease in triglyceride-rich lipoproteins leads to the potential to treat genetic dyslipidemias involving both cholesterol and triglycerides. A novel peptide and a formulation that reduces localized irritation are in development and will be used in future clinical studies of apoE mimetics.

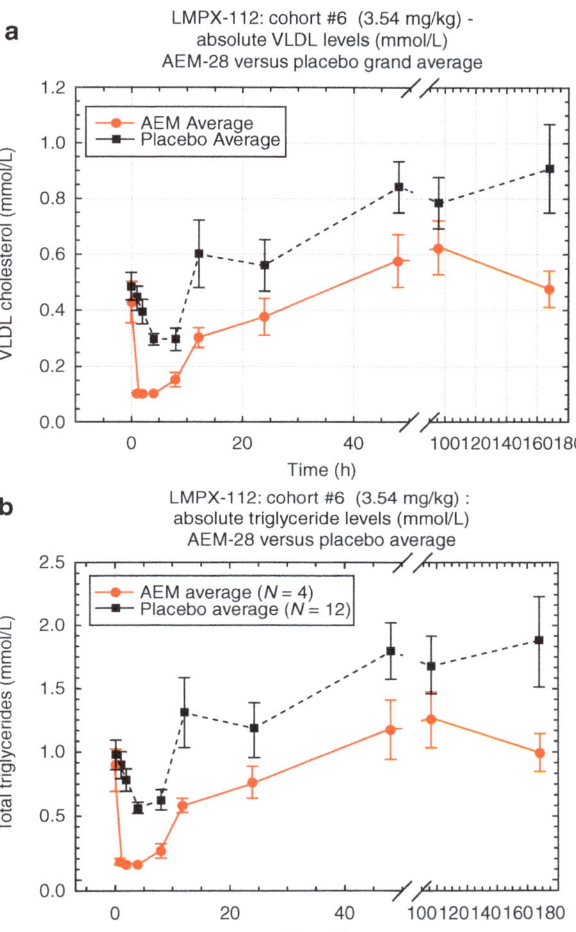

Fig. 5 Effect of AEM-28 on VLDL and triglycerides in cohort 6, 3.54 mg/kg dose. There were two placebo and four active subjects in each of the six cohorts in the SAD limb. The placebos for all six cohorts were combined. (**a**) Effect of AEM-28 on VLDL cholesterol. (**b**) Effect of AEM-28 on total triglycerides

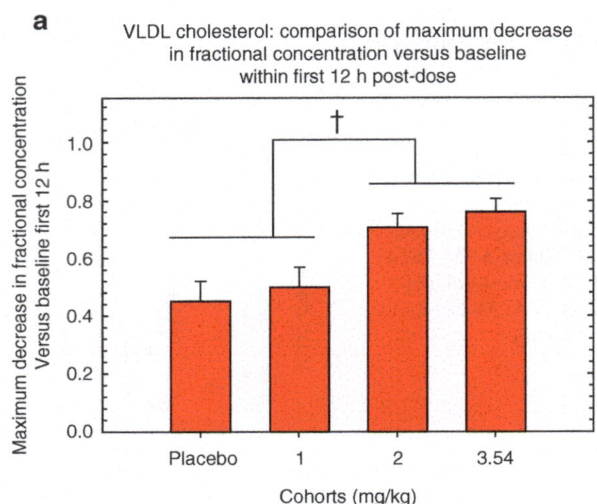

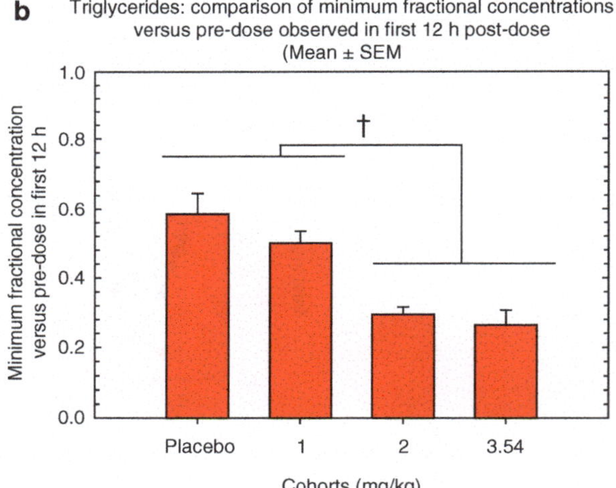

Fig. 6 Effect of AEM-28 on VLDL cholesterol (**a**) and total triglycerides (**b**) in all cohorts from the MAD limb of LPX-112. The decrease from baseline in all cohorts is displayed. Placebo VLDL cholesterol and total triglycerides declined during the treatment and follow-up fasting period (2 h post dose). The decreases in active drug recipients in cohorts 8 and 9 (2.0 and 3.54 mg/kg) were significantly greater ($^{\dagger}p<0.05$) than placebo and cohort 7 (1.0 mg/kg)

Conclusions

ApoE mimetics have shown promise in reducing plasma cholesterol levels rapidly in all of the animal studies and in the human trials, reducing VLDL cholesterol and total triglycerides. In addition, both in animal and human studies, the effect appears to last for a long period, even past the peptide administration period. This sustained effect is analogous to the cholesterol-independent effects of apoE which has been shown to control cellular signaling in cells of the immune system. Analogous to apoE, the apoE mimetics exert effects on suppressing systemic and vascular inflammation in animal models such as mice and rabbits. In addition, in vitro and animal studies have also shown peptide-mediated release of apoE. Considering failed therapeutic trials of HDL-raising drugs and recombinant HDL clinical studies and lack of progress in the clinical trials of apoA-I mimetic peptides, targeting apoE and its cell signaling functions to control human atherosclerosis and other lipid-mediated inflammatory disorders is expected to have potential for the amelioration of these diseases.

References

Abifadel M, Varret M, Rabès J-P, Allard D, Ouguerram K, Devillers M, Cruaud C, Benjannet S, Wickham L, Erlich D, Derré A, Villéger L, Farnier M, Beucler I, Bruckert E, Chambaz J, Chanu B, Lecerf J-M, Luc G, Moulin P, Weissenbach J, Prat A, Krempf M, Junien C, Seidah NG, Boileau C (2003) Mutations in PCSK9 cause autosomal dominant hypercholesterolemia. Nat Genet 34:154–156

Anantharamaiah GM, Jones JL, Brouillette CG, Schmidt CF, Chung BH, Hughes TA, Bhown AS, Segrest JP (1985) Studies of synthetic peptide analogs of the amphipathic helix. Structure of complexes with dimyristoyl phophatidylcholine. J Biol Chem 260:10248–10255

Ason B, Tep S, Davis HR Jr, Xu Y, Tetzloff G, Galinski B, Soriano F, Dubinina N, Zhu L, Stefanni A, Wong KK, Tadin-Strapps M, Bartz SR, Hubbard B, Ranalletta M, Sachs AB, Flanagan WM, Strack A, Kuklin NA (2011) Improved efficacy for ezetimibe and rosuvastatin by attenuating the induction of PCSK9. J Lipid Res 52:679–687

Ason B, van der Hoorn JWA, Chan J, Lee E, Pieterman EJ, Nguyen KK, Di M, Shetterly S, Tang J, Yeh W-C, Schwarz M, Jukema JW, Scott R, Wasserman SM, Princen HMG, Jackson S (2014) PCSK9 inhibition fails to alter hepatic LDLR, circulating cholesterol and atherosclerosis in the absence of ApoE. J Lipid Res 55:2370–2379

Avila EM, Holdsworth G, Sasaki N, Jackson RL, Harmony JAK (1982) Apoprotein E suppresses phytohemagglutinin-activated phospholipid turnover in peripheral blood mononuclear cells. J Biol Chem 257:5900–5909

Blom DJ, Hala T, Bolognese M, Lillestol MJ, Toth PD, Burgess L, Ceska R, Roth E, Koren MJ, Ballantyne CM, Monsalvo ML, Tsirtsonis K, Kim JB, Scott R, Wasserman SM, Stein EA, for the DESCARTES Investigators (2014) A 52-week placebo-controlled trial of evolocumab in hyperlipidemia. N Engl J Med 370:1809–1819

Bradley WA, Hwang SL, Karlin JB, Lin AH, Prasad SC, Gotto AM Jr, Gianturco SH (1984) Low-density lipoprotein receptor binding determinants switch from apolipoprotein E to apolipoprotein B during conversion of hypertriglyceridemic very-low-density lipoprotein to low-density lipoproteins. J Biol Chem 259:14728–14735

Brandeis R, Brandys Y, Yehuda S (1989) The use of the Morris Water Maze in the study of memory and learning. Int J Neurosci 48:29–69

Brown MS, Goldstein JL (1986) A receptor-mediated pathway for cholesterol homeostasis. Science 240:34–47

Clay MA, Anantharamaiah GM, Mistry MJ, Balasubramaniam A, Harmony JAK (1995) Localization of a domain in apolipoprotein E with both cytostatic and cytotoxic activity. Biochemistry 34:11142–11151

Danielsson B, Ekman R, Johansson BG, Nilsson-Ehle P, Petersson BG (1978) Isolation of a high density lipoprotein with high contents of arginine-rich apoprotein (apoE) from rat plasma. FEBS Lett 86:299–302

Datta G, Chaddha M, Garber DW, Chung BH, Tytler EM, Dashti N, Bradley WA, Gianturco SH, Anantharamaiah GM (2000) The receptor binding domain of apolipoprotein E, linked to a model Class A amphipathic helix, enhances internalization and degradation of LDL by fibroblasts. Biochemistry 39:213–220

Datta G, Garber DW, Chung BH, Chaddha M, Dashti N, Bradley WA, Ginaturco SH, Anantharamaiah GM (2001a) Cationic domain 141–150 of apoE covalently linked to a class A amphipathic helix enhances atherogenic lipoprotein metabolism in vitro and in vivo. J Lipid Res 42:959–966

Datta G, Chaddha M, Hama S, Navab M, Fogelman AM, Garber DW, Mishra VK, Epand RM, Epand RF, Lund-Katz S, Phillips MC, Segrest JP, Anantharamaiah GM (2001b) Effects of increasing hydrophobicity on the physical-chemical and biological properties of a class A amphipathic helical peptide. J Lipid Res 42:1096–1104

Datta G, Epand RF, Epand RM, Chaddha M, Kirksey MA, Garber DW, Lund-Katz S, Phillips MC, Hama S, Navab M, Fogelman AM, Palgunachari MN, Segrest JP, Anantharamaiah GM (2004) Aromatic residue position on the nonpolar face of class A amphipathic helical peptides determines biological activity. J Biol Chem 279:26509–26517

Datta G, White CR, Dashti N, Chaddha M, Palgunachari MN, Gupta H, Handattu SP, Garber DW, Anantharamaiah GM (2010a) Anti-inflammatory and recycling properties of an apolipoprotein mimetic peptide, Ac-hE18A-NH_2. Atherosclerosis 2085:134–141

Datta G, Chaddha M, Handattu SP, Palgunachari MN, Nayyar G, Garber DW, Gupta H, White CR, Anantharamaiah GM (2010b) ApoE mimetic peptide reduces plasma lipid hydroperoxide content with a concomitant increase in HDL paraoxonase activity. Exp Med Biol 660:1–4

Davignon J (2005) Apolipoprotein E and atherosclerosis: beyond lipid effect. Arterioscler Thromb Vasc Biol 25:267–269

Dyer CA, Curtiss LK (1991) A synthetic peptide mimic of plasma apolipoprotein E that binds the LDL receptor. J Biol Chem 266:22803–22806

Dyer CA, Cistola DP, Perry GC, Curtiss LK (1995) Structural features of synthetic peptides of apolipoprotein E that bind the LDL receptor. J Lipid Res 36:80–88

Endo A (1992) The discovery and development of HMG-CoA reductase inhibitors. J Lipid Res 33:1569–1582

Fitzgerald K, Frank-Kamenetsky M, Mant T, Ritter J, Chiesa J, Munasamy M, Hutabarat R, Clausen V, Watkins D, Smith K, Sutherland J, Cehelsky J, Kretschmer M, Nechev L, Karsten V, Nochur S, Binne L, Vaishnaw A, Simon A (2012) Pharmacodynamic results for ALN-PCS, a novel RNAi therapeutic for the treatment of hypercholesterolemia. Arterioscler Thromb Vasc Biol 32:A67

Garber DW, Kulkarni KR, Anantharamaiah GM (2000) A sensitive and convenient method for lipoprotein profile analysis of individual mouse plasma samples. J Lipid Res 41:1020–1026

Garber DW, Handattu S, Aslan I, Datta G, Chaddha M, Anantharamaiah GM (2003) Effect of an arginine-rich amphipathic helical peptide on plasma cholesterol in dyslipidemic mice. Atherosclerosis 168:229–237

Gianturco SH, Gotto AM Jr, Hwang S-LC, Karlin JB, Lin AHY, Prasad SC, Bradley WA (1983) Apolipoprotein E mediates uptake of S_f 100–400 hypertriglyceridemic very low density lipoproteins by the low density lipoprotein receptor pathway in normal human fibroblasts. J Biol Chem 258:4526–4533

Goldberg DI, Nayyar G, Garber DW, Handattu SP, Anantharamaiah GM (2013) Sustained effects of apolipoprotein E mimetic peptides on established lesions in apoE null mice. Circulation 128:A10759

Gonzsales JC, Gordts PI, Foley EM, Esko JD (2013) Apolipoproteins E and AV mediate lipoprotein clearance by hepatic proteoglycans. J Clin Invest 135:2742–2751

Gordon T, Kannel WB, Castelli WP, Dawber TR (1981) Lipoproteins, cardiovascular disease, and death. The Framingham Heart Study. Arch Intern Med 141:1128–1131

Gupta H, White CR, Handattu S, Garber DW, Datta G, Chaddha M, Dai L, Gianturco SH, Bradley WA, Anantharamaiah GM (2005) Apolipoprotein E mimetic peptide dramatically lowers plasma cholesterol and restores endothelial function in Watanabe Heritable Hyperlipidemic rabbits. Circulation 111:3112–3118

Handattu SP, Datta G, Epand RM, Epand RF, Palgunachari MN, Mishra VK, Monroe CE, Keenum TD, Chaddha M, Anantharamaiah GM, Garber DW (2010) Oral administration of L-mR18L, a single domain cationic amphipathic helical peptide, inhibits lesion formation in apoE null mice. J Lipid Res 51:3491–3499

Handattu SP, Nayyar G, Garber DW, Palgunachari MN, Monroe CE, Keenum TD, Mishra VK, Datta G, Anantharamaiah GM (2013a) Two apolipoprotein E mimetic peptides with similar cholesterol reducing properties exhibit differential atheroprotective effects in apo E null mice. Atherosclerosis 227:58–68

Handattu SP, Monroe CE, Nayyar G, Palgunachari MN, Kadish I, van Groen T, Anantharamaiah GM, Garber DW (2013b) In vivo and in vitro effects of an apolipoprotein E mimetic peptide on amyloid-β pathology. J Alzheimers Dis 36:335–347

Hooper AJ, Burnett JR (2013) Anti-PCSK9 therapies for the treatment of hypercholesterolemia. Expert Opin Biol Ther 13:429–435

Innerarity TL, Friedlander EJ, Rall SC Jr, Weisgraber KH, Mahley RW (1983) The receptor-binding domain of human apolipoprotein E. Binding of apolipoprotein E fragments. J Biol Chem 258:12341–12347

Kelly ME, Clay MA, Mistry MJ, Hsieh-Li H-M, Harmony JAK (1994) Apolipoprotein E inhibition of proliferation of mitogen-activated T lymphocytes: production of interleukin 2 with reduced biological activity. Cell Immunol 159:124–139

Kita T, Brown MS, Watanabe Y, Goldstein JL (1981) Deficiency of low density lipoprotein receptors in liver and adrenal gland of the WHHL rabbit, an animal model of familial hypercholesterolemia. Proc Natl Acad Sci U S A 78:2268–2272

Lagace TA (2014) PCSK9 and LDLR degradation: regulatory mechanisms in circulation and in cells. Curr Opin Lipidol 25:387–393

Linton MF, Atkinson JB, Fazio S (1995) Prevention of atherosclerosis in apolipoprotein E-deficient mice by bone marrow transplantation. Science 267:1034–1037

Ma PTS, Gil G, Sudhof TC, Bilheimer DW, Goldstein JL, Brown MS (1986) Mevinolin, an inhibitor of cholesterol synthesis, induces mRNA for low density lipoprotein receptor in livers of hamsters and rabbits. Proc Natl Acad Sci U S A 83:8370–8374

Mahley RW (1988) Apolipoprotein E: cholesterol transport protein with expanding role in cell biology. Science 240:622–630

Mahley RW, Ji Z-S (1999) Remnant lipoprotein metabolism: key pathways involving cell-surface heparan sulfate proteoglycans and apolipoprotein E. J Lipid Res 40:1–16

Mims MP, Darnule AT, Tovar RW, Pownall HJ, Sparrow DA, Sparrow JT, Via DP, Smith LC (1994) A nonexchangeable apolipoprotein E peptide that mediates binding to the low density lipoprotein receptor. J Biol Chem 269:20539–20547

Mistry MJ, Clay MA, Kelly ME, Steiner MA, Harmony JAK (1995) Apolipoprotein E restricts interleukin-dependent T lymphocyte proliferation at the G1A/G1B boundary. Cell Immunol 160:14–23

Nayyar G, Handattu SP, Monroe CE, Chaddha M, Datta G, Mishra VK, Keenum TD, Palgunachari MN, Garber DW, Anantharamaiah GM (2010) Two adjacent domains (141-150 and 151-160) of apoE covalently linked to a class A amphipathic helical peptide exhibit opposite atherogenic effects. Atherosclerosis 213:449–457

Nayyar G, Garber DW, Palgunachari MN, Monroe CE, Keenum TD, Handattu SP, Mishra VK, Anantharamaiah GM (2012) Apolipoprotein E mimetic is more effective than apolipoprotein A-I mimetic in reducing lesion formation in older female apo E null mice. Atherosclerosis 224:326–331

Nikoulin IR, Curtiss LK (1998) An apolipoprotein E synthetic peptide targets to lipoproteins in plasma and mediates both cellular lipoprotein interactions in vitro and acute clearance of cholesterol-rich lipoproteins in vivo. J Clin Invest 101:223–234

Pepe MG, Curtiss LK (1986) Apolipoprotein E is a biologically active constituent of the normal immunoregulatory lipoprotein, LDL-In. J Immunol 136:3716–3723

Pham T, Kodvawala A, Hui DY (2005) The receptor binding domain of apolipoprotein E is responsible for its antioxidant activity. Biochemistry 44:7577–7582

Plump AS, Smith JD, Hayek T, Aalto-Setala K, Walsh A, Verstuyft JG, Rubin EM, Breslow JL (1992) Severe hypercholesterolemia and atherosclerosis in apolipoprotein E-deficient mice created by homologous recombination in ES cells. Cell 71:343–353

Poirier S, Mayer G, Poupon V, McPherson PS, Desjardins R, Ly K, Asselin M-C, Day R, Duclos FJ, Witmer M, Parker R, Prat A, Seidah NG (2009) Dissection of the endogenous cellular pathways of PCSK9-induced low density lipoprotein receptor degradation: evidence for an intracellular route. J Biol Chem 284:28856–28864

Ramprasad MP, Anantharamaiah GM, Garber DW, Katre NV (2002) Sustained-delivery of an apolipoproteinE-peptidomimetic using multivesicular liposomes lowers serum cholesterol levels. J Control Release 79:207–218

Roth EM, Taskinen M-R, Ginsberg HN, Kastelein JJP, Colhoun HM, Robinson JG, Merlet L, Pordy R, Baccara-Dinet MT (2014) Monotherapy with the PCSK9 inhibitor alirocumab versus ezetimibe in patients with hypercholesterolemia: results of a 24 week double-blind, randomized Phase 3 trial. Int J Cardiol 176:55–61

Sharifov OF, Nayyar G, Garber DW, Handattu SP, Mishra VK, Goldberg D, Anantharamaiah GM, Gupta H (2011) Apolipoprotein E mimetics and cholesterol-lowering properties. Am J Cardiovasc Drugs 11:371–381

Sharifov OF, Nayyar G, Ternovoy VV, Palgunachari MN, Garber DW, Anantharamaiah GM, Gupta H (2014) Comparison of anti-endotoxin activity of apoE and apoA mimetic derivatives of a model amphipathic peptide 18A. Innate Immun 20:867–880

Shore VG, Shore B (1973) Heterogeneity of human plasma very low density lipoproteins. Separation of species differing in protein components. Biochemistry 12:502–507

Sparrow JT, Sparrow DA, Culwell AR, Gotto AM Jr (1985) Apolipoprotein E: phospholipid binding studies with synthetic peptides containing the putative receptor binding region. Biochemistry 24:6984–6988

Tytler EM, Segrest JP, Epand RM, Nie SQ, Epand RF, Mishra VK, Venkatachalapathi YV, Anantharamaiah GM (1993) Reciprocal effects of apolipoprotein and lytic peptide analogs on membranes. Cross-sectional molecular shapes of amphipathic alpha-helixes control membrane stability. J Biol Chem 268:22112–22118

Van Lenten BJ, Wagner AC, Jung C-L, Ruchala P, Waring AJ, Lehrer RI, Watson AD, Hama S, Navab M, Anantharamaiah GM, Fogelman AM (2008) Anti-inflammatory apoA-I-mimetic peptides bind oxidized lipids with much higher affinity than human apoA-I. J Lipid Res 49:2302–2311

Weisgraber KH (1994) Apolipoprotein E: structure-function relationships. Adv Protein Chem 45:249–302

Weisgraber KH, Innerarity TL, Harder KJ, Mahley RW, Milne RW, Marcel YL, Sparrow JT (1983) The receptor-binding domain of human apolipoprotein E. Monoclonal antibody inhibition of binding. J Biol Chem 258:12348–12354

White CR, Garber DW, Anantharamaiah GM (2014) Anti-inflammatory and cholesterol-reducing properties of apolipoprotein mimetics: a review. J Lipid Res 55:2007–2021

Zaiou M, Arnold KS, Newhouse YM, Innerarity TL, Weisgraber KH, Segall ML, Phillips MC, Lund-Katz S (2000) Apolipoprotein E – low density lipoprotein receptor interaction: influences of basic residue and amphipathic a-helix organization in the ligand. J Lipid Res 41:1087–1095

Zhang SH, Reddick RL, Piedrahita JA, Maeda N (1992) Spontaneous hypercholesterolemia and arterial lesions in mice lacking apolipoprotein E. Science 258:468–471

Zhang D-W, Lagace TA, Garuti R, Zhao Z, McDonald M, Horton JD, Cohen JC, Hobbs HH (2007) Binding of proprotein convertase subtilisin/kexin type 9 to epidermal growth factor-like repeat A of low density lipoprotein receptor decreases receptor recycling and increases degradation. J Biol Chem 282:18602–18612

Zhu Y, Bellosta S, Langer C, Bernini F, Plas RE, Mahley RW, Assmann G, von Eckardstein A (1998) Low-dose expression of a human apolipoprotein E transgene in macrophages restores cholesterol efflux capacity of apolipoprotein E-deficient mouse plasma. Proc Natl Acad Sci U S A 95:7585–7590

Apolipoprotein E and Mimetics as Targets and Therapeutics for Alzheimer's Disease

Michael P. Vitek, Fengqiao Li, and Carol A. Colton

Abstract After age, the APOE4 genotype is the largest risk factor for Alzheimer's disease (AD). We have developed a series of novel "COG" peptides that mimic the actions of full-length apolipoprotein-E3. Using multiple approaches, we show that COG1410 crosses the blood-brain barrier to provide anti-inflammatory and neuroprotective activities similar to those associated with APOE2- and APOE3-carrying individuals. Like holo-apoE3, COG112 and COG1410 stimulate neurite outgrowth and provide inhibition of inflammatory cytokine release that is independent of APOE-genotype of the treated cells. Using our CVN mouse model of AD that develops behavioral deficits, neuronal loss, amyloid plaques, and neurofibrillary tangle in a time-dependent manner, treatment with COG1410 significantly improves learning and memory behaviors, while decreasing neuronal loss, decreasing amyloid plaques, and decreasing neurofibrillary tangles. This desirable spectrum of disease ameliorating activities after COG treatments suggests a new approach for the treatment of Alzheimer's and other APOE4-associated diseases.

M.P. Vitek (✉)
Department of Neurology and Duke University Medical Center, Cognosci, Inc., Durham, NC, USA
e-mail: mikevitek@cognosci.com

F. Li
Cognosci, Inc., Durham, NC, USA

C.A. Colton
Department of Neurology, Duke University Medical Center, Durham, NC, USA

G.M. Anantharamaiah, D. Goldberg (eds.), *Apolipoprotein Mimetics in the Management of Human Disease*, DOI 10.1007/978-3-319-17350-4_11

Introduction

Humans are the only species to express multiple isoforms of apolipoprotein E (apoE). The most common isoforms of the protein, apoE2, apoE3, and apoE4, are encoded by polymorphisms in the single APOE gene located on human chromosome 19. The importance of these polymorphisms to the human population was made clear with the breakthrough discovery that the APOE4 gene was highly associated with Alzheimer's disease (AD) patients (Saunders et al. 1993; Mayeux et al. 1993). An intense research effort over the ensuing years has confirmed and extended these initial results. In contrast to the healthy population where APOE3 is represented in about 77 % and APOE4 is represented in about 16 % of the younger population, APOE4 is displayed in 45–85 % of the Alzheimer's population, depending upon the study population tested (Mahley and Huang 2012; Michaelson 2014). Furthermore, patients carrying one APOE4 gene (heterozygous for APOE4) have an earlier onset of Alzheimer's symptomatology ranging from 10 years before non-APOE4 carriers, while patients carrying two APOE4 genes (homozygous for APOE4) typically show onset about 20 years before non-APOE4 carriers (Corder et al. 1993). The severe cognitive impairment in APOE4 patients with AD can be explained, at least in part, by the extensive synaptic damage and neuronal death found in APOE4 postmortem brains (Camicioli et al. 1999; Koffie et al. 2012).

The enhanced association between APOE4 and AD has led to numerous additional studies on the potential association of other brain diseases with the APOE4 genotype. Specifically, patients carrying an APOE4 gene with traumatic brain injury (TBI) suffered worse outcomes than those carrying the APOE3 gene (Friedman et al. 1999; Crawford et al. 2002). Similarly, reports on Parkinson's disease (PD), amyotrophic lateral sclerosis (ALS), stroke, and cerebral hemorrhage find that outcomes are worse in APOE4 carriers than in APOE3 carriers (Schmidt et al. 2010; Praline et al. 2011; Kester et al. 2014; Wagle et al. 2009). These combined observations point to a neuroprotective role, where apoE2 and apoE3 may be more potent neuroprotective agents than apoE4. Alternatively, apoE4 may play a destructive role in neurodegenerative diseases, serving as a dominant gain of a negative function. In either case, the end result is similar, synaptic and neuronal loss is increased, and the course and severity of outcomes in APOE4 carriers is worsened.

A precise answer to the question of how the APOE4 gene and the apoE4 protein contribute to neurological disease is open. Several lines of evidence, however, support a loss of a protective function. We and others have shown that levels of the holo-apoE protein are lower in APOE4 carriers than in non-APOE4 carriers (Vitek et al. 2009; Gupta et al. 2011). This difference in holo-apoE protein levels persists between APOE4 carriers and their non-APOE4 counterparts even during aging when a global decline in holo-apoE protein levels occurs (Simon et al. 2012). Additional studies with primary neuronal cultures showed that apoE3, but not apoE4 protein isoforms, supported neurite outgrowth, suggesting a neurotrophic function for apoE3 (Nathan et al. 1994). Studies on primary neuronal cultures also show that apoE3 protects against excitotoxicity-mediated cell death with more potency than apoE4 proteins (Buttini et al. 2010). We and others have also shown that apoE3 proteins are reasonable anti-inflammatory agents compared to apoE4 proteins in immune cells in culture and in whole animals (Brown et al. 2002; Colton et al. 2004; Zhu et al. 2012; Vitek et al. 2009). Following a variety of inflammatory challenges including injections with lipopolysaccharide (LPS) or in models of human disease, the presence of APOE3 and its apoE3 protein product is associated with lower levels of inflammatory mediators like tumor necrosis factor alpha (TNFα), interleukin-6 (IL-6), and nitric oxide (NO) compared to their APOE4/apoE4 counterparts (Colton et al. 2002; Zhu et al. 2012). When viewed as a whole, these reports strongly support that apoE3 delivers anti-inflammatory and neuroprotective effects that are much less evident with apoE4. Combined with lower levels of apoE4 protein, this lower potency of apoE4 could begin to explain the unchecked, more rapid progression and more severe outcomes of neurodegenerative diseases.

To address the pathological state in APOE4 carriers, we reasoned that addition of apoE2 or apoE3 would compensate for the neuroprotective function that was missing with apoE4. If true, one simple solution would be to add apoE2 or apoE3 to the brain. However, as shown by Linton (Linton et al. 1991), moving a protein containing 299 amino acids per monomeric subunit of the apoE dimer across the blood-brain barrier into the brain is unlikely. In Linton's study, liver transplants where the donated liver was a different APOE genotype than the host resulted in the liver-specific donor apoE protein isoform only being present in the blood. The brain continued to express only the host apoE protein isoform. These findings discouraged the idea that exogenous holo-apoE2 or holo-apoE3 proteins could be administered peripherally and find their way into the brains of APOE4 carriers to augment the low neuroprotective actions of the apoE4 protein isoform. More recently, several groups have engineered adenoviral vectors to express human apoE2 or apoE3 proteins, and clinical trials are planned to inject these viral vectors into the brain to increase the levels of apoE2 and/or apoE3 proteins through local production and release in the brain (Feng et al. 2004; Evans et al. 2011).

Peptides as Mimetics of Holo-ApoE Proteins

We have taken a different approach to increase the functional equivalents of apoE2 and/or apoE3 in the brain. To circumvent the problems with holo-proteins, we created peptides containing amino acid residues 133–149 from the receptor-binding region of the apoE protein, a region that is conserved between all of the apoE protein isoforms. Interestingly, despite having the same binding region structure as the apoE3 and apoE4 isoforms, apoE2 shows decreased binding to the LDL receptor, a common receptor that is involved in the clearance of lipoprotein particles from the blood (Rall et al. 1983). These characteristics strongly argue that the three-dimensional structure of apoE2 dimers inhibits exposure of this receptor-binding region to apoE receptors and/or changes the regional secondary alpha-helical structure of this region. The changed binding of apoE2 results in hyperlipoproteinemia, a lipid disorder commonly found in APOE2 carriers.

The original peptide made to mimic the binding region was named COG133, and multiple analogs of COG133 with enhanced cell penetration have now been

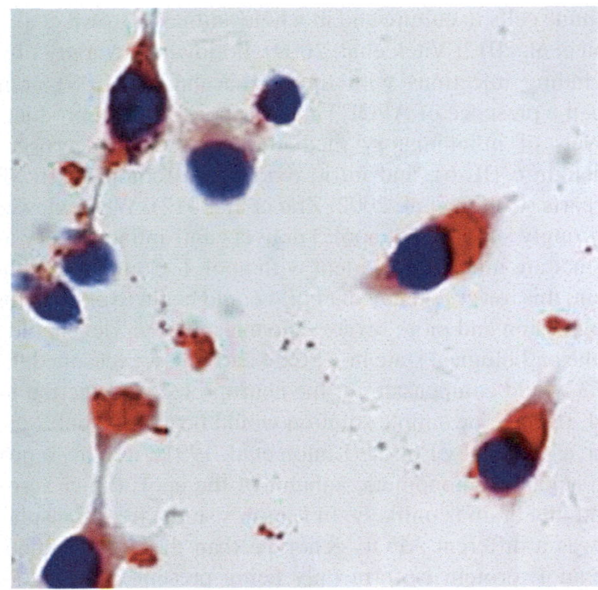

Fig. 1 COG133 penetrates cells and accumulates in the cytoplasm. Adherent BV2 microglia cells were treated with 5 μM biotin-COG133 conjugate for 1 h before cells were washed, fixed, and permeabilized. Avidin-Cy3 dye (*red*) (Rockland Immunochemicals, Umerick, PA) was added for 2 h followed by extensive washing to remove unbound dye. Cell nuclei with counterstained with Hoechst stain (*blue*). In parallel, additional BV2 cells were treated with COG133 alone lacking a biotin conjugate. Images were taken with fluorescence and with white light, and the images merged electronically. Cells stained with COG133 alone did not display red staining. Cells stained with biotin-COG133 featured avidin-Cy3 staining that was mainly found in the cytoplasm, indicating that the biotin-COG133 conjugate crossed the plasma membrane

made. Cell-based studies clearly demonstrated that these peptides entered cells and were capable of altering cellular functions (Fig. 1). Our data from a number of different studies have now also shown that these peptides (a) mimic the anti-inflammatory action of holo-apoE2 and/or holo-apoE3 proteins (Table 1, Figs. 4 and 5, and Christensen et al. 2011), (b) cross the blood-brain barrier in pharmacologically relevant quantities (Figs. 2 and 3 and Lynch et al. 2003), and (c) promote functional changes such as neurite outgrowth (Fig. 6). Using macrophagic cell lines, we tested these compounds for anti-inflammatory potency and the results are shown in Table 1. COG112 displays significantly enhanced anti-inflammatory potency owing to its fusion with a 17 amino acid prefix derived from the protein transduction domain (PTD) known as antennapedia (Li et al. 2006). Like apoE-mimetic peptides, PTDs are amphipathic α-helices that enhance the receptor independent uptake of peptides and proteins. COG449 is a dimer of COG112 that is chemically cross-linked through a single cysteine residue found on each COG112 monomer that resides between the antennapedia prefix and the apoE-133–149 domain. COG1410 is an engineered version of COG133 where amino-iso-butyric acids (aibs) were used to enhance the α-helicity and potency of this analog

Table 1 COG compounds and related peptides used in these studies

Name	Sequence	NO IC_{50} (μM)	TNF-α IC_{50} (μM)	LD_{50} by MTS (μM)
COG112 (antp + apoE 133–149)	Acetyl-RQIKIWFQNRRMKWKKCLRVRLASHLRKLRKRLL-amide	0.8	0.9	5.1
COG133 (apoE 133–149)	Acetyl-LRVRLASHLRKLRKRLL-amide	8.8	2.8	>25
Antennapedia (antp = penetratin®)	Acetyl-RQIKIWFQNRRMKWKKC	16.8	11	>25
COG449 (BMOE covalently cross-linked dimer of COG112)	Acetyl-RQIKIWFQNRRMKWKKCLRVRLASHLRKLRKRLL-amide | Bis-maleimide-ethane | Acetyl-RQIKIWFQNRRMKWKKCLRVRLASHLRKLRKRLL-amide	0.6	0.8	2.1
ApoE-141–149 dimer	Acetyl-LRKLRKRLLLRKLRKRLL-amide	>25	>25	>25
VR55	Acetyl-VSRRR-amide	>30	>30	>30
COG1410	Acetyl-AS(aib)LRKL(aib)KRLL-amide	2.8	3.8	17.5
COG197 (reverse of 1410)	Acetyl-LLRK(aib)LKRL(aib)SA-amide	>25	>25	>25
COG125 (negative control = apoE 133–147)	Acetyl-LRVRLASHLRKLRKR-amide	>25	>25	>25

Primary sequences of apoE-mimetic compounds using standard single-letter amino acid abbreviations with the exception of "aib" for aminoisobutyric acid. Anti-inflammatory measures were determined from a murine BV2 microglial cell line stimulated with 100 ng/ml LPS and treated with increasing concentrations of each of the COG/apoE-mimetics listed. After an overnight incubation, conditioned media were removed, and released levels of TNF-α were measured with an Invitrogen Mouse TNF-α ELISA assay kit. Viability of adherent cells remaining in the microtiter plates was measured using a Promega MTS assay kit. For cell viability assays to assess LD50's, cells grown in complete growth medium with no additions were considered to have 100% signal for viability, and media alone were considered to have 0% signal. IC_{50} values for TNF-α inhibition were calculated under the assumption that LPS-only (no peptide added) cultures exhibit a 100 % response and no-LPS (no peptide added) cultures exhibit a 0 % response (typically below the limit of detection of the kit). IC_{50} and LD_{50} were empirically determined after plotting using the Prism program (GraphPad Software, Inc.)

(Laskowitz et al. 2006). VR55 is another engineered version of COG133 that lacks anti-inflammatory activity (Dawson et al. 2014). Minami et al. (2010) used a head to tail dimer of apoE-141–149 to increase levels of the secreted amyloid peptide precursor alpha (sAPPα) fragment with a concomitant reduction of amyloid beta peptide (Aß), which may have applications in Alzheimer's therapies. Unlike the COG series of compounds, the apoE-141–149 dimer (Table 1) does not display anti-inflammatory activity in BV2 microglial cell cultures. In all cases, the percentage of viable cells treated with apoE141–149 dimer at the IC_{50} concentrations of each peptide was greater than 90 %. From the literature, another apoE-mimetic peptide called Ac-hE18A-NH2 is a 28-residue fusion peptide that contains residues 141–150 fused to a carboxy-terminal 4F peptide and also displays anti-inflammatory activities (Handattu et al. 2013).

ApoE-Mimetic Peptides Cross the BBB

Many different proteins and peptides are given to patients as therapeutic agents, and some of them cross the blood-brain barrier (BBB). Using specialized methods, including a capillary depletion technique, insulin was shown to be saturably transported across the BBB into the brain parenchyma (Duffy and Pardridge 1987; Triguero et al. 1990). Using a different mechanism of passive diffusion, neuropeptide-Y (NPY) was also found to cross the BBB into the brain parenchyma (Kastin and Akerstrom 1999). These and additional studies demonstrate that selected proteins and peptides can move from the blood, cross the BBB, and enter the brain parenchyma to have biological and/or therapeutic activities.

Although holo-apoE proteins do not cross the BBB (Linton et al. 1991), apoE-mimetic peptides can move into the brain parenchyma and the amount and rate of entry can be measured using various techniques. In association with Zlokovic and Deane, we have studied the uptake of apoE-derived peptides into the brain parenchyma using their brain perfusion technique as described by Deane et al. (2004) and LaRue et al. (2004). A tyrosinated derivative of COG1410 (Y-COG1410 = acetyl-YAS(aib)LRKL(aib)KRLL-amide) was synthesized, radiolabeled with sodium-^{125}I by the lactoperoxidase method, quenched with an excess of free tyrosine, and purified using two sequential G10 sephadex columns equilibrated in phosphate-buffered saline (PBS). Ringer's solution was gassed continuously at 37 °C with 5 % CO_2/95 % O_2 followed by addition of ^{125}I-Y-COG1410 (50 nM) plus ^{14}C-inulin as a reference molecule for extracellular space or ^{99m}Tc-albumin as a marker of vascular space. To determine BBB penetration, we cannulated the right common carotid artery in anesthetized mice with a fine polyethylene tube that was connected to an extracorporeal perfusion circuit as described by LaRue et al. (2004). Brains were initially perfused with an artificial plasma solution (123 mM NaCl, 4 mM KCl, 2.5 mM $CaCl_2$, 1.8 mM $MgCL_2$, 25 mM $NaHCO_3$, 1.2 mM KH_2PO_4, 5.5 mM D-glucose, and 6 % dextran) containing 20 % washed sheep red blood cells. Perfusion solutions were gassed with 95 % O_2/5 % CO_2 and warmed to 37 °C to recreate normal brain conditions. At the start of perfusion, the contralateral common carotid artery was ligated and both jugular veins were severed to allow free drainage of perfusate and prevent re-circulation of the blood. Brains were then perfused via the cannulated right common carotid artery with the gassed Ringer's containing the labeled peptides and reference markers using a peristaltic pump. At 1, 5, and 10 min after the start of perfusion, animals were decapitated, their brains quickly removed, and ipsilateral cortex dissected, weighed, and homogenized. Aliquots of the homogenate and perfusion fluid were counted in a gamma counter (Wallac, Perkin Elmer) to quantify ^{125}I-label, and another aliquot was solubilized in Soluene (Packard) at 50 °C for 2 h, mixed with scintillation fluid (Picofluor, Packard), and counted in a scintillation counter (Packard Tricarb) to quantify ^{14}C-inulin. When ^{99m}Tc label was used, it was quantified by measurement in a gamma counter. Volume of distribution V_d was calculated as disintegrations per minute (dpm) per gram (g) of brain tissue divided by dpm per milliliter (ml) of perfusate. The values of the V_d for ^{125}I-peptide in the brain homogenate were corrected for the ^{99m}Tc-albumin that is a marker of the vascular space. Thus, the corrected V_d for brain ^{125}I-peptide was equal to V_d for brain ^{125}I-peptide minus the V_d for brain ^{99m}Tc-albumin (LaRue et al. 2004) since the TCA precipitation showed that most (94 %) of ^{125}I-label and ^{99m}Tc-label were precipitable, indicating that they were not significantly degraded. The plot of V_d versus time for ^{125}I-Y-COG1410 and ^{14}C-inulin as corrected for albumin space is shown in Fig. 2. Using this perfusion method with three animals at each time point, we showed that the V_d of brain ^{125}I-Y-COG1410 increased with time, while the V_d of brain ^{14}C-inulin did not increase with time (Fig. 2), which is consistent with parenchymal uptake of ^{125}I-Y-COG1410.

Because of the importance of accurately detecting brain uptake of COG peptides, we also used biological methods. This approach demonstrates BBB penetrance by demonstrating a change in a specific brain-based mechanism when a drug is perfused into the periphery. For these experiments we used the method of Rousselle et al. (2003). This assay is based on the brain-specific analgesic activity of dalargin (YaGLFR = D-Ala2, Leu4, Arg6-enkephalin), an opiate peptide. Dalargin does not cross the BBB by itself so that peripheral administration does not confer analgesia, while direct administration to the brain does confer analgesia. When dalargin is coupled to a molecule that crosses the BBB into the brain, the conjugated dalargin binds

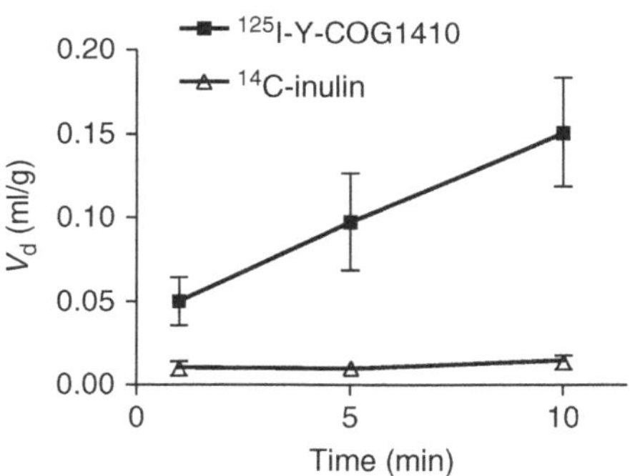

Fig. 2 Time-dependent transport of ^{125}I-Y-COG1410 across the blood-brain barrier. We used the vascular brain perfusion method as described in the text above. We observed that V_d for COG1410 increased over time, while inulin, an extracellular space marker, did not increase over time and has been previously reported (Deane et al. 2004)

opiate receptors within the brain to alter peripheral responses to pain. As shown by Rouselle, the changed physiological response was not due to inactivation of dalargin by linking it to a brain-penetrating agent. Dalargin alone or dalargin fused to the protein transduction domain known as SynB1 (dalargin-SynB1) equally competed for binding of the ligands ^{3}H-DAMGO, ^{3}H-DADLE, or ^{3}H-DPDPE to opiate receptors in a bovine brain opiate radioreceptor binding assay. He then showed that dalargin alone had a V_d of about 15 μl/g, while the dalargin-SynB1 fusion greatly increased the V_d to 300 μl/g. This robust change for V_d in the brain parenchyma occurred even though the volume in the vasculature, V_v, of dalargin alone or the dalargin-SynB1 fusion peptide are both 17 μl/g. As an in vivo test of BBB transport, he then used intravenous administration of dalargin or dalargin-SynB1 fusion into mice and put them on a hot plate to stimulate sensory and pain receptors. A time-dependent increase in analgesic activity was observed in the dalargin-SynB1-treated mice that was significantly greater than the analgesic activity in dalargin-treated mice (Rousselle et al. 2003) and matches the physical method showing the brain penetrance of dalargin-SynB.

We used Rouselle's novel approach as described above to test uptake of COG peptides across the BBB in mice. Rather than a hot plate, however, we have used the Hargreaves test (Hargreaves et al. 1988) to measure latency of foot withdrawal from an infrared radiant beam as an in vivo measure of analgesic activity. One of the advantages of this method is that repeated testing does not contribute to the development of hyperalgesia (Hargreaves et al. 1988). Briefly, each mouse was placed in a clear plastic chamber to acclimate for 10 min. A radiant heat source was positioned directly under the plantar surface of the hind paw to deliver an infrared light beam at 40 % active intensity (Plantar Test Apparatus model 390, IITC Life Science, Woodland Hill, CA). When the animal withdraws the paw, a timer is stopped, and the heat source automatically switches off. To prevent thermal injury, a cutoff time of 10 s was also set. The mean paw withdrawal latency (in seconds) was measured at the indicated times after injection of dalargin alone or dalargin-COG fusion peptides and plotted as shown in Fig. 3. Groups of ten mice were dosed with a single compound and the mean ± SDs are plotted for each time point. Compared to dalargin alone, dalargin-SynB1 fusion peptide-treated mice showed a significant increase in foot withdrawal latency within 5 min of intraperitoneal (IP) injection of dalargin-SynB1 fusion peptide ($p<0.05$). Similarly, dalargin-112 (dalargin linked to COG112 through a peptide bond) and dalargin-1410 (dalargin linked to COG1410 through a peptide bond) showed a significant increase in foot withdrawal latency within 5 min of IP administration ($p<0.05$). In contrast, treatment with dalargin-THRLPRRRRR conjugate as a negative control, and with COG1410 alone, failed to show an increase in foot withdrawal latency ($p>>0.05$). These data strongly support that peripherally administered dalargin-peptide conjugates cross the BBB to bind to brain opiate receptors and induce analgesic activity that results in slower times of foot withdrawal from a radiant heat source. The combination of results from the classical perfusion method and this biological activity method clearly demonstrates that COG compounds cross the blood-brain barrier where they may accumulate to biologically active concentrations (also see Lynch et al. 2003).

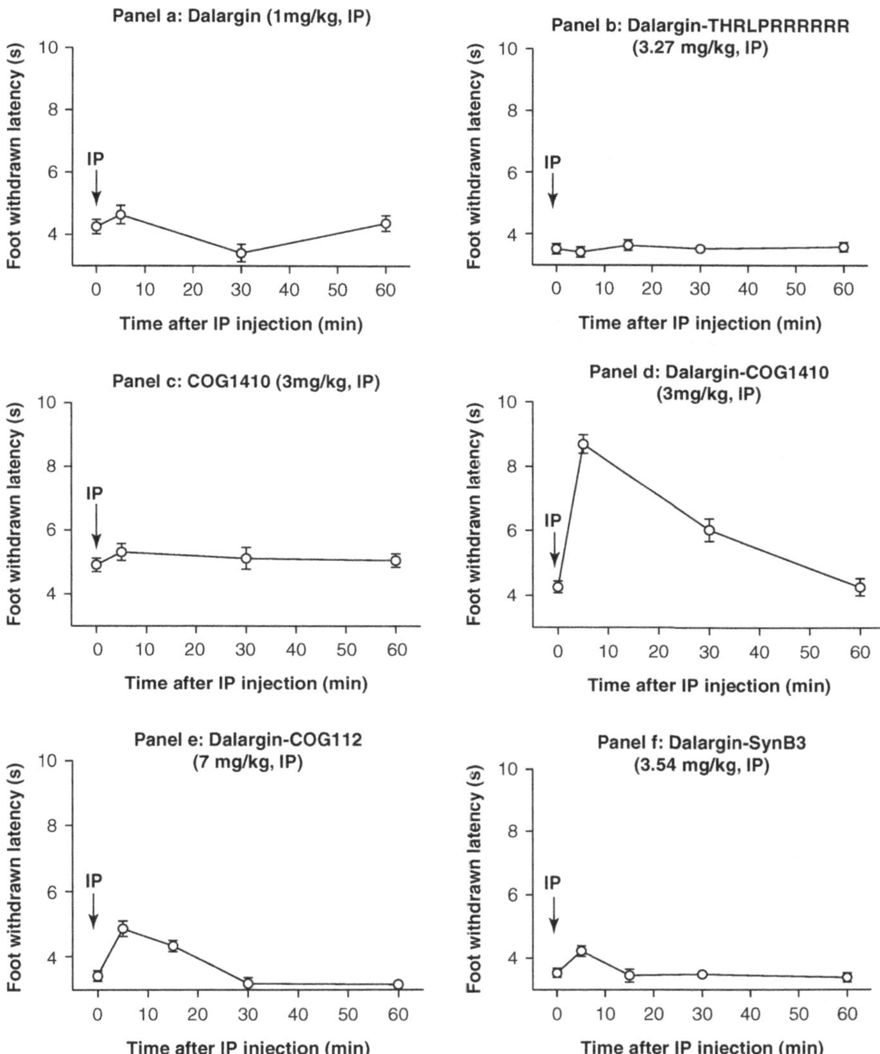

Fig. 3 Time-dependent transport of apoE-mimetic-dalargin fusion peptides across the blood-brain barrier. As described above, the opiate peptide known as dalargin was synthesized together with the indicated peptide partners. Equimolar amounts were administered by intraperitoneal injection at time = 0, and the time-dependent response to a radiant heat source was measured at different time points and plotted. Data show that dalargin alone (Panel **a**), dalargin fused to a negative control peptide that does not cross the BBB (Panel **b**), and COG1410 alone (Panel **c**) are not associated with a significant increase in foot withdrawal in response to a radiant heat source (Hargreaves' test). In contrast, dalargin-COG1410 (Panel **d**), dalargin-COG112 (Panel **e**), and dalargin-SynB3 fusion peptides (Panel **f**) all show a transient and significant increase in foot withdrawal latencies ($p<0.05$ versus time 0), indicating the transport of active dalargin across the BBB by the fusion partner peptide

ApoE Has an Anti-inflammatory Activity in Humans

To better understand the anti-inflammatory activity of apoE-mimetic peptides in humans, we have employed an ex vivo human blood assay (Thurm and Halsey 2005). Briefly, human blood from seven volunteers (four males, three females) was collected by venipuncture using sodium citrate as an anticoagulant. Triplicate 150 μL samples of citrated blood were treated with increasing concentrations of lipopolysaccharide (LPS, 10 μL per sample). After incubation at 37 °C with gentle shaking for 3 h, the samples were centrifuged and plasma fractions were collected. Plasma was diluted 1:10 in phosphate-buffered saline (PBS, pH 7.4), and TNF-α levels in the diluted plasma were quantified with Invitrogen's Human TNF-α ELISA kit. The relationship between the secreted levels of TNF-α and LPS concentration was then used to determine the EC_{90}, defined as the LPS dose that produces 90 % of the maximum secreted level of TNF-α. Using the EC_{90} concentration of LPS determined for each individual, we then defined the dose-response curves (DRC) of COG112 and COG143. Blood samples were pretreated with serial concentrations of COG112 or COG143 and corresponding controls for 30 min prior to addition of the EC_{90} concentration of LPS. Plasma fractions were collected by centrifugation at 3 h after LPS addition, followed by TNF-α ELISA analysis. In this manner we were able to determine the IC_{50} for COG112/COG143 inhibition of LPS-induced TNF-α release for each individual. The composite average values are shown in Fig. 4. We also performed a complete blood count (CBC) on each sample before and after 3 h of incubation with increasing concentrations of COG112/COG143 and did not find any changes in measured hematological parameters with exposure to apoE-mimetic peptides. Extending our previous findings (Christensen et al. 2011), these data clearly show that COG112

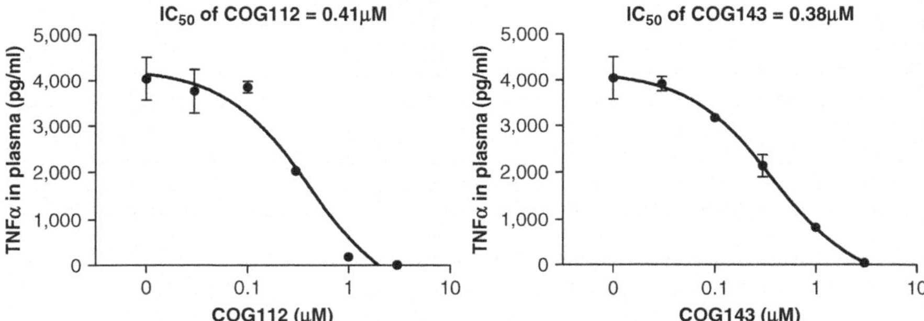

Fig. 4 COG112 and COG143 are effective anti-inflammatory agents in human blood. As described in the text, blood samples from seven volunteers were collected and treated with increasing concentrations of lipopolysaccharide (*LPS*) to determine the LPS concentration for each individual that would give 90 % of the maximal response as measured by TNF-α release (known as the EC_{90}). Using this EC_{90}-LPS value for each individual, additional blood was drawn and treated with LPS plus increasing concentrations of COG112 or COG143 as indicated. TNF-α release into the media was measured and the average secreted values (± SEM) of all seven individuals were plotted. IC_{50} values were then empirically determined for each apoE-mimetic peptide

and COG143 are anti-inflammatory agents with potencies in the sub-μM range in human primary blood samples that normally express human holo-apoE proteins.

The Anti-inflammatory Activity Ex Vivo in Peritoneal Macrophages Is Dependent on ApoE Genotype

To determine whether APOE genotype influences the anti-inflammatory activity of apoE-mimetic peptides, we measured the LPS-stimulated TNF-α response of primary peritoneal macrophages isolated from mice expressing APOE3/3, APOE3/0, APOE4/4, APOE4/0, or APOE0/0 genotypes (where APOE0/0 is a homozygous APOE knockout mouse). Mice were primed by intraperitoneal injection of sodium periodate followed by peritoneal lavage with PBS 72 h later. Lavage fluid was centrifuged and the recovered cells were plated into 48-well microtiter plates. After an overnight incubation at 37 °C in a tissue culture incubator, media and nonadherent cells were removed and fresh media added. Replicate wells ($n=4$ for each treatment) received LPS or LPS plus 5 μM COG1410. Cells were then incubated overnight, conditioned media removed for measurement of TNF-α (Invitrogen Mouse TNF-α ELISA kit), and viability of adherent cells measured with a Promega MTS viability kit. In all cases, cell viability was 90 % or greater. As shown in Fig. 5, treatment with

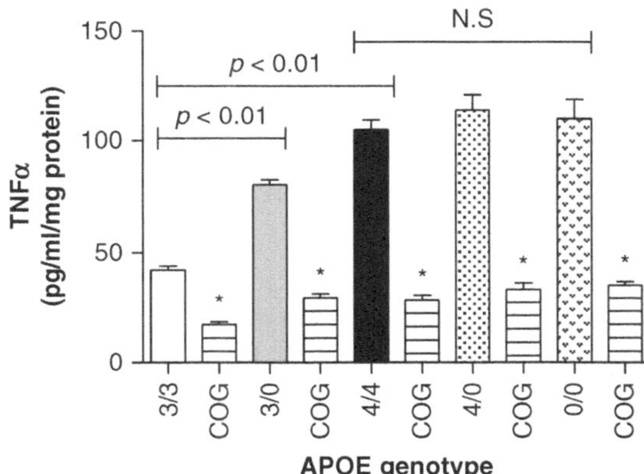

Fig. 5 COG1410 inhibits TNF-α release from peritoneal macrophages of different APOE genotypes. Peritoneal macrophages were harvested as described from APOE3/3 (homozygous APOE3), APOE3/0 (heterozygous APOE3 and heterozygous APOE knockout), APOE4/4, APOE4/0, and APOE0/0 mice. Macrophages were stimulated with LPS ± 5 μM COG1410 overnight and TNF-α levels measured in conditioned media. Total cellular protein was also measured. In each genotype, COG1410 significantly reduced TNF-α release ($p<0.01$). APOE3/3 cells treated with LPS alone had the lowest amount of TNF-α release, which was significantly less than all other genotypes ($p<0.01$). APOE3/0 cells treated with LPS alone had significantly more TNF-α release than APOE3/3 and significantly less TNF-α release than APOE4/4 cultures ($p<0.01$). TNF-α release was not significantly different between APOE4/4, APOE4/0, and APOE0/0 cultures ($p>0.05$)

COG1410 significantly reduced TNF-α release in all APOE genotypes tested. This result shows that supplementation with an apoE-mimetic peptide can significantly reduce inflammatory responses independent of the APOE genotype of the host cell. It is also interesting to note that the highest production of TNF-α was found in LPS-treated cultures from APOE0/0 (homozygous APOE knockout) mice, heterozygous APOE4/0 or homozygous APOE4/4 cells, which were not significantly different from each other. In contrast, homozygous APOE3/3 cells had the lowest levels of TNF-α release, while heterozygous APOE3/0 cells had an intermediate level of TNF-α release. Zhu et al. (2012) found similar outcomes in their experiments using the same mice strains used here. They further showed that LPS treatment of whole animals resulted in significant increases in markers of brain inflammation including IL-1ß, IL-6, TNF-α, GFAP, and F4/80. Like our results, they found that the magnitude of each of these inflammatory markers increased as a function of APOE genotype such that APOE0/0 ≥ APOE4/4 > APOE3/3 > APOE2/2. Importantly, Zhu and colleagues also found that the loss of synaptic markers such as PSD-95, drebin, and synaptophysin shared the same genotype-specific pattern. Overall, analysis of genotypic responses clearly shows that apoE3 protein is a more potent anti-inflammatory mediator than apoE4 protein and that the anti-inflammatory potency of apoE4 protein is equivalent to the lack of apoE protein (i.e., homozygous APOE0/0 knockout cells). It is also important to note that the reduction in TNF-α release depended upon the dose of apoE3 protein. Mice that expressed two APOE3 genes (homozygous APOE3/3 mice) released less TNF-α than heterozygous APOE3/0 cells that express only one APOE3 gene. Supplementation with the apoE-mimetic peptide further reduced TNF-α release in all cells tested, further supporting the idea that apoE3 protein/mimetic peptides are anti-inflammatory agents.

APOE Regulates Neurite Outgrowth

Adding to the multifunctional nature of holo-apoE, Nathan et al. (1994) found that apoE3 protein supported neurite outgrowth of dorsal root ganglion (DRG) neurons, while apoE4 protein was much less supportive. In Fig. 6, we show that COG112 and COG1410 can synergize with nerve growth factor (NGF) to facilitate neurite outgrowth in primary DRG cultures and hippocampal neuronal cultures. DRG neurons were cultured according to Li et al. (2010). Briefly, primary rat DRG from P2 Sprague-Dawley rat pups were cultured in DMEM/Neurobasal A medium with B27 supplement, 0.5 % FBS, and 5 ng/ml of NGF. Cells were plated onto poly-D-lysine-coated coverslips and treated with specific COG compounds. After 3 days, the cells were fixed in 4 % formaldehyde, blocked with goat serum, and permeabilized. Cells were immunoreacted with rabbit anti-neuron-specific beta III tubulin (Abcam, Inc.), washed, and detected with an ABC Elite horseradish peroxidase kit with 3,3′-diaminobenzidine chromophore. Primary rat P2 hippocampal cells were similarly prepared, again in the presence of 5 ng/ml of NGF plus the indicated treatments with COG compounds. A separate well was treated with a high concentration of NGF

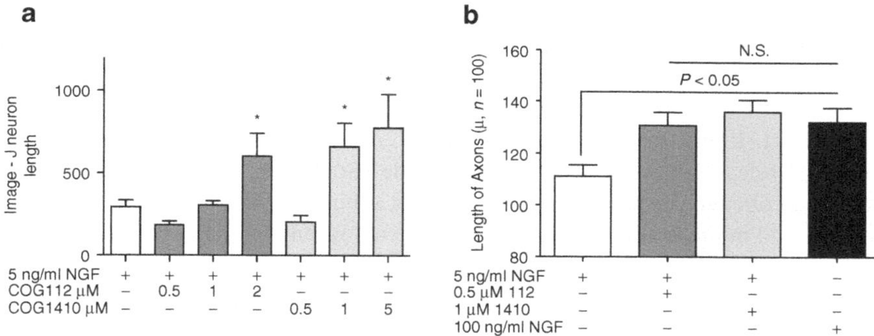

Fig. 6 (**a**) Neurite outgrowth increases in cultured dorsal root ganglion treated with COG112 or COG1410. DRGs were cultured as described in the text in the presence of a suboptimal amount of NGF (5 ng/ml) plus increasing concentrations of COG112 or COG1410 as indicated. Both COG112 and COG1410 at the doses indicated by the *asterisk* were significantly greater than controls ($p<0.05$). (**b**) Neurite outgrowth increases in cultured hippocampal neurons treated with COG112 or COG1410. Primary hippocampal cultures were treated with a suboptimal amount of NGF (5 ng/ml) plus COG112, COG1410, or an optimal dose of NGF (100 ng/ml). Compared to the suboptimal NGF dose, COG112, COG1410, and larger amounts of NGF significantly increase axonal length ($p<0.05$). Compared to an optimal dose of NGF, COG112 and COG1410 do not significantly change axonal length ($p>0.05$)

(100 ng/mL) as a positive control for enhanced neurite extension. After fixing and staining, the length of the axons for each neuron was measured with NIS-Elements imaging software using a Nikon inverted microscope. As shown in Fig. 6a, both COG112 and COG1410 treatment significantly increased the length of axons in DRG cultures compared to the negative controls which contained only a basal (sub-optimal for neurite extension) level of NGF (5 ng/mL). In Fig. 6b, hippocampal cultures stimulated with COG112 or COG1410 plus 5 ng/ml of NGF grew axons to a length that was not significantly different from the increased neurite extension observed in cultures treated with a high level of NGF (100 ng/mL, positive control). These data support that COG112 and COG1410 demonstrate synergistic neurotrophic effects with NGF on axon growth, which may help to stimulate neuronal recovery after insults from injury or disease.

COG112/COG1410 as Supplementation Therapy for Tg2576/NOS2 Knockout Alzheimer's Mice

In more recent studies, we have begun to address how apoE-mimetic peptides function within the brain. We have previously reported that apoE3 and apoE-mimetic peptides specifically bind to a protein found in brain lysates called SET, also known as Inhibitor #2 of Protein Phosphatase 2A or I2PP2A (Christensen et al. 2011). Normally, SET would bind to PP2A and decrease its phosphatase activity. In the presence of apoE-mimetic peptides, SET binding to PP2A is antagonized so that SET/apoE-mimetic peptide complexes are formed and unbound PP2A levels increase, as does PP2A-mediated phosphatase activity. PP2A is well known to dephosphorylate neurofibrillary tangles in Alzheimer's brains (Matsuo et al. 1994; Sontag et al. 1996). In more recent work, PP2A activity was also associated with decreased release of the amyloid beta peptide (Sontag et al. 2007). Importantly, Iqbal and colleagues showed that the catalytic subunit of PP2A was reduced more than twofold in the brains of Alzheimer's patients when compared to age-matched, healthy control brains (Vogelsberg-Ragaglia et al. 2001). Furthermore, SET (aka Inhibitor #2 of PP2A or I_2PP2A) is an endogenous PP2A inhibitor that is increased by about 30 % in AD brains as compared to age-matched controls (Tanimukai et al. 2005). The combination of these effects in AD results in significantly lowered levels of brain PP2A-mediated phosphatase activity. Iqbal and others have shown that PP2A is the main enzyme that dephosphorylates phospho-tau proteins in neurofibrillary tangles (Liang et al. 2008). Iqbal further showed that treatment of brain slices with okadaic acid, a potent inhibitor of PP2A, caused a robust increase in phospho-tau which, in many respects, forms structures highly reminiscent of neurofibrillary tangles (Gong et al. 2000). Under these conditions, inhibition of phosphatase activity permits the accumulation of phosphorylated tau, which then appears to form neurofibrillary tangle-like (NFT-like) structures.

Based on these activities of PP2A in AD brains, we have studied the actions of apoE-mimetic peptide treatment in mouse models of Alzheimer's disease. We recently reported that two different Alzheimer's mouse models, the Tg2576/NOS2$^{-/-}$ and APP-SwDI/NOS2$^{-/-}$ (CVN-AD) mouse strains, both displayed extensive amyloid plaque-like deposits, neurofibrillary tangle-like deposits, neuronal loss, and behavioral deficits (Colton et al. 2006, 2014; Wilcock et al. 2009). With the availability of these improved mouse models of Alzheimer's disease, we focused upon the ability of COG1410 and COG112 (more potent analogs of COG133 that also cross the blood-brain barrier) to alter the AD-like pathology in the brains of these double-transgenic mice. Briefly, 9-month-old animals were treated three times weekly for 3 months with lactated Ringer's vehicle (LR) or COG112 in LR by subcutaneous injection of 100 μl volume of LR or 4 mg/Kg of COG112 in LR buffer. A third group of animals were treated three times weekly with subcutaneous COG1410 in LR buffer at 4 mg/kg. Following treatment for 3 months, the mice were tested for changes in learning and memory and sacrificed. Brains were perfused with PBS, removed, and then fixed in 4 % paraformaldehyde. Frozen brain sections were cut, and sections were then immunostained using a polyclonal anti-amyloid-ß-peptide antibody (Biosource #44-338-100) to stain amyloid plaque-like structures, a monoclonal AT8 anti-phospho-tau antibody (ThermoScientific, Waltham, MA) to stain neurofibrillary tangle-like structures, and an anti-NeuN antibody (Chemicon, MAB377, Temecula, CA) to stain all neurons. Immunopositive cells were detected using the VECTASTAIN (ABC) kit (Vector Laboratories, Burlingame, CA) and photographed on a Nikon microscope. Objects consisting of amyloid plaques, neurofibrillary tangles, and neuronal cell bodies were counted using the optical fractionator method with Stereo Investigator 9 software package (MicroBrightField, Williston, VT) interfaced with a Nikon microscope with a computer-controlled mechanical stage (Colton et al. 2014). Further analysis of images was performed with Image-Pro Plus software (Media Cybernetics, Inc., Bethesda, MD).

Overall, we found that treatment with COG112 or COG1410 significantly reduced the pathology and improved the learning and memory behavior of Tg2576/NOS2$^{-/-}$ mice. As shown in Fig. 7, amyloid plaques were significantly higher in vehicle-treated animals (Panel 7a) compared to those treated with COG1410 (Panel 7b) or with COG112 (Panel 7c) ($p<0.01$ by pairwise *t*-tests). This result compares favorably to our recent publication showing that COG1410 treatment of CVN-

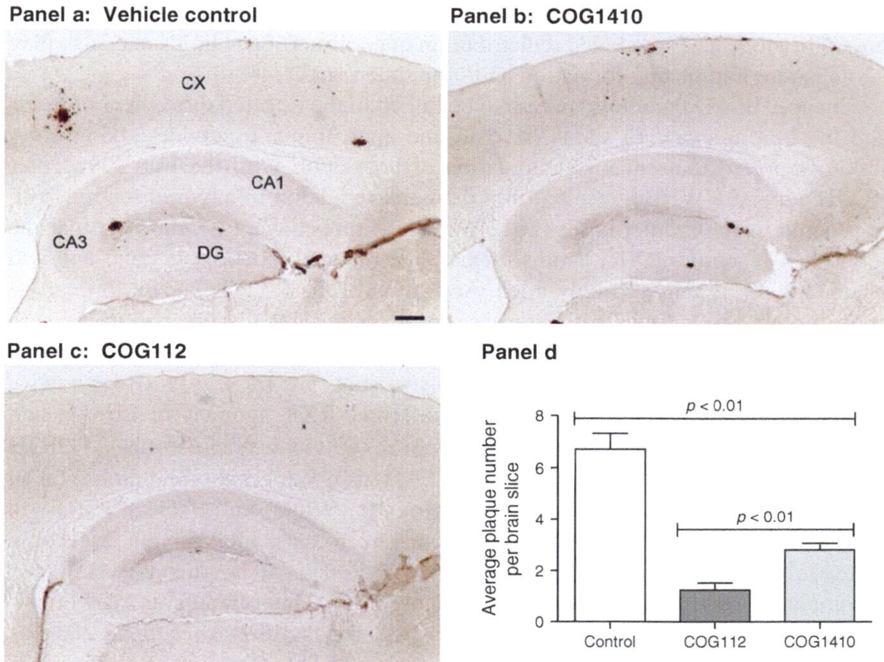

Fig. 7 Treatment with COG112 or COG1410 reduces amyloid plaque burden in Tg2576/NOS2$^{-/-}$ mice. Representative brain slices from double-transgenic mice treated 3× weekly over months 10, 11, and 12 with lactated Ringer's buffer (Panel **a**), COG1410 (Panel **b**), or COG112 (Panel **c**) were stained for amyloid beta peptide. Each plaque structure was counted on every 10th slice from a brain hemisphere and the average ± SEM is plotted in (Panel **d**). The number of plaques in the control-treated mice was significantly greater than in the COG112- or COG1410-treated mice ($p<0.01$). The number of plaques in the COG112-treated mice was significantly less than those from the COG1410 treated mice ($p<0.01$)

Alzheimer's mice reduces amyloid plaque density and significantly reduces both soluble and insoluble Aß 1–40 and Aß 1–42 (Vitek et al. 2012). Similar to our data, Minami et al. (2010) showed a dimer of apoE-141–149 reduced Aß release from cells. COG112 contains this exact protein sequence and COG1410 contains an engineered version of this 141–149 region of apoE. Both of the COG peptides reduce Aß-containing amyloid plaques when subcutaneously injected as described above. Since apoE-141–149 dimers did not display anti-inflammatory activity in our BV2 assay (Table 1), the ability of apoE-mimetic peptides to reduce Aß production and reduce amyloid plaque formation may not be a strict function of anti-inflammatory activity. On the other hand, Handattu et al. (2013) showed that a fusion peptide called Ac-hE18A-NH_2 containing apoE-141–150 linked to the amphipathic 18A peptide does possess anti-inflammatory activity (Datta et al. 2010). This peptide also reduced amyloid plaque burden in an AD mouse model, in this case, the APP/PS1Δ9 mouse strain. Since the Ac-hE18A-NH_2 peptide was also shown to reduce plasma cholesterol and atherosclerotic plaque formation, this finding raises the possibility that apoE-mediated redistribution of cholesterol and lipids may also play a role in amyloid plaque formation and/or maintenance.

Changes in AD pathology may also be linked to the targeted movement of lipids and the lipid-association status of apoE and apoE-mimetic peptides. Jiang et al. (2008) reported that enhanced lipidation of holo-apoE with the liver-X-receptor (LXR) agonist GW3965 resulted in a dramatic reduction in amyloid load in APP transgenic mice. Cramer et al. (2012) furthered this concept by showing that the retinoid-X-receptor (RXR) agonist bexarotene reduced Abeta levels and amyloid plaque burden in amyloid-only mice. Activation of the RXR is known to increase apoE protein levels by increasing transcription of the APOE gene and to increase the apoE lipidation state by increasing ABCA1 and ABCG1, membrane-based transporters for lipid. In contrast, an extensive study by Tai et al. (2014) shows a very complex pattern of effects of two different RXR agonists in EFAD3 and EFAD4 Alzheimer's mice (EFAD3 is a 5xFAD amyloid mouse on an APOE3/3 transgenic replacement background, and EFAD4 is a 5xFAD amyloid mouse on an APOE4/4 transgenic replacement background). While universal increases in ABCA1 were observed following RXR agonist treatments, apoE protein levels only increased in EFAD4 mice with short-term RXR agonist treatments which was accompanied by significant decreases in soluble Aß42 and oligomeric Aß. Longer-term treatment with RXR agonists, however, abrogated these beneficial changes and, in the case of EFAD3, may actual increase Aß levels. Tai goes on to speculate that the significant hepatomegaly associated with RXR agonist treatment may, in the long term, reverse the initial beneficial effects of short-term gains in apoE protein levels and lipidated apoE levels. While these and other RXR agonist studies continue, the observed increases in apoE protein levels and in apoE lipidation status appear to confer a protective effect in transgenic amyloid-only mice that further supports the concept that supplementation with apoE/mimetics may be an effective therapeutic strategy in AD.

Our findings that apoE-mimetic peptides reactivate PP2A (Christensen et al. 2011) also provide a reasonable mechanism for the reduction in Aß production observed in AD mice treated with apoE/mimetics (see Fig. 7). Sontag et al. (2007) reported that overexpression of the catalytic subunit of PP2A (PP2Ac) decreased Aß release from cells while overexpression of a dominant negative catalytic subunit of PP2A increased Aß release from cells in culture. Going further, Liu et al. (2013) used lentiviral-anti-SET-siRNA vectors in APP-Tg2576 mice to show that activation of PP2A activity levels in the brain was associated with a decrease in amyloid plaque structures as well as decreased Aß 1–40 and 1–42 levels. Liu also showed that simultaneous inhibition of PP2A with a lentiviral-anti-PP2A-siRNA vector abolished all of the reductions observed with anti-SET-siRNA vectors. These combined results suggest that some aspect of APP processing into Aß may require activation through a kinase, which is opposed by the PP2A phosphatase.

Phosphorylated Tau and Neurofibrillary Tangles

An increase in the number of phosphate groups per tau protein is associated with the formation of aggregates of tau known as neurofibrillary tangles, which are one of the defining pathologies in the brains of AD patients. Neurons containing hyperphosphorylated tau protein are commonly identified using antibodies generated against specific disease-associated phosphorylation sites. As shown in Fig. 8, immunostaining using an antibody (called AT8) directed against ser202/thr205 of phosphorylated tau in NFT-like structures was greatest in cortical brain regions of vehicle-treated animals (Panels 8a and 8c) compared to those treated with COG1410 (Panel 8b) or treated with COG112 (Panel 8d). These results are consistent with our mechanism of action where apoE-mimetic peptides increase the levels of PP2A-mediated phosphatase activity (Christensen et al. 2011). We previously reported that COG1410 treatment of CVN-AD mice also significantly reduced phospho-tau and NFT-like structures in this different strain of transgenic AD models (Vitek et al. 2012). Using an entirely different type of AD mouse model, Ghosal et al. (2013) showed that treatment of AICD-Alzheimer's mice with COG112 also reduced levels of phospho-tau and NFT-like structures. Wang et al. (2010) showed that overexpression of SET would decrease levels of PP2A-mediated phosphatase activity in the brain, resulting in increased levels of phosphorylated tau and NFT-like structures in rat brains, which indirectly supports the findings we present in Fig. 8. Liu et al. (2013) went further by using a lentiviral-anti-SET-siRNA approach to decrease SET levels in transgenic mouse brain and found that levels of phosphorylated tau and NFT-like structures were reduced, results that directly support our mechanism of action with apoE-mimetic peptides. Collectively, these data strongly indicate that the abnormal phosphorylation of tau as typically found in AD can be reduced by treatment with apoE-mimetic peptides.

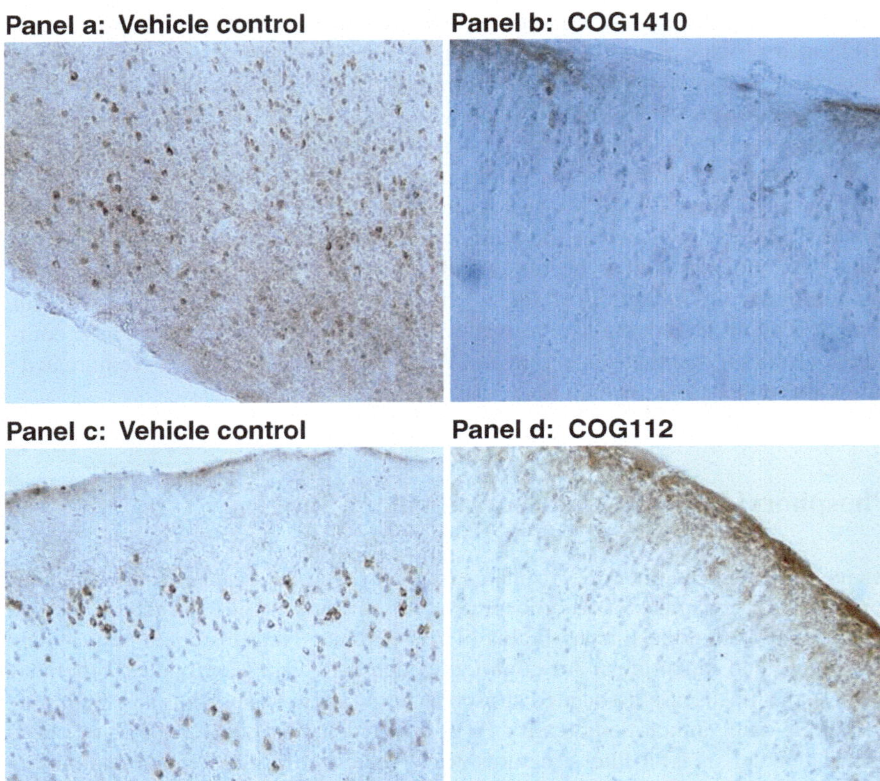

Fig. 8 Treatment with COG112 or COG1410 reduces neurofibrillary tangle burden in Tg2576/NOS2$^{-/-}$ mice. Representative brain slices from double-transgenic mice treated 3× weekly over months 10, 11, and 12 with lactated Ringer's buffer (Panel **a**), COG1410 (Panel **b**), lactated Ringer's buffer (Panel **c**) or COG112 (Panel **d**) were stained for phosphorylated tau with the AT8 monoclonal antibody. Cortical brain regions are displayed

Neuronal Loss

Perhaps the most overlooked but significant pathological characteristic of Alzheimer's disease is the loss of functional neurons in the brains of patients. While many mouse models of AD display pathological lesions and some behavioral deficits, very few models demonstrate significant neuronal loss. One of the key features of Tg2576/NOS2$^{-/-}$ and CVN-AD mice is that they display significant neuronal loss that progresses with the age of the animal (Wilcock et al. 2008; Colton et al. 2014). Using NeuN staining of neurons in the CA2/3 region of the hippocampus and unbiased stereological counting, we showed that treatment of these mouse models with COG112 (Panel 9a) or COG1410 (Panel 9b) resulted in significantly more neurons than in animals treated with vehicle alone (Panel 9c) ($p < 0.001$ by pairwise t-test). Interestingly, the number of neurons in the COG112-treated animals was not significantly different from those treated with COG1410 ($p > 0.05$ by t-test), even though the number of amyloid plaques was lower in COG112-treated than in COG1410-treated animals (Fig. 7). Ghosal et al. (2013) used amyloid precursor protein intracellular domain (AICD)-overexpressing mice to show that treatment with COG112 rescued the impaired neurogenesis associated with the AICD mice. Although the number of bromodeoxyuridine (BrdU)-labeled neurons was higher in the COG112-treated mice, this result still leaves open the question as to whether COG112 treatment inhibited the death of neurons or whether it promoted the birth and maturation of new neurons as a way to preserve neuronal numbers in the face of amyloid plaque and neurofibrillary tangle pathologies. Additional staining of immature neurons with doublecortin (DCX) was also greater in the COG112-treated animals, suggesting that the treatment may be encouraging enhanced neuron proliferation (Ghosal et al. 2013). All of these findings together suggest that treatments designed to reduce amyloid plaques and reduce neurofibrillary tangles may be effective in reducing neuronal loss in an Alzheimer's mouse model (Fig. 9).

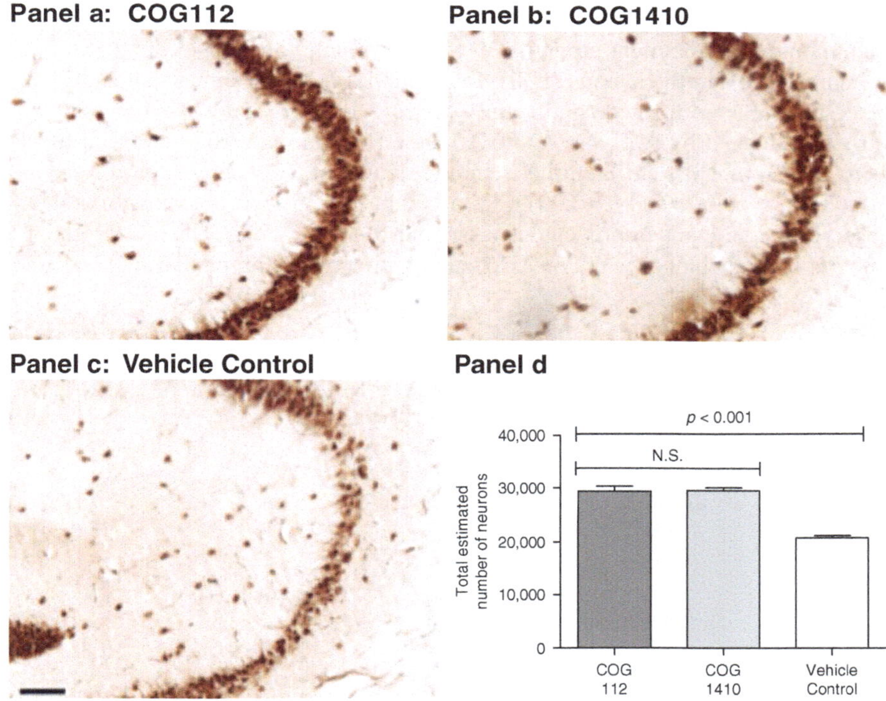

Fig. 9 Treatment with COG112 or COG1410 reduces neuron loss in Tg2576/NOS2$^{-/-}$ mice. Representative brain slices from double-transgenic mice treated 3× weekly over months 10, 11, and 12 with COG112 (Panel **a**), COG1410 (Panel **b**), or lactated Ringer's buffer (Panel **c**) were stained for neurons with NeuN antibody. The number of neurons in the CA2/3 region of the hippocampus of three mice per treatment was counted using unbiased stereological methods. The average (± SEM) number of neurons is shown in Panel d. The number of neurons in the control-treated mice was significantly less than in the COG112- or COG1410-treated mice ($p<0.001$). The number of neurons in the COG112-treated mice was not significantly different than those from the COG1410-treated mice ($p>0.05$)

Behavioral Deficits

The development of amyloid plaque and neurofibrillary tangle-like pathologies coupled with neuronal loss in Tg2576/NOS2$^{-/-}$ mice also leads to deficits in spatial memory performance in the radial arm water maze (Colton et al. 2006). We treated Tg2576/NOS2$^{-/-}$ mice with COG112 (3 mg/Kg, subcutaneous in 100 μl lactated Ringer's buffer) three times per week for 3 months (months 10, 11, and 12) and then performed our standard radial arm water maze. Briefly, mice are placed into different arms of a six-arm water maze and allowed to swim to an escape platform for each trial. For the first 10 trials on day 1 of testing, the escape platform is alternated between visible and hidden just below the surface as part of the acquisition phase of learning the maze. The remaining five trials on day 1 and the 15 trials on day 2 employ a hidden platform. For each trial, an entry into an arm that lacks the escape platform is scored as an error. The total number of errors before the animal finds the escape platform is recorded for each trial. Trials are grouped into blocks of three consecutive trials. For each trial block, the errors for each mouse in a treatment group (COG112 vs. vehicle) on each of the three trials are combined, and the average ± SEM is plotted. Figure 10 shows that COG112-treated animals performed significantly better than their vehicle-treated counterparts as analyzed by two-way ANOVA where interaction, errors, and trial block were all significantly different between the treatment and vehicle control groups ($p<0.036$, $p<0.001$ and $p<0.001$). Using eight mice per group, we were able to observe a significant improvement in spatial memory with COG112 treatment. The improved behavior was also associated with a reduction in neuronal loss and

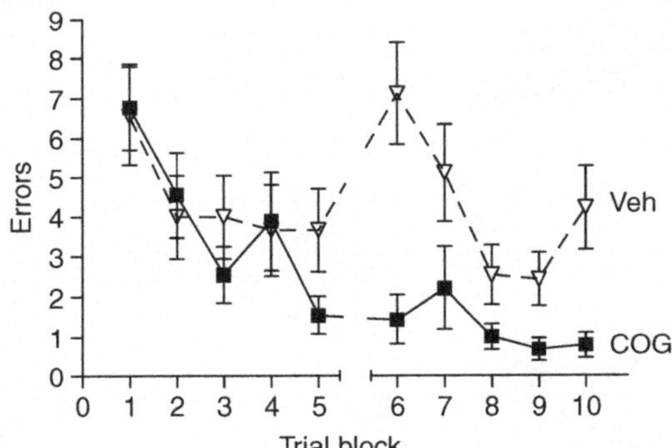

Fig. 10 Tg2576/NOS2−/− mice treated with COG112 perform significantly better than their vehicle-treated counterparts. Double-transgenic mice were treated 3× weekly over months 10, 11, and 12 with lactated Ringer's buffer (Veh) or COG112 (COG). Mice were then tested in the radial arm water maze and the number of errors counted for each trial block. The average number of errors ± SEM was plotted for the vehicle control (*dashed line* with *open triangles*) or the COG112 treatment (*solid lines* with filed *boxes*). $n=8$ mice per group. Performance of COG112-treated animals was significantly better (less errors) than controls when analyzed by two-way ANOVA (interaction $p<0.05$, errors $p<0.01$, trial block $p<0.01$)

in plaque- and tangle-like structures as we detailed above. Since COG112 antagonizes SET, our data also supports the importance of SET protein as a pathological factor. This concept is strongly re-enforced by Liu et al. (2013) who used a lentiviral-anti-SET-siRNA approach to decrease SET levels in Tg2576 mice. Their study clearly demonstrated that lentiviral induced reduction in SEt also produced improved spatial memory performance in this mouse model of AD. Essentially, Liu's experiment provides a more direct molecular approach to show what we have found with COG apoE peptide treatment. Similarly, Handattu et al. (2013) used transgenic amyloid-only mice to show that their Ac-hE18A-NH_2 apoE-mimetic peptide also reduced behavioral deficits in a classical water maze. Cramer et al. (2012) showed that increased apoE protein levels associated with bexarotene treatment improved behavioral performance in transgenic amyloid-only mice. The diverse nature of testing paradigms using apoE-mimetic peptides and pharmacological strategies to increase apoE protein levels strongly support that supplementation to increase brain "apoE functional units" results in improved behavioral performance, one of the outcomes of primary importance to patients with Alzheimer's.

Conclusions

The strong association between the presence of an APOE4 gene allele and its apoE4 protein product with the presence of Alzheimer's disease implores us to better understand the mechanism of action by which APOE genes and/or apoE proteins contribute to the disease state. Through these studies, we can clearly point to the superior anti-inflammatory and neurotrophic actions of apoE3 protein isoforms over apoE4 protein isoforms as contributors to brain health. Our findings that supplementation with apoE-mimetic peptides like COG112 and COG1410 produces an anti-inflammatory state in spite of an APOE4 genetic background strongly argue for the concept that APOE4 carriers suffer from the lack of a protective function that is afforded by APOE2 and/or APOE3 gene products. Further supporting this concept is our findings that peripheral supplementation with apoE-mimetic peptides that cross the blood-brain barrier increases the amount of apoE-directed protective functions in the brain. This point is further reinforced by our extensive studies in animal models of traumatic brain injury (TBI), stroke, intracranial hemorrhage, subarachnoid hemorrhage, peripheral nerve crush, and spinal cord injury, where supplementation with apoE-mimetic peptides yielded significant improvements in behavioral outcomes, pathology-based outcomes, and survival (Hoane et al. 2007; Tukhovskaya et al. 2009; James et al. 2009; Gao et al. 2006; Li et al. 2010; Wang et al. 2014). Interestingly, the gain of anti-inflammatory function may be specific to the receptor-binding region of holo-apoE, as peptides outside of the receptor-binding region do not display anti-inflammatory activity nor binding to SET (Vitek, unpublished). As we previously published in CVN-Alzheimer's mice (Vitek et al. 2012), our new data show that COG112 and COG1410 also reduce amyloid plaques, NFTs, and neuronal loss while improving learning and memory behaviors in another Alzheimer's mouse model, the Tg2576/NOS2$^{-/-}$ double-transgenic mice. The COG112/COG1410-mediated gain of these protective functions in multiple animal models of AD lays the groundwork for future studies to evaluate the effectiveness of apoE supplementation in human patients suffering from Alzheimer's disease.

Acknowledgments and Disclosures Michael P. Vitek, Ph.D., is an Associate Professor of Neurology at Duke University Medical Center, Chief Executive Officer and a stockholder of Cognosci, Inc., and Interim Chief Executive Officer and a stockholder of Oncotide Pharmaceuticals, Inc. Matters pertaining to any institutional or individual conflict of interest are managed by the DUMC Conflict of Interest Committee. Dr. Fengqiao Li is Chief Scientific Officer and a stockholder of Cognosci, Inc. Dr. Carol A. Colton is a Professor of Neurology at Duke University Medical Center where matters pertaining to institutional or individual conflict of interest are managed by the DUMC Conflict of Interest Committee. We would like to thank Ms. M. Jansen for her expert assistance with some experiments presented in this chapter.

References

Brown CM, Wright E, Colton CA, Sullivan PM, Laskowitz DT, Vitek MP (2002) Apolipoprotein E isoform mediated regulation of nitric oxide release. Free Radic Biol Med 32(11):1071–1075, Access. No's.: 12031891

Buttini M, Masliah E, Yu GQ, Palop JJ, Chang S, Bernardo A, Lin C, Wyss-Coray T, Huang Y, Mucke L (2010) Cellular source of apolipoprotein E4 determines neuronal susceptibility to excitotoxic injury in transgenic mice. Am J Pathol 177(2):563–569, Access. No's.: 20595630 2913361

Camicioli R, Kaye J, Payami H, Ball MJ, Murdoch G (1999) Apolipoprotein E epsilon4 is associated with neuronal loss in the substantia nigra in Alzheimer's disease. Dement Geriatr Cogn Disord 10(6):437–441, Access. No's.: 10559556

Christensen DJ, Ohkubo N, Oddo J, Van Kanegan MJ, Neil J, Li F, Colton CA, Vitek MP (2011) Apolipoprotein E and peptide mimetics modulate inflammation by binding the SET protein and activating protein phosphatase 2A. J Immunol 186(4):2535–2542, Access. No's.: 21289314

Colton CA, Brown CM, Czapiga M, Vitek MP (2002) Apolipoprotein-E allele-specific regulation of nitric oxide production. Ann N Y Acad Sci 962:212–225, Access. No's.: 12076977

Colton CA, Needham LK, Brown C, Cook D, Rasheed K, Burke JR, Strittmatter WJ, Schmechel DE, Vitek MP (2004) APOE genotype-specific differences in human and mouse macrophage nitric oxide production. J Neuroimmunol 147(1–2):62–67, Access. No's.: 14741429

Colton CA, Vitek MP, Wink DA, Xu Q, Cantillana V, Previti ML, Van Nostrand WE, Weinberg JB, Dawson H (2006) NO synthase 2 (NOS2) deletion promotes multiple pathologies in a mouse model of Alzheimer's disease. Proc Natl Acad Sci U S A 103(34):12867–12872, Access. No's.: 16908860 1550768

Colton CA, Wilson JG, Everhart A, Wilcock DM, Puolivali J, Heikkinen T, Oksman J, Jaaskelainen O, Lehtimaki K, Laitinen T, Vartiainen N, Vitek MP (2014) mNos2 deletion and human NOS2 replacement in Alzheimer disease models. J Neuropathol Exp Neurol 73(8):752–769, Access. No's.: 25003233 4131941

Corder EH, Saunders AM, Strittmatter WJ, Schmechel DE, Gaskell PC, Small GW, Roses AD, Haines JL, Pericak-Vance MA (1993) Gene dose of apolipoprotein E type 4 allele and the risk of Alzheimer's disease in late onset families. Science 261(5123):921–923, Access. No's.: 8346443

Cramer PE, Cirrito JR, Wesson DW, Lee CY, Karlo JC, Zinn AE, Casali BT, Restivo JL, Goebel WD, James MJ, Brunden KR, Wilson DA, Landreth GE (2012) ApoE-directed therapeutics rapidly clear beta-amyloid and reverse deficits in AD mouse models. Science 335(6075): 1503–1506, Access. No's.: 22323736 3651582

Crawford FC, Vanderploeg RD, Freeman MJ, Singh S, Waisman M, Michaels L, Abdullah L, Warden D, Lipsky R, Salazar A, Mullan MJ (2002) APOE genotype influences acquisition and recall following traumatic brain injury. Neurology 58(7):1115–1118, Access. No's.: 11940706

Datta G, White CR, Dashti N, Chaddha M, Palgunachari MN, Gupta H, Handattu SP, Garber DW, Anantharamaiah GM (2010) Anti-inflammatory and recycling properties of an apolipoprotein mimetic peptide, Ac-hE18A-NH(2). Atherosclerosis 208(1):134–141, Access. No's.: 19656510 2813354

Dawson HN, Kolls B, Laskowitz DT (2014) Peptide compounds for suppressing inflammation. US Patent Application WO2012129077 A2

Deane R, Zheng W, Zlokovic BV (2004) Brain capillary endothelium and choroid plexus epithelium regulate transport of transferrin-bound and free iron into the rat brain. J Neurochem 88(4):813–820, Access. No's.: 14756801 3980859

Duffy KR, Pardridge WM (1987) Blood-brain barrier transcytosis of insulin in developing rabbits. Brain Res 420(1):32–38, Access. No's.: 3315116

Evans VC, Graham IR, Athanasopoulos T, Galley DJ, Jackson CL, Simons JP, Dickson G, Owen JS (2011) Adeno-associated virus serotypes 7 and 8 outperform serotype 9 in expressing atheroprotective human apoE3 from mouse skeletal muscle. Metabolism 60(4):491–498, Access. No's.: 20580777

Feng X, Eide FF, Jiang H, Reder AT (2004) Adeno-associated viral vector-mediated ApoE expression in Alzheimer's disease mice: low CNS immune response, long-term expression, and astrocyte specificity. Front Biosci 9:1540–1546, Access. No's.: 14977565

Friedman G, Froom P, Sazbon L, Grinblatt I, Shochina M, Tsenter J, Babaey S, Yehuda B, Groswasser Z (1999) Apolipoprotein E-epsilon4 genotype predicts a poor outcome in survivors of traumatic brain injury. Neurology 52(2):244–248, Access. No's.: 9932938

Gao J, Wang H, Sheng H, Lynch JR, Warner DS, Durham L, Vitek MP, Laskowitz DT (2006) A novel apoE-derived therapeutic reduces vasospasm and improves outcome in a murine model of subarachnoid hemorrhage. Neurocrit Care 4(1):25–31, Access. No's.: 16498192

Ghosal K, Stathopoulos A, Thomas D, Phenis D, Vitek MP, Pimplikar SW (2013) The apolipoprotein-E-mimetic COG112 protects amyloid precursor protein intracellular domain-overexpressing animals from Alzheimer's disease-like pathological features. Neurodegener Dis 12(1):51–58, Access. No's.: 22965147

Gong CX, Lidsky T, Wegiel J, Zuck L, Grundke-Iqbal I, Iqbal K (2000) Phosphorylation of microtubule-associated protein tau is regulated by protein phosphatase 2A in mammalian brain. Implications for neurofibrillary degeneration in Alzheimer's disease. J Biol Chem 275(8):5535–5544, Access. No's.: 10681533

Gupta VB, Laws SM, Villemagne VL, Ames D, Bush AI, Ellis KA, Lui JK, Masters C, Rowe CC, Szoeke C, Taddei K, Martins RN, A. R. Group (2011) Plasma apolipoprotein E and Alzheimer disease risk: the AIBL study of aging. Neurology 76(12):1091–1098, Access. No's.: 21422459

Handattu SP, Monroe CE, Nayyar G, Palgunachari MN, Kadish I, van Groen T, Anantharamaiah GM, Garber DW (2013) In vivo and in vitro effects of an apolipoprotein e mimetic peptide on amyloid-beta pathology. J Alzheimers Dis 36(2):335–347, Access. No's.: 23603398 4120251

Hargreaves K, Dubner R, Brown F, Flores C, Joris J (1988) A new and sensitive method for measuring thermal nociception in cutaneous hyperalgesia. Pain 32(1):77–88, Access. No's.: 3340425

Hoane MR, Pierce JL, Holland MA, Birky ND, Dang T, Vitek MP, McKenna SE (2007) The novel apolipoprotein E-based peptide COG1410 improves sensorimotor performance and reduces injury magnitude following cortical contusion injury. J Neurotrauma 24(7):1108–1118, Access. No's.: 17610351

James ML, Sullivan PM, Lascola CD, Vitek MP, Laskowitz DT (2009) Pharmacogenomic effects of apolipoprotein e on intracerebral hemorrhage. Stroke 40(2):632–639, Access. No's.: 19109539 2699752

Jiang Q, Lee CY, Mandrekar S, Wilkinson B, Cramer P, Zelcer N, Mann K, Lamb B, Willson TM, Collins JL, Richardson JC, Smith JD, Comery TA, Riddell D, Holtzman DM, Tontonoz P,

Landreth GE (2008) ApoE promotes the proteolytic degradation of Abeta. Neuron 58(5):681–693, Access. No's.: 18549781 2493297

Kastin AJ, Akerstrom V (1999) Nonsaturable entry of neuropeptide Y into brain. Am J Physiol 276(3 Pt 1):E479–E482, Access. No's.: 10070013

Kester MI, Goos JD, Teunissen CE, Benedictus MR, Bouwman FH, Wattjes MP, Barkhof F, Scheltens P, van der Flier WM (2014) Associations between cerebral small-vessel disease and Alzheimer disease pathology as measured by cerebrospinal fluid biomarkers. JAMA Neurol 71(7):855–862, Access. No's.: 24818585

Koffie RM, Hashimoto T, Tai HC, Kay KR, Serrano-Pozo A, Joyner D, Hou S, Kopeikina KJ, Frosch MP, Lee VM, Holtzman DM, Hyman BT, Spires-Jones TL (2012) Apolipoprotein E4 effects in Alzheimer's disease are mediated by synaptotoxic oligomeric amyloid-beta. Brain 135(Pt 7):2155–2168, Access. No's.: 22637583 3381721

LaRue B, Hogg E, Sagare A, Jovanovic S, Maness L, Maurer C, Deane R, Zlokovic BV (2004) Method for measurement of the blood-brain barrier permeability in the perfused mouse brain: application to amyloid-beta peptide in wild type and Alzheimer's Tg2576 mice. J Neurosci Methods 138(1–2):233–242, Access. No's.: 15325132

Laskowitz DT, Fillit H, Yeung N, Toku K, Vitek MP (2006) Apolipoprotein E-derived peptides reduce CNS inflammation: implications for therapy of neurological disease. Acta Neurol Scand Suppl 185:15–20, Access. No's.: 16866906

Li FQ, Sempowski GD, McKenna SE, Laskowitz DT, Colton CA, Vitek MP (2006) Apolipoprotein E-derived peptides ameliorate clinical disability and inflammatory infiltrates into the spinal cord in a murine model of multiple sclerosis. J Pharmacol Exp Ther 318(3):956–965, Access. No's.: 16740622

Li FQ, Fowler KA, Neil JE, Colton CA, Vitek MP (2010) An apolipoprotein E-mimetic stimulates axonal regeneration and remyelination after peripheral nerve injury. J Pharmacol Exp Ther 334(1):106–115, Access. No's.: 20406857 2912037

Liang Z, Liu F, Iqbal K, Grundke-Iqbal I, Wegiel J, Gong CX (2008) Decrease of protein phosphatase 2A and its association with accumulation and hyperphosphorylation of tau in Down syndrome. J Alzheimers Dis 13(3):295–302, Access. No's.: 18430997 2655351

Linton MF, Gish R, Hubl ST, Butler E, Esquivel C, Bry WI, Boyles JK, Wardell MR, Young SG (1991) Phenotypes of apolipoprotein B and apolipoprotein E after liver transplantation. J Clin Invest 88(1):270–281, Access. No's.: 2056122 296029

Liu GP, Wei W, Zhou X, Shi HR, Liu XH, Chai GS, Yao XQ, Zhang JY, Peng CX, Hu J, Li XC, Wang Q, Wang JZ (2013) Silencing PP2A inhibitor by lenti-shRNA interference ameliorates neuropathologies and memory deficits in tg2576 mice. Mol Ther 21(12):2247–2257, Access. No's.: 23922015 3863796

Lynch JR, Tang W, Wang H, Vitek MP, Bennett ER, Sullivan PM, Warner DS, Laskowitz DT (2003) APOE genotype and an ApoE-mimetic peptide modify the systemic and central nervous system inflammatory response. J Biol Chem 278(49):48529–48533, Access. No's.: 14507923

Mahley RW, Huang Y (2012) Apolipoprotein e sets the stage: response to injury triggers neuropathology. Neuron 76(5):871–885, Access. No's.: 23217737

Matsuo ES, Shin RW, Billingsley ML, Van deVoorde A, O'Connor M, Trojanowski JQ, Lee VM (1994) Biopsy-derived adult human brain tau is phosphorylated at many of the same sites as Alzheimer's disease paired helical filament tau. Neuron 13(4):989–1002, Access. No's.: 7946342

Mayeux R, Stern Y, Ottman R, Tatemichi TK, Tang MX, Maestre G, Ngai C, Tycko B, Ginsberg H (1993) The apolipoprotein epsilon 4 allele in patients with Alzheimer's disease. Ann Neurol 34(5):752–754, Access. No's.: 8239575

Michaelson, D. M. (2014). "ApoE4: The most prevalent yet understudied risk factor for Alzheimer's disease." Alzheimers Dement 10:861–8. Access. No's.: 25217293

Minami SS, Cordova A, Cirrito JR, Tesoriero JA, Babus LW, Davis GC, Dakshanamurthy S, Turner RS, Pak D, Rebeck GW, Paige M, Hoe HS (2010) ApoE mimetic peptide decreases Abeta production in vitro and in vivo. Mol Neurodegener 5:16, Access. No's.: 20406479 2890633

Nathan BP, Bellosta S, Sanan DA, Weisgraber KH, Mahley RW, Pitas RE (1994) Differential effects of apolipoproteins E3 and E4 on neuronal growth in vitro. Science 264(5160):850–852, Access. No's.: 8171342

Praline J, Blasco H, Vourc'h P, Garrigue MA, Gordon PH, Camu W, Corcia P, Andres CR, French ALSSG (2011) APOE epsilon4 allele is associated with an increased risk of bulbar-onset amyotrophic lateral sclerosis in men. Eur J Neurol 18(8):1046–1052, Access. No's.: 21251163

Rall SC Jr, Weisgraber KH, Innerarity TL, Mahley RW (1983) Identical structural and receptor binding defects in apolipoprotein E2 in hypo-, normo-, and hypercholesterolemic dysbetalipoproteinemia. J Clin Invest 71(4):1023–1031, Access. No's.: 6300187 436959

Rousselle C, Clair P, Smirnova M, Kolesnikov Y, Pasternak GW, Gac-Breton S, Rees AR, Scherrmann JM, Temsamani J (2003) Improved brain uptake and pharmacological activity of dalargin using a peptide-vector-mediated strategy. J Pharmacol Exp Ther 306(1):371–376, Access. No's.: 12682214

Saunders AM, Strittmatter WJ, Schmechel D, George-Hyslop PH, Pericak-Vance MA, Joo SH, Rosi BL, Gusella JF, Crapper-MacLachlan DR, Alberts MJ et al (1993) Association of apolipoprotein E allele epsilon 4 with late-onset familial and sporadic Alzheimer's disease. Neurology 43(8):1467–1472, Access. No's.: 8350998

Schmidt S, Kwee LC, Allen KD, Oddone EZ (2010) Association of ALS with head injury, cigarette smoking and APOE genotypes. J Neurol Sci 291(1–2):22–29, Access. No's.: 20129626 2840700

Simon R, Girod M, Fonbonne C, Salvador A, Clement Y, Lanteri P, Amouyel P, Lambert JC, Lemoine J (2012) Total ApoE and ApoE4 isoform assays in an Alzheimer's disease case-control study by targeted mass spectrometry (n=669): a pilot assay for methionine-containing proteotypic peptides. Mol Cell Proteomics 11(11):1389–1403, Access. No's.: 22918225 3494189

Sontag E, Nunbhakdi-Craig V, Lee G, Bloom GS, Mumby MC (1996) Regulation of the phosphorylation state and microtubule-binding activity of Tau by protein phosphatase 2A. Neuron 17(6):1201–1207, Access. No's.: 8982166

Sontag E, Nunbhakdi-Craig V, Sontag JM, Diaz-Arrastia R, Ogris E, Dayal S, Lentz SR, Arning E, Bottiglieri T (2007) Protein phosphatase 2A methyltransferase links homocysteine metabolism with tau and amyloid precursor protein regulation. J Neurosci 27(11):2751–2759, Access. No's.: 17360897

Tai LM, Koster KP, Luo J, Lee SH, Wang YT, Collins NC, Ben Aissa M, Thatcher GR, LaDu MJ (2014). "Amyloid-beta Pathology and APOE Genotype Modulate Retinoid X Receptor Agonist Activity in vivo." J Biol Chem 289:30538–55. Access. No's.: 25217640

Tanimukai H, Grundke-Iqbal I, Iqbal K (2005) Up-regulation of inhibitors of protein phosphatase-2A in Alzheimer's disease. Am J Pathol 166(6):1761–1771, Access. No's.: 15920161 1602412

Thurm CW, Halsey JF (2005). "Measurement of cytokine production using whole blood." Curr Protoc Immunol, Volume 66, Chapter 7: Unit 7 18B, pages 1–12. Access. No's.: 18432956

Triguero D, Buciak J, Pardridge WM (1990) Capillary depletion method for quantification of blood-brain barrier transport of circulating peptides and plasma proteins. J Neurochem 54(6):1882–1888, Access. No's.: 2338547

Tukhovskaya EA, Yukin AY, Khokhlova ON, Murashev AN, Vitek MP (2009) COG1410, a novel apolipoprotein-E mimetic, improves functional and morphological recovery in a rat model of focal brain ischemia. J Neurosci Res 87(3):677–682, Access. No's.: 18803296 2752425

Vitek MP, Brown CM, Colton CA (2009) APOE genotype-specific differences in the innate immune response. Neurobiol Aging 30(9):1350–1360, Access. No's.: 18155324 2782461

Vitek MP, Christensen DJ, Wilcock D, Davis J, Van Nostrand WE, Li FQ, Colton CA (2012) APOE-mimetic peptides reduce behavioral deficits, plaques and tangles in Alzheimer's disease transgenics. Neurodegener Dis 10(1-4):122–126, Access. No's.: 22326991 3363346

Vogelsberg-Ragaglia V, Schuck T, Trojanowski JQ, Lee VM (2001) PP2A mRNA expression is quantitatively decreased in Alzheimer's disease hippocampus. Exp Neurol 168(2):402–412, Access. No's.: 11259128

Wagle J, Farner L, Flekkoy K, Wyller TB, Sandvik L, Eiklid KL, Fure B, Stensrod B, Engedal K (2009) Association between ApoE epsilon4 and cognitive impairment after stroke. Dement Geriatr Cogn Disord 27(6):525–533, Access. No's.: 19494491

Wang X, Blanchard J, Kohlbrenner E, Clement N, Linden RM, Radu A, Grundke-Iqbal I, Iqbal K (2010) The carboxy-terminal fragment of inhibitor-2 of protein phosphatase-2A induces Alzheimer disease pathology and cognitive impairment. FASEB J 24(11):4420–4432, Access. No's.: 20651003 3229424

Wang R, Hong J, Lu M, Neil JE, Vitek MP, Liu X, Warner DS, Li F, Sheng H (2014) ApoE mimetic ameliorates motor deficit and tissue damage in rat spinal cord injury. J Neurosci Res 92(7):884–892, Access. No's.: 24633884

Wilcock DM, Lewis MR, Van Nostrand WE, Davis J, Previti ML, Gharkholonarehe N, Vitek MP, Colton CA (2008) Progression of amyloid pathology to Alzheimer's disease pathology in an amyloid precursor protein transgenic mouse model by removal of nitric oxide synthase 2. J Neurosci 28(7):1537–1545, Access. No's.: 18272675 2621082

Wilcock DM, Gharkholonarehe N, Van Nostrand WE, Davis J, Vitek MP, Colton CA (2009) Amyloid reduction by amyloid-beta vaccination also reduces mouse tau pathology and protects from neuron loss in two mouse models of Alzheimer's disease. J Neurosci 29(25):7957–7965, Access. No's.: 19553436 2871319

Zhu Y, Nwabuisi-Heath E, Dumanis SB, Tai LM, Yu C, Rebeck GW, LaDu MJ (2012) APOE genotype alters glial activation and loss of synaptic markers in mice. Glia 60(4):559–569, Access. No's.: 22228589 3276698

The manufacturer's authorised representative in the EU is Springer Nature Customer Service Centre GmbH, Europaplatz 3, 69115 Heidelberg, Germany. If you have any concerns regarding our products, please contact ProductSafety@springernature.com

Printed and bound by CPI Group (UK) Ltd, Croydon, CR0 4YY
15/07/2026
02167618-0001